THE CONTINUING CARE
OF TERMINAL CANCER PATIENTS

THE CONTINUING CARE OF TERMINAL CANCER PATIENTS

Proceedings of an International Seminar on
Continuing Care of Terminal Cancer Patients
Milan, 19-20 October 1979

Editors

ROBERT G. TWYCROSS, MA, DM, FRCP

Consultant Physician
Sir Michael Sobell House
The Churchill Hospital
Headington, Oxford, England

VITTORIO VENTAFRIDDA, MD

Director
Division of Pain Therapy and Rehabilitation
Istituto Nazionale per lo Studio e la Cura dei Tumori
Milan, Italy

PERGAMON PRESS

OXFORD · NEW YORK · TORONTO · PARIS · SYDNEY · FRANKFURT

U.K.	Pergamon Press Ltd., Headington Hill Hall, Oxford OX3 0BW, England
U.S.A.	Pergamon Press Inc., Maxwell House, Fairview Park, Elmsford, New York 10523, U.S.A.
CANADA	Pergamon of Canada, Suite 104, 150 Consumers Road, Willowdale, Ontario M2J 1P9, Canada
AUSTRALIA	Pergamon Press (Aust.) Pty. Ltd., P.O. Box 544, Potts Point, N.S.W. 2011, Australia
FRANCE	Pergamon Press SARL, 24 rue des Ecoles, 75240 Paris, Cedex 05, France
FEDERAL REPUBLIC OF GERMANY	Pergamon Press GmbH, 6242 Kronberg-Taunus, Hammerweg 6, Federal Republic of Germany

First edition 1980

British Library Cataloguing in Publication Data

International Seminar on Continuing care of Terminal Cancer Patients, *Milan, 1979*
The continuing care of terminal cancer patients
1. Cancer patients - Congresses
2. Terminal care - Congresses
I. Title II. Twycross, Robert Geoffrey
III. Ventafridda, Vittorio
362.1'9'6994   RC262   80-49926

ISBN 0-08-024943-4

In order to make this volume available as economically and as rapidly as possible the authors' typescripts have been reproduced in their original forms. This method has its typographical limitations but it is hoped that they in no way distract the reader.

Printed in Great Britain by A. Wheaton & Co. Ltd, Exeter

CONTENTS

VI – MANAGEMENT AND ORGANIZATION

PREFACE

Out of an estimated 50 million deaths annually in the world, more than 5 million are attributed to cancer (World Health Organization, 1979). In Europe and North America about one-fifth of the population die of cancer. It is estimated that by the year 2000 the number of cancer deaths will have risen to 8 million annually. Most of those dying of cancer will have distressing symptoms of one kind or another; about 60% will experience severe pain. It is generally agreed that current health care systems do not cater adequately for the varied needs of the patient with terminal cancer. In addition to good symptom control, the patient needs psychological support. This includes the friendship and companionship of trained health-care personnel. People who can explain what is happening to the patient, answer with authority questions about the likely pattern of future events, and encourage and help the patient achieve his maximum physical capability.

In order to elucidate the physical and psychological needs of the patient with terminal cancer, an International Seminar was held in Milan in October 1979, and was attended by about 150 doctors. The papers presented at the seminar comprise the contents of this book. As the list of contents shows, many aspects of terminal care were discussed. It would be foolish, however, to claim that the subject has been covered fully. There are a number of obvious omissions; for example, there are no contributions by nurses. This is because the seminar concentrated on the role and responsibility of the doctor in this area of care. As the authors come from a variety of clinical backgrounds and cultures, the book may at times appear disjointed. It does, however, have a unifying principle, namely that the dying cancer patient is worth caring about. Where differences exist, they relate to differences of opinion as to what constitutes appropriate care.

The first section of the book discusses the moral and legal aspects of terminal care. The advent of palliative, anti-neoplastic treatments has not only resulted in an improved prognosis for many patients but, for others, has led to a situation in which the treatment is in many respects worse than the disease. In an age when traditional moral values are either ignored or repudiated, there is a real need for specific guidelines for the medical and other caring professions. The second section deals with the fundamentally important area of communication between the doctor and the patient, and emotional aspects of terminal illness. The next sections cover the relief of pain, the control of other symptoms, and the often neglected areas of physical therapy and rehabilitation. The fifth section discusses the benefit, in suitably selected patients, of more intensive

nutritional support. In the final chapters, the management and organization of
terminal cancer care is discussed, in the light of three programmes already
operative in North America. The need for a team approach is emphasized, as is the
need for a radical reorientation in the doctor's objectives.

This book will, we believe, provide doctors with a greater insight into the needs
of the patient with terminal cancer and his family. It will also act as a
valuable resource and reference book, and so enable the doctor to deal more
effectively with his patient's distressing symptoms. We should like to record our
gratitude to the Floriani Foundation for their sponsorship. The seminar was held
under the auspices of the International Union Against Cancer (UICC), the International Association for the Study of Pain (IASP), the Associazione Italiana per
lo Studio del Dolore (AISD), the Istituto Nazionale per lo Studio e la Cura dei
Tumori, and the Lega Italiana per la lotta contro i Tumori.

We also acknowledge with gratitude the patronage extended to the seminar by His
Excellency Sandro Pertini, President of the Italian Republic.

Robert G Twycross

Vittorio Ventafridda

REFERENCE

Cancer Statistics, *Technical Report Series*, *No 632*. World Health Organization,
Geneva, 1979.

LIST OF SPEAKERS

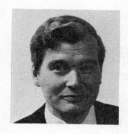

ROBERT G. TWYCROSS, MA, DM, FRCP
*Consultant Physician, Sir Michael Sobell House, The Churchill Hospital,
Headington, Oxford - England*

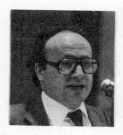

SANTE BASSO-RICCI, M.D.
*Assistant Professor, Department of Radiology, Istituto Nazionale per lo
Studio e la Cura dei Tumori, Milan - Italy*

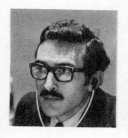

FEDERICO BOZZETTI, M.D.
*Assistant, Division Clinical Oncology, Istituto Nazionale per lo Studio e la
Cura dei Tumori, Milan - Italy*

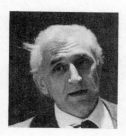

GIOVANNI CAIZZI
Deputy Attorney-General, Milan - Italy

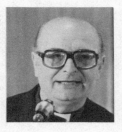

P. LUIGI MARIO CATTORETTI, o.p.
Co-Edtior Res Medicae - Ex editor Sacra Doctrina, journal of Phylosophy & Theology, Milan - Italy

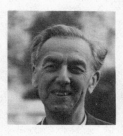

GORDON R. DUNSTAN, The Reverend Cannon, MA, DD, FSA
Professor of Moral and Social Theology, King's College, University of London, London - England

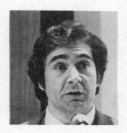

CHARLES A. GARFIELD, Ph.D.
Research Psychologist and Assistant Clincial Professor, Cancer Research Institute, University of California School of Medicine, S. Francisco, USA

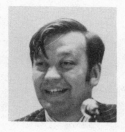

E. RICHARD HILLER, M.D.
Consultant Physician in Continuing Care, Countess Mountbatten House, Southampton - England

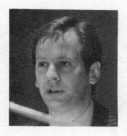

IAN McC. KENNEDY, LLM
Barrister, Reader in English Law - King's College, University of London, London - England

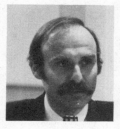

SILVIO MONFARDINI, M.D.
Assistant Professor, Division of Clinical Oncology, Istituto Nazionale per lo Studio e la Cura dei Tumori, Milan - Italy

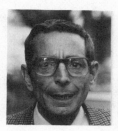

GUIDO MORICCA, M.D.
Professor and Director, Department of Anesthesiology, Resuscitation and Pain Therapy, Istituto Regina Elena, Rome - Italy

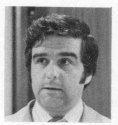

BALFOUR M. MOUNT, MD., F.R.C.S. (C)
Associate Professor, McGill University - Director of Palliative Care, Royal Victoria Hospital, Montreal - Quebec

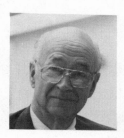

WILLIAM NORTON, M.D.
Associate Physician, Hospice, New Haven, Conn. - USA

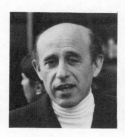

FRANCO PANNUTI, M.D.
Director, Division of Chemotherapy, Ospedale Malpighi, Bologna - Italy

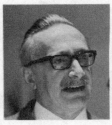

ROMEO POZZATO, M.D.
Director, Forensic Medicine Institute, Università degli Studi, Milan - Italy

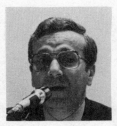

BRUNO SALVADORI, M.D.
*Director, Division of Clinical Oncology - Istituto Nazionale per lo Studio e
la Cura dei Tumori, Milan - Italy*

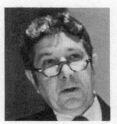

ARTHUR H. SCHMALE, M.D.
*Assistant Professor Medicine, University of Rochester Cancer Center,
Rochester N.Y. - USA*

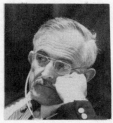

MAURICE E. SHILS, M.D., Sc.D.
*Director of Nutrition, Attending Physician, Memorial Sloan-Ketting Cancer
Center New York - USA*

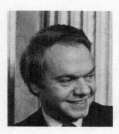

JEAN SIEGFRIED, M.D. Priv. Doz.
*Professor, Department of Neurosurgery, Universitatssital Zurich,
Zurich -Switzerland*

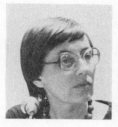

AVERIL STEDEFORD, MRC
Psychiatrist, Sir Michael Sobell House, The Churchill Hospital, Headington, Oxford - England

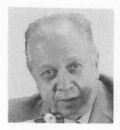

MARIO TIENGO, M.D.
Professor and Chairman of Anesthesiology and Resuscitation, Università degli Studi, Milan - Italy

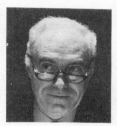

VITTORIO VENTAFRIDDA, M.D.
Director, Division of Pain Therapy and Rehabiliation, Istituto Nazionale per lo Studio e la Cura dei Tumori, Milan - Italy

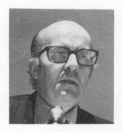

CARLO VETERE, M.D.
General Director, Ministry of Health, office for the establishment of the N.H.S., Rome - Italy

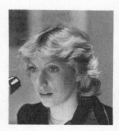

RITA ZANOLLA, M.D.
Physiatrist, Department of Pain Therapy and Rehabilitation, Istituto Nazionale per lo Studio e la Cura dei Tumori, Milan - Italy

OPENING REMARKS

Virgilio Floriani, The Floriani Foundation

The aim of the Floriani Foundation is to promote studies and research in the field of medicine in order to discover new techniques that may help improve the quality of life for people suffering from debilitating chronic diseases. In 1978, we organized a symposium in Venice on advanced cancer pain. As a result of this, we thought it worthwhile to consider the patient as a human being in the last months of his life.

He who, like me, has reached the age of reflection about the many questions of our existence, finds particularly fascinating the study of the emotions and feelings experienced by a person aware that his death is close. When we talk of certain problems it is part of our nature to think of others and never of ourselves. This leads to a distorted vision of reality. To avoid this I have imagined myself a terminally ill patient. I do not know the probability of this happening, but certainly the possibility exists.

Having thought deeply and lived through some sad experiences, I should like to underline the help that I would like to receive and the requests I will make to those who assist me. First, as soon as medicines and other treatments become useless, I shall want to be taken away from the big hospitals. These structures which, as we all know, have very important functions to perform, would become a nightmare to me and I should no longer feel a human being but only a number among many and a pitiful case; an example of a disease that has defeated science. Second, I should like everything to be done to relieve physical pain. Then I should like to go back to my family but, if my relatives cannot help me sufficiently or if they become exhausted, I should wish to be admitted to some small institution where I may still feel at home. There are many interesting examples of such small and specialized institutions in other countries.

Human nature reinforces itself as the body surrenders. Relieved from pain and close to my family, I should like to be invited and helped to deal actively with the human and material problems posed by my imminent death. I shall have much advice and many suggestions for the people I love and that I am going to leave. There will be many matters to discuss. In this way the time will go swiftly by in what could become the most humanly interesting period of my life. After having settled my affairs, I should like to be helped to appreciate that my life has reached completion and not to consider death as tragic but natural.

I am not a physician, nor a psychologist; I am just a human being who has expressed his feelings and has emphasized the need for all kinds of help. On behalf of the Floriani Foundation, I welcome you all to this seminar. I am certain that during our time together, advances will be made in the understanding of scientific and praftical ways of assisting terminally ill patients and so help them reach the end as serenely as possible.

Umberto Veronesi, Director of Istituto Nazionale Tumori and President of International Union against Cancer (UICC)

He who knows how jealous the International Union Against Cancer (UICC) is of its name and how carefully it examines such requests, will understand the importance of having received the patronage of UICC. The Union offers its name to no more than five international meetings a year, and the fact that unanimously both the executive committee and scientific board decided to support this Seminar, witnesses not only to the high standard of the programme and of the organization, but also to the importance of the subject.

Terminal cancer care is a difficult subject that cannot be ignored any longer, and UICC has recognized it as one area in which studies and research should be concentrated in the next few years. The UICC hopes to support such studies directly. Further, I anticipate that an edition of our quarterly review will shortly be devoted almost entirely to the problem of pain control and to the care of the patient with terminal cancer.

Cardinal Giovanni Colombo, Archdiocese of Milan

The mission of the physician — the protection and the promotion of human life — has been considered since time immemorial a most noble task because it concerns a fundamental, holy and inviolable value. Christianity incorporates this humanistic interpretation of medicine but gives, as its own contribution, a higher and more binding vision of life: it is a "gift" from God, protected by Him with the commandment "Thou shalt not kill" and entrusted by Him to man who is both responsible and accountable for it.

The promotion and protection of life are important throughout the whole of a person's existence, from conception to death. The Church shares in the admiration and gratitude of all humanity for the amazing and continuing advances in medical science and for technical developments that have helped to sustain life when threatened by one of a number of serious illnesses. In this seemingly limitless field, similar advances in relation to terminal illness are also to be welcomed. This extraordinary progress, that affects life at all its stages, renders the practice of euthanasia even more unjustified and disquieting. The Catholic Church has no doubts about condemning euthanasia — the deliberate and direct suppression of the life of any person — even if affected by a painful and incurable disease (*Gaudium et Spes*, 27).

Neither the individual, on his own initiative or if requested, nor the Government have the "right" to bring about the death of a human being voluntarily and directly. In relation to the care of patients with terminal cancer, this means that the use of treatments, including the administration of drugs, must not lead to a form of freely wanted or imposed euthanasia. Between this extreme, always morally illicit, and certain other interventions that in themselves aim at relieving pain but inexorably affect the length of life, doubts and ethical perplexities will arise that only a competent and cautious physician can resolve. The physician will operate within the limits bounded by the absolute respect for human life and the right of every human being to die with dignity and serene awareness.

The words of Pope Paul VI, spoken by Cardinal Villot to the French Medical Catholic Association on October 3, 1970, provide clarification and consolation for all doctors:

> "The duty of the physician consists more in striving to relieve pain than in prolonging as long as possible with every available means a life that is no longer fully human and that is naturally coming to its conclusion."

I
THERAPEUTIC STRATEGY: DECISION MAKING

Clarifying the Issues

G. R. DUNSTAN

Faculty of Theology and Religious Studies, King's College, London, UK

The morality concerning death and dying is in confusion. Confusion hinders good
professional practice when it disturbs mutual expectations. It is important that
doctor, patient and the community should know what to expect of one another in
roughly comparable situations. Uncertainty breeds indecision in the practitioner;
it engenders fear, hostility and litigiousness among patients. To clarify the
issues in terminal care may, therefore, help towards a practice that is well
grounded, more confident, and better understood.

There is bound to be confusion at a time of uneven medical advance. In England
and elsewhere the most notable advances in terminal care have been in hospices
created for the purpose. New skills have been developed and tested in the
pharmacological control of pain, delirium and other distressing symptoms attending
terminal cancer especially. A new understanding has been developed of the social,
emotional and spiritual needs of patients, and the hospice has been created as a
community designed to meet these needs. For patients being nursed at home, family
doctors and domiciliary nurses are being taught the same understanding and skills.
Teaching and practice are finding their way into medical schools and general
hospitals, but slowly. The advance in terminal care, in serving the interest of
the patient in his dying, is uneven.

Confusion enters, meanwhile, from other areas of medical practice. The popular
misunderstanding (though not the reality) of the intensive care unit is of the
application of advanced technology for keeping people artificially alive, to deny
them the boon of death. The coincidence of this with the development of cadaveric
transplants for renal failure brings further fear: that the patient is not
treated for himself alone, but as a means to some further end, to which his
interests may be sacrificed.

Even death itself is problematical: when it was a "mystery" it had at least a
certain finality; now that it has become a process, scientifically studied and
monitored, uncertainty enters: in popular fear, no one is quite sure what being
dead means.

It is not death so much as dying that is popularly feared. The word "cancer"
still evokes widespread fear of "dying in agony"; and the only alternative, in the
popular imagination, is to hasten the process of dying, to kill. It is not that
life is held cheaper today, despite the more open practice and legitimation of
abortion, and despite the extent of terrorism and political murder. The increasing

3

rejection of the death penalty, exemplified in the 1979 campaign in France, is
evidence of a higher moral value put upon life, even that of violent criminals.
The ambivalence of today comes from a weighing of values one against another: the
value of life set against some degree of pain, some degree of hardship or of
handicap. Those who campaign for "euthanasia" wish, either to make the physician
the arbiter, the judge, in that comparison, or to licence him to execute it if a
patient should choose for himself that he would rather be killed than live.

Imprecision confuses the arguments, and weakens resolution. The paraphrase of
euthanasia, "the painless inducement of death", is itself deceptive. "To induce"
commonly means in English "to prevail upon, to persuade"; it is used with an agent,
a person, not a process or an event, like death. Candidates for euthanasia vary
according to the sympathies of the euthanasist: from the child born severely
deformed to the incurably ill and the aged or demented.   It is more honest to
use words like infanticide, aegricide, senicide, dementicide (or amenticide) -
all compounded from the root -cido, and telling the truth that some specific
person is being killed. "Euthanasia" for the chronic sick would then be either
homicide by request, or professionally assisted suicide, according to the means
employed. It is for doctors and for society itself - not one or the other - to
decide whether such a role is compatible with the doctor's profession; whether
killing patients who present difficulties will advance therapy as effectively as
meeting the challenge until the difficulties are overcome.

During the years when "human rights" has become the most popular slogan in
political and social campaigning, the advocates of euthanasia have invented and
exploited "the right to die". There is indeed a "right to die", grounded in our
natural mortality: just as the right to marry is grounded in our sexuality, as
the right to move about, write and speak freely and to associate is grounded in
our sociability - and so on. A man is denied his right to die if he is kept
"alive" improperly by inept medical intervention when nature should be allowed to
take its course and he might die in peace. But the duties attached to these
rights are limited: they are protective only, not causative, not such as to make
the right effective. The law should properly protect the right of the subject to
marry, or to move or write or speak freely - but not compel him to. Similarly, it
should protect (if necessary) a man's right to die - but it may impose on no one a
duty on that account to kill him. The misuse of a slogan of this sort adds
further to the prevalent confusion over death and dying, and complicates the
circumstances in which physicians have to make medical and moral decisions.

It may be, indeed, that insensitive or over-zealous medical action in the prolonging of dying invites just fears and justified resentment. That a doctor's
duty is limited in this respect was recognised early in the Hippocratic corpus and
has been confirmed by the highest Christian authorities in recent times. (Pius XII,
1957). The discussion is conducted in the terms of "ordinary" and "extraordinary"
means of medical care: ordinary care, the patient is under obligation to request
and the physician to provide; extraordinary intervention, which would impose on
the patient hardship disproportionate to foreseeable benefit, he is not bound
either to request or to accept, and the physician is not bound to provide.
Definitions of what is "ordinary" and "extraordinary" vary widely; but the intent
of the distinction is clear. It is to insist that it is the patient's ultimate
interest which should determine the treatment he receives, that interest being
seen in relation to his unique being and his unique human and social condition or
environment. (Duncan, Dunstan and Welbourn, 1977; Linacre Centre, 1979). The
motives which might prompt a doctor to impose improper restraints upon his dying -
by surgical, pharmacological or mechanical intervention beyond what is required
for symptom control - are several and varied. Uncertainty; fear of appearing
incompetent; fear of litigation; undue deference to the feelings of relatives or
of nurses; a will to experiment in method or technique; pride in technical

achievement; genuine mistake or miscalculation - for nothing is certain in this field; all or any of these might intervene, to cause a patient's dying to be prolonged beyond its proper term. And most of them, it may be observed, spring from that confusion of expectations to which this paper has drawn attention. The remedy lies in better mutual understanding among all persons involved - though the tension inherent in decision in any particular case cannot be, and ought not to be, minimized or removed.

We may best consider the duties, and the relevant decisions, in terms of the interests to be served. By definition, a patient in terminal care has no longer an interest in being cured. His condition may be ameliorated for a while - the phase which R.G.Twycross, differing slightly from Calman and Paul, (Calman and Paul, 1978) has termed "palliative" - by "the modification of the pathological process by treatment in order to delay the otherwise inevitable consequences of that process" (Twycross).   But after that his interest is in dying, in achieving his natural mortal end with the minimum of distress and the maximum capacity to enjoy or even repair such human relationships as he might choose. The relevant duties are not those of the physician only; they attach to a whole community of persons attendant upon the patient in his dying: his relatives and friends, his nurses, his priest or spiritual adviser or the hospital chaplain, and other persons in the hospital community. Insofar as the physician is "in charge" of the case, his own attitude may well determine how far he is an enabler of those other persons to do their respective duties, to contribute their respective parts, and certainly he has specific duties of his own.

The relief of the patient from distressing symptoms is the aim and product of the total medical and nursing care. Much of it is reducible to good routine. Medical decisions are required in the assessment of distress - pain, breathlessness, delirium - and their appropriate management by pharmaceutical means. There is no alternative here to the highest technical competence in the doctor. Only sound knowledge and competent prescription will deliver him, for instance, from a paralysing fear of making his patient dependent on analgesic drugs, so leaving the patient to suffer pain from which a more assured doctor would readily relieve him.

The time may come when an increased dosage, necessary to control distress, may depress respiration and cough and so hasten the development of pneumonia from which the patient may die. Propagandists for euthanasia term this "the lethal analgesic dose"; they then conclude that "doctors are killing patients already; it would therefore be no departure in principle if euthanasia were legally permitted". The argument is false. The two practices stand on different principles. In euthanasia the direct intent is to kill, and the means employed would be specific to that end. In proper analgesic care the direct intention is to relieve pain or distress, and the means employed are specific to that intent. They are also effective to that end - the primary effect is to relieve the symptom complained of. They may also have a secondary effect, unintended but inevitable, in the processes which result in the death of the patient. The physician is not held culpable, in law or morals, for this secondary effect, no less drastic remedy being available.

This principle of "double effect" is of high importance in this context, though it is by no means confined to it. For instance, a ship's hull may be damaged by a collision and water begins to pour in. The captain orders alarm bells to be sounded and watertight doors to be closed. The speed of the operation must be determined by the speed of the intake of water and the degree of threat to the ship. If a member of the ship's company is trapped on the wrong side of the watertight door and drowned, his death is consequent upon the captain's order - a

6 G.R. Dunstan

secondary consequence or effect of it - but the captain is not culpable for the
death of his seaman, no less drastic remedy being available to him for ensuring
the safety of his crew.

But - reverting from the nautical to the medical instance - should not the
pneumonia also be controlled? There are antibiotic medicines specific for
pneumonia; is the doctor not under obligation to use them, and so to relieve the
patient's pain while not also shortening his life? The answer to the question
lies in the answer to another: is good medical treatment specific to particular
diseases or to particular patients? If to the disease, then the process of dying
will be prolonged; the patient's interest in dying would be denied, subordinated
to a pharmacological process, the technical activity of combating a particular
disease; he would, in fact, be denied his right to die. If good medical care is
specific to the patient, then - in the given circumstances, and with all other
duties done and relationships set in order - the patient is served in his interest
in dying by being allowed to die.

In fact, therapeutic progress, as developed in the Hospices, has made "the lethal
analgesic dose" an obsolete and unnecessary concept. A right understanding and
treatment of pain can give patients the necessary relief with little or no risk of
the secondary effect- and the common obligation to use the least drastic remedy
would indicate this as the appropriate management in most cases. There is no
place in such management for the language of "euthanasia", "active" or "passive" -
a useless distinction in any case - or of "withdrawal of treatment" or "allowing
to die". The management offered is active and appropriate to the patient at every
stage.

If we allow that the object of terminal care is this positive one, to serve the
interest of the patient in his dying, we can overturn the generally negative view
which often prevails about the nursing and medical care of the dying. It is a
positive activity to the end. A small linguistic distinction may be useful here
between two Latin words which have influenced our common speech. The normal Latin
word for "to heal, cure, or make sound or healthy", is sanare. The word from
which we derive our verb "to cure" is curare - which means simply "to care for,
to look after, to take charge of". If we regard the medical and nursing task as
always "to cure" - ad sanandum, as the Latins would say - then terminal care must
always end in defeat; death is a denial of cure. But if the task is properly ad
curandum, to take care of, to cherish even when sanare is no longer possible,
then we can see a positive end, requiring positive skills, chosen and applied as
each patient, at each changing moment of time, has need.

REFERENCES

Calman, K.C., and Paul, J. (1978). An Introduction to Cancer Medicine. London:
    Macmillan. p. 182.
Duncan, A.S., Dunstan, G.R. and Welbourn, R.B. (1977), Dictionary of Medical
    Ethics, London: Darton, Longman and Todd. s.v. Prolongation of Life.
Linacre Centre (1979), Paper no. 3, Ordinary and Extraordinary Means of Prolonging
    Life. London, 60 Grove End Road, NW8 9NH.
Pius XII, Pope (1957). Allocution of 24 Nov. 1957 to anaesthetists. Acta
    Apostolicae Sedis, xxxxix, pp. 1027-33.
Twycross, R.G. (1979) - in private correspondence.

Moral Aspects

L. M. CATTORETTI

Res Medicae, Milan, Italy

When caring for a patient with terminal cancer two fundamental problems demand attention. First, the issue of truthfulness in our dealings with the patient and, second, euthanasia.

COMMUNICATING THE TRUTH

In spite of extensive discussions during the last twenty years, controversy and uncertainty remains. The choice is between *saying*, *not saying*, or *lying*. From the anthropological point of view, both moralists and jurists agree that man has a fundamental right to know the truth about his condition. In the case of the patient with terminal cancer, however, right to truth should not mean "idolatry of truth". It is claimed that truth does not stultify but liberates, that it reveals hitherto untapped mental resources. It is said that truth can never be brutal or traumatic. Yet there is no doubt that "exactitude" can do irreparable psychological damage. The patient can be "struck by lightning" by a physician who mistakes exactitude for truth, and who acts because of a supposed obligation to information at all costs.

From the ethical point of view, persistent deep perplexities exist, and relate to reluctance to *say* the truth, *how* to say it, and to uncertainty about the balance between the advantages and disadvantages deriving from the communication of the truth. Though there appears to be a consensus in favour of telling the patient when he is terminal, this does not seem to happen in practice. Moreover, there is still controversy about *who* should tell the patient; whether it should be the physician, priest, another member of the hospital staff, or the relatives.

A seminar with thirty-five doctors from nearly every Western country has recently been held in Turin under the aegis of the International Union Against Cancer and Lega Italiana Per la Lotta Contro i Tumori, on the theme "Does the Physician Know How to Talk to the Patient About Cancer?". The conclusions reached were rather pessimistic and, in most cases, mainly negative. In a Round Table on the same subject held early in 1979 in the Faculty of Medicine and Surgery at the Catholic University of Rome, "empathy" was considered to be the best arbiter when deciding whether or not to tell the patient the truth.

Communication by means of non-verbal or indirect verbal means should not be forgotten — a glance, an adjective, an indirect question. Such means are used repeatedly by the physician throughout the time that elapses between diagnosis and the death of his patient. They are methods of communication which cannot be avoided and which need to be used well. But how capable are doctors of dealing with the intricacies of non-verbal dialogue?

The tacit understanding whereby cancer is kept secret is still deeply rooted in many countries. In France, Germany, and Italy it is still the rule that physicians communicate the diagnosis of cancer to the patient's relatives but not to the patient himself, as it is considered that the knowledge of such a diagnosis is intolerable for anyone. It is commonly said by leading oncologists that less than a tenth of their patients know they have got cancer. In contrast, in North America everybody knows. This is partly because of the fear of litigation but it has had the result that the doctor is much more explicit with his patients. On the other hand, the largest cancer hospital in the United States sends patients' bills and other communications in envelopes without any indication of the sender, just in case the patient wishes to conceal his illness from his relatives.

While Catholic moralists are unanimous in affirming the doctor's general duty to speak the truth, there is only one circumstance in which there is an absolute responsibility to do so, namely, when, on the one hand, the adjective "Christian" is added to the physician, priest, hospital staff or relative and, on the other, when the terminally ill patient is also a "Christian" patient. In this case it is necessary to say the whole truth as the Christian caregiver has a duty to inform the Christian patient about his real condition. It is an obligation from which the Christian cannot escape, because death is the most important moment in life, a moment which should be approached with both awareness and serenity. However, even this clear cut moral directive has been contradicted by an entire excursus of ecclesiastic teaching, even papal. Since the contribution on this subject by Pope Pius XII, and despite the general acceptance of the moral obligation for Christians to be truthful to each other, a number of exceptions have been put forward. For example, if it is anticipated that the patient's health is likely to be endangered further by the traumatic effect of receiving unbearable news, then the truth need not be revealed as no advantage would result even in the religious sphere, as the patient would probably be driven further away from God.

Even so, despite the ethical uncertainty, it is possible to offer a few guidelines. We can be unanimous in affirming our common obligation to avoid deliberate lying as this may lead to irreversible despair in the patient when he discovers the web of deceit in which he has been ensnared. Two guiding principles are suggested in this connection which appear to have general support among patients, doctors and priests.

1. Communication of the truth should always be with the good of the patient in mind.

2. At all costs maintain respect for the authentic wishes of the terminally ill patient.

There are many ways in practice of not respecting a patient. For example, enclosing him in an exclusively technical world which is suitable only for the initated, a world in which he cannot find any room for himself and his rights, and in which he is unable to influence the course of events. Alternatively, surrounding the patient with religious ritual which does more to tranquillize the healthy ones around him, rather than being a genuine expression of the patient's own faith. Or, destroy him psychologically by an overdose of information which he does not want to hear, and then perhaps prevent him from talking about his death with those around him, or not allow him to reveal his fears, his anguish, his wishes, and his residual hopes.

In view of Catholic teaching, telling the truth to the patient with terminal cancer provokes concrete and disquieting questions in all those who surround the one who is dying — doctors, nurses, other hospital personnel, relatives, and even the priest.

We are all unprepared, both culturally and spiritually, to cope with the death of
one of our fellows. For this reason alone it is necessary to reject any routine
or absolute attitude in the matter of the communication of the truth. Such attitudes would simply serve to reveal our own internal poverty.

EUTHANASIA

The ethical aspects of this subject are thoroughly described in Professor Dunstan's
contribution. I wish only to stress how euthanasia is a concept still in evolution.
The word is used to describe a number of different courses of action and to avoid
the confusion of ambiguity a variety of semi-descriptive terms have been introduced,
such as: *euthanasia of agony, medico-thanasia, passive euthanasia, assisted
suicide, active euthanasia.* Although consistently opposed to active euthanasia (a
kind of assisted suicide), the moral law suffers from interpretative excursuses,
often contradictory, with regard to passive euthanasia. These range from the
problems caused by *therapeutic abstention* to those of *therapeutic suspension*, from
extraordinary means in therapy to *indirect* and *concealed* euthanasia. In spite of
the unreserved condemnation of active euthanasia by Catholic teaching, from Pope
Pius XII to Pope John Paul II, a ferment of tension and thought surrounds the
various forms of morally acceptable passive euthanasia.

In contrast to past generations, it is the current prevailing conviction that a
good death — desirable and to be envied — is a sudden death in full well-being.
Better still if we are unconscious or asleep. It is deemed irrelevant if death
comes unexpectedly to a man, not giving him time to adjust to it, to accept it, or
to give it significance. By contrast, the patient with terminal cancer is seen to
be left with a double sentence of having to live his own *physical* death together
with his own *personal* death, which marks, at least for believers, the passage from
time to eternity.

The right "to die with dignity" is dogmatically asserted by many, including the
Catholic Church in both pontifical and episcopal teaching. Yet a conference of
Bishops concluded that "everything conspires to prevent us from overcoming the
anguish, diffuse and often unconscious, that we feel when confronted by our personal death. And it is in order to mask this anguish that often the doctor will
start pointless therapies to give him the illusion that he can win against death,
or at least not to take part in it; that the priest will seek protection in his
liturgies and bestowal of sacraments; that the family will lavish money that each
one may say 'everything possible was done'."

All these technical, religious and social rites protect only the healthy ones from
their anguish. As long as men inhabit this world they will no doubt continuously
invent new ones. The problem is to know whether these rites are supportive or
whether they simply serve to reject brutally the one who is dying.

Meanwhile, in so much darkness, Christian moralists cannot but ask for divine
enlightenment. If I had to suggest an appropriate prayer, I would whisper to them
to repeat what a non-believer, Salvatore Quasimodo, the 1959 Nobel Prizewinner for
literature, composed in 1949 in a moment of inspiration:

> *And so should we deny you, God
> of the tumors, God of the live flower,
> and begin with a "no" to the sombre
> stone "I am" and consent to death
> and on each grave write our
> only certitude: "thànatos athànatos"?*

Without a name to recall the dreams,
tears and furies of this man
defeated by still unanswered questions?
Our dialogue changes; the absurd
now becomes possible. There,
beyond the fog curtain, inside the trees,
the power of leaves keeps watch,
true is the river that presses its banks.
Life is not dream. True is man
and so is his crying, jealous of silence.
God of silence, open the solitude.

REFERENCES

AAVV: Il morire come tema di prassi ecclesiale, in *Concilium* 4, 1974.

AAVV: Diritto di vivere, diritto di morire, in *Vita e Pensiero*, May-June 1974.

AAVV: Rencontre avec les mourants, in *Cahiers Laennec* 2, 1974.

AAVV: Respect de la vie, respect de la mort, in *Cahiers Laennec* 4, 1974.

AAVV: Therapeutiques des souffrances terminales, in *Cahiers Laennec* 1, 1975.

AAVV: Problèmes éthiques posés aujourd'hui par la mort et le mourir. *Conférence épiscopale francaise*, March 1976.

AAVV: *Morire si, ma quando?* (a cura di P. Beretta), Ed. Paoline, 1977.

AAVV: La mort, problèmes et approches, in *Lumière et vie*, XXVII, 138, 1978.

AAVV: L'etica medica di fronte all'agonia: "Rendere possibile une morte dignitosa", in *I.S.I.S.* 19, 1979, p. 18.

AAVV: Confronto ISIS tra deontologia medica e teologia morale sul moderno concetto di morte, in *I.S.I.S.* 23, 1979, p. 5.

Aldovrandi, M.: Di fronte alla diversità dei principi (dovuta alla differenza di civiltà, di cultura, di religione, ecc.), il medico deve seguire la propria coscienza o quella del malato, in *Medicina e morale*, II, *1969, pp. 73-85.

Bolech, P. and Huber, J.: Die Kommunikation der Wahrheit am Krankenbett, in *Arzt und Christ* 2, 1976, pp. 97-102. Trad. It. in *Res Medicae* 4, 1978.

Bronzetti, E.: Come muore l'uomo? ogni risposta non fa regola, in *I.S.I.S.* 25, 1979, pp. 16-18.

Bruaire, C.: *Une éthique pour la médecine.* Fayard, 1978.

Draper, E. and Collum, J.: Psicologia dell'invecchiamento: il processo della morte, in *La Clinica osteotrica e ginecologica*, IV, 3, 1979, pp. 691-695.

Duffy, J.C.: *Emotional issues in the lives of the physicians.* Springfield, Illinois, 1979. Trad. Itl. I problemi emotivi del medico, ed. Il pensiero scientifico, 1973.

*ediz. Orizzonte Medico

Engelmeier, M.P.: Terapie in punto di morte, in *L'ancora nella unita di salute*, July-August 1970, pp. 316-334.

Ferland, J. Esquisse d'une politique morale dur les soins des mourants dans les milieux hospitaliers, in *L'Hopital Catholique*, Vol. 7, 1, 1979, pp. 15-17. Trad. It. in *Res. Medicae*, 1980, in prep.

Gennari, G.: Teologia della morte per l'uomo d'oggi, in *Medicina e morale*, VI, *1973, pp. 179-221.

Kubler-Ross, E. *On death and Dying*, McMillan. Trad. It. ed. Cittadella, 1976.

Lentrodt, K.W.: Gedanken über den Tod, in *Arzt und Christ*, 1, 1976, pp. 12-22. Trad. It. in *Res. Medicae*, 6, 1979, in prep.

Marcozzi, V.: Morte e vita umana (problemi medico-morale) in *Medicina e Morale*, VI, *1973, pp. 145-178.

Mathe', G.: *Dossier Cancer*, ed. Stock, 1977. Trad. It. Inchiesta sul cancro, Rizzoli, 1979.

Mehta, M.: *Intractable Pain*, W.B. Saunders. Trad. It. ed. Manapese, 1975.

Perico, G.: Diritto di morire? in *Aggiornamenti sociali*, anno XXVI, 12, 1975, pp. 665-682.

Signorati, L. Un progetto per migliorare la qualità di vita dei malati in fase terminale al Centro ospedaliero Hotel-Dieu di Sherbrooke (Canada), in *Anime e corpi*, 82, 1979, pp. 251-262.

SCHWARTZENBURG, L. and Viansson-Ponte', P.: *Changer la mort*, ed. Albin Michel, 1977. Trad. It. Mondadori, 1979.

Sontag, S. *Illness as Metaphor*, New York, 1977. Trad. It. Einaudi, 1979.

Szekely, A.: Suizid: ethische und pastorale Aspekte, in *Arzt und Christ* 1, 1977, pp. 35-42. Trad. It. in *Res. Medicae*, 4, 1979.

Thomas, L.V.: *Anthropologie de la mort*, Payot, 1975. Trad. It. Garzanti, 1976.

Visser, G. Il rispetto della vita propria ed altrui e i principi della morale, in *Medicina e Morale*, I, *1968, pp. 88-95.

Visser, G. Lo sviluppo della scienza può modificare dei principi ritenuti perenni? in *Medicina e Morale*, II, *1969, pp. 39-49.

Zalba, M. La distinzione tra mezzi ordinari e straordinari nella scienza medica e i problemi morali connessi, in *Medicina e Morale*, II, *1969, pp. 51-72.

---

*ediz. Orizzonte Medico

When to Stop Anti-Cancer Treatment

S. MONFARDINI

Division of Clinical Oncology, Istituto Nazionale Tumori, Milano, Italy

ABSTRACT

In recent years the medical treatment for various forms of neoplastic disease has markedly improved in terms of strategy, number of effective drugs, and incidence of objective responses. Since the achievement of a significant response is generally translated into an improved survival compared to that of non-responders, a patient should not be considered terminal as long as there is a reasonable possibility of inducing an objective response in that patient. Previous unsuccessful treatment is only a relative contraindication, since second- or third-line treatments may yield significant rates of response in tumours sensitive to chemotherapy. In a border-line situation, the choice between anticancer treatment or terminal care is made after considering the possible therapeutic advantage in the light of the psychological attitude of the patient towards therapy.

INTRODUCTION

To the medical oncologist it is quite important that he recognizes the moment when anticancer chemotherapy is becoming irrelevant to the needs of a particular patient. Such a decision has been made increasingly difficult by recent advances in the medical treatment of various forms of neoplasm, and the fact that there is an increasing overlap between control of tumour on one hand and the simple control of symptoms of uncontrollable tumour on the other (Saunders, 1978). It is evident that stopping of anticancer treatment in a particular patient should be considered only after careful consideration of the relative value of available single anti-tumour drugs or combinations. For this reason a brief review of the progress achieved in the field of anticancer chemotherapy is inlcuded.

PRESENT ACHIEVEMENT OF CANCER CHEMOTHERAPY

In recent years the medical treatment of various forms of neoplasm has improved markedly in terms of strategy, number of effective drugs and incidence of objective responses (Monfardini and co-workers, 1979). The response is considered significant when a complete (CR) or partial (PR) response is demonstrated objectively by the regression of measurable lesions. Table 1 shows the average response rate obtained with various drug combinations in the principal solid tumours.

13

S. Monfardini

TABLE 1   Average Expected Response Rate with Various Drug Combinations
                         in Advanced Solid Tumours

Neoplasm	CR (%)	CR + PR (%)
Hodgkin's disease	70-80	85-95
Non-Hodgkin's lymphomas	50-60	60-80
Wilms' tumour	60-70	70-80
Testicular cancer	60-70	85-95
Ovarian cancer	25-30	70-80
Breast cancer	12-20	50-70
Soft tissue sarcomas		
children	30-40	70-80
adults	<10	25-35
Lung cancer		
small cell	30-40	70-90
other	20-30	40-60
Bladder cancer	<20	50-60
Head and neck cancer	20-30	40-60
Ewing sarcoma	<20	50-60
Gastric cancer	<15	20-35
Colorectal cancer	<10	20-30
Endometrial cancer	10-20	40-60
Epidermoid cancer (cervix, oesophagus)	<20	30-40
Malignant melanoma	<10	20-30

In comparison with the use of a single agent, combination chemotherapy has proved
to be definitely superior in a number of tumours, though in an equal number greater
efficacy with multiple agents has not yet been demonstrated (Table 2). Hodgkin's
disease is an important example of the progress obtained by combination chemotherapy (Table 3). In this disorder, chemotherapy with single agents has produced
CR in only 10-30% of cases, while the introduction of intermittent intensive combination chemotherapy (MOPP) has increased the CR rate to 60-70%. In those who remit
completely, about 65% are still free of disease after 10 years (Bonadonna, 1978).
Patients relapsing on MOPP still have a good chance of a complete response with
different drug combinations. As in Hodgkin's disease, so in many other types of
tumour the achievement of a significant response is generally translated into
improved survival. The primary criteria used for comparing treatment regimens
remains median survival and the percentage of the treated population that achieve
long-term survival. The percentage of the population showing CR and duration of CR
are secondary criteria; and PR ranks as a tertiary criterion.

DECISION BETWEEN ANTICANCER THERAPY AND TERMINAL CARE

This summary of current results of anticancer chemotherapy is necessary in order
to understand why, in a given patient, as long as there is a reasonable possibility
of inducing an objective response, with a potential increase in survival, the
patient should not be considered terminal. The rationale in favour of continuing
anticancer treatment is, however, not only the possible achievement of an objective
response, but also the fact that the patient feels the difference between anti-
cancer and terminal care. Both for physician and patient anticancer therapy means
there is still a possibility of obtaining a clinically useful response even if,
after each cycle of treatment, side-effects temporarily lower the quality of life
(Table 4). In the majority of cases the toxic effects of antitumour chemotherapy
appear to be an acceptable price to pay if one thinks of the psychological benefit
of an active attitude towards the disease. On the other hand, the tendency towards

TABLE 2   Comparison of Combination Chemotherapy and Single Agent
Chemotherapy in the Major Tumour Types

Tumour type	Combination Chemotherapy
Hodgkin's disease Non-Hodgkin's lymphomas Acute lymphocytic leukaemia Acute myelocytic leukaemia Multiple myeloma Breast carcinoma Testicular carcinoma Small cell carcinoma of the lung Soft tissue sarcomas	Definitely superior
Gastric carcinoma Colon carcinoma Ovarian carcinoma Lung carcinoma (other than small cell) Head and neck carcinoma Neuroblastoma Osteosarcoma Ewing sarcoma Chronic lymphocytic leukaemia	Possibly superior
Melanoma Cervix carcinoma	Not superior

TABLE 3   Response Rates for Single Agents and Principal
Combination Chemotherapy Regimens Used in Hodgkin's Disease

Drugs	Complete remission
Nitrogen mustard	15%
Vinblastine	30%
Vincristine	15%
Adriamycin	10%
Bleomycin	10%
Bis-chloroethyl-nitrosourea	10%
Chloroethyl-cyclohexyl-nitrosourea	20%
Prednisone	5%
Procarbazine	20%
Imidazole carboxamide	10%
MOPP Nitrogen mustard Vincristine Procarbazine Prednisone	70-80%
ABVD Adriamycin Bleomycin Vinblastine DTIC	75%

S. Monfardini

TABLE 4   The Effect of Anticancer Agents on the Quality of Life

Target	Toxicity	Drug
Bone marrow	Leukopenia Thrombocytopenia	All drugs except: Steroids Bleomycin L-Asparaginase
GI tract	Stomatitis	Adriamycin Bleomycin Methotrexate 5-Fluorouracil Actinomycin D
	Gastritis	Corticosteroids Methotrexate
	Diarrhoea Paralytic ileus	5-Fluorouracil Vincristine
Skin	Hyperpigmentation Alopecia	Bleomycin Busulfan Adriamycin Cyclophosphamide Actinomycin D Vinblastine Vincristine
Nervous system	Paraesthesiae Peripheral neuropathy Deafness Lethargy	Vincristine Vinblastine cis-Platinum L-Asparaginase
Heart	Cardiac failure* Hypertension*	Adriamycin Daunomycin Corticosteroids
Lungs	Fibrosis*	Bleomycin Busulfan Methotrexate Cyclophosphamide
Pancreas	Pancreatitis	L-Asparaginase
GU system	Uterine bleeding Cystitis	Oestrogens Cyclophosphamide
Liver	Abnormal liver function tests (fibrosis)	Methotrexate Cytosine arabinoside L-Asparaginase
Kidney	Abnormal kidney function tests (tubulonecrosis)	Methotrexate cis-Platinum Mithramycin

*Long term side effects

an aggressive approach should be tempered by consideration of those factors which may limit anticancer treatment in patients with far-advanced cancer (Table 5).

TABLE 5 Limits to the Continuation of Anticancer Treatment

Life expectancy less than 2 months
Performance status less than 40
Organ failure: Pulmonary, remal or hepatic
Lack of patient and family cooperation
Tumour resistance to anticancer chemotherapy

The risk/benefit ratio should receive careful evaluation before dismissing the prospect of further anticancer treatment. Previous unsuccessful chemotherapy is only a relative contraindication since second- or third-line treatments may yield significant response rates in tumours sensitive to chemotherapy.

A schematic approach to the determination of the boundary between anticancer chemotherapy and terminal care has been attempted (Table 6). Three groups of neoplastic diseases can be identified:

1) neoplasms where several therapeutic alternatives are available before cessation of anticancer therapy;

2) neoplasms where initial chemotherapy failure can be followed by some therapeutic alternatives;

3) tumour types where little space exists before cessation of anticancer therapy.

TABLE 6   Schematic Outline of the Boundary between Anticancer Chemotherapy and Terminal Care in the Principal Tumour Types

	Tumour types	Useful sequential treatment	Terminal care
I	Wilms' tumour Hodgkin's disease Non-Hodgkin's lymphoma	1st line combination ↓	
	Acute lymphoblastic and myeloblastic leukaemia Testicular carcinoma Breast carcinoma	2nd line combination with non cross-resistant drugs ↓	
	Small cell carcinoma of the lung Soft tissue sarcomas Multiple myeloma Ovarian carcinoma	Single agents sequentially	Stop anticancer treatment if the possibility of inducing an objective response becomes negligible
II	Gastric and colo-rectal carcinoma Lung carcinoma (other than small cell)	1st line combination ↓	
	Head and neck carcinoma Neuroblastoma Osteosarcoma Ewing sarcoma Bladder carcinoma	Single agents sequentially	
III	Malignant melanoma Cervix carcinoma	Single agents sequentially	

Considering this schematic distinction, an active attitude is more justified in groups I and II and less in group III. The present conventional treatment may, of course, be supplemented by the use of potentially new useful agents at present under investigation. Despite this schematic approach, great difficulties may be encountered in assessing individual cases. When this occurs the following guide-lines are recommended:

1) Since continued assessment is the key to appropriate care, regular review may allow aggressive antitumour measures to be reinstituted should the patient's general condition improve spontaneously.

2) Because of the difficulty of the problem and of the fluidity of clinical situations, a second opinion may at times be necessary (Calman, 1978).

3) In border-line situations, the decision should result from a consideration of possible therapeutic advantage in the light of the psychological attitude of the patient towards therapy.

REFERENCES

Saunders, C.M. (1978) Appropriate treatment, appropriate death. In: *The Management of Terminal Disease* (Ed. C.M. Saunders), pp. 1-9. Edward Arnold, London.

Monfardini, S., Brunner, K., Crowther, D. and Olive, D. (1979) *Postgraduate Courses on Clinical Cancer Chemotherapy. Manual for Course Participants.* Vol. 47, 2nd ed. UICC Technical Report Series. Geneva.

Bonadonna, F. (1978) Hodgkin's disease: chemotherapy. In: *Current Therapy 1978* (Ed. H.F. Conn). W.B. Saunders, Philadelphia, London, Toronto.

Calman, K.C. (1978). Physical aspects. In: *The Management of Terminal Disease* (Ed. C.M. Saunders), pp. 33-43. Edward Arnold, London.

Legal Aspects

I. KENNEDY

Reader in English Law, King's College, London, UK

INTRODUCTION

When a lawyer is invited to comment on the continuing care of those
dying from cancer, the first reaction of many is surprise. The
assumption is commonly made that the decisions to be taken in
caring for such patients, the therapeutic strategy to be adopted,
are wholly medical matters and thus wholly for doctors to make,
with or without discussion with the patient. Of course, such
decisions are medical matters in that they arise in the context of
the professional relationship of doctor and patient and they are
for doctors to make in that the doctor is the professional "on the
spot" caring for the patient. But, it cannot be stated too empha-
tically that the principles by reference to which decisions are
made are not within the unique prerogative of doctors to lay down.
The word strategy, for example, implies that choices are available
and choices if they are to be rationally defensible must be made
by reference to known and accepted principles. Such principles are
those which have been worked out by the larger society, not doctors
alone, and which embody the moral, philosophical and spiritual
assumptions of that society. The law is one source of such principles. Indeed, in so far as the law represents the embodiment of
those rules deemed so important by society as to warrant setting
them out formally with appropriate sanctions for non-observance,
legal principles are the most important regulator of the doctors
decisions. This is so even though explicit reference to the law
is rarely, if ever, made, since the law establishes the pattern
with which other normative principles, to which the doctor may more
readily refer, his professional code of ethics, his or society's
code of morality, by and large conform.

In the case of the dying, as in all other areas of medicine, therefore, the doctor must pay due heed to the law. He must act within
the law: he is never above it. The law, or more correctly stated,

19

those who make the law, has a corresponding obligation to ensure
that the principles and rules laid down meet certain criteria.
First, the law must be clear. Secondly, it must be sensitive to
the particular circumstances it seeks to regulate, for example,
the realities of modern medical practice, and the availability
and use of new technology and medicines. Thirdly, it must strike
an appropriate balance between the interests of the various parties involved without putting in jeopardy certain fundamental
commitments, such as, for example, the protection of the individual
and the absolute prohibition on the taking of another's life.

Some argue that the law in England does not meet the first of these
criteria and thus cannot satisfy ex hypothesi the other two.
This is because in England there is no statute nor code setting
out the law governing the continuing care of the terminally ill, nor
are there more than a couple of cases decided by the Courts.[1] Nonetheless legal principles undoubtedly do exist and obviously condition the choices taken by doctors. The fact, however, that the
law is not well-documented has produced at least three unfortunate
effects. First, it has led to doubts as to the precise legal obligations of a doctor in a particular case. This has in turn
helped to foster the view that there is really no law at all, indeed that the law is an irrelevance. Alternatively, the practice
has grown up that if the law is not clear, then, given that the
possibility of being prosecuted for a crime or sued to recover
damages may exist, albeit as a remote possibility in England, it is
better always for the doctor to err on the side of caution and
follow the most conservative or restrictive view of the law. This
practice, which is much more common in the United States, has acquired its own descriptive term, defensive medicine, a term suggestive of the notion that an unnecessary and destructive tension
exists between what the doctor thinks is good medicine and what the
law requires of him.

It is my submission that the law of England relating to the care
of terminally ill patients can be stated with sufficient clarity
to dispel these criticisms. I further submit that when properly
understood it is sufficiently sensitive to the varying realities
it would seek to regulate as to make unnecessary any recourse to
defensive medicine. The law is to be found in the general corpus
of English law and in the writings of commentators.

PRINCIPLE UNDERLYING THE LAW

Before setting out the law, it is important to discover to what
extent there exists any unifying principle or premise which draws
together the individual legal rules. Such a principle not only

---

[1]Re Potter, The Times, July 26, 1963; R v Bodkin Adams, 1957,
Criminal Law Review.

adds rational coherence to what would otherwise be a set of unrelated rules, but also supplies the reference point whereby novel
dilemmas may be resolved. One such principle, often referred to in
Continental Europe and the United States is that of contract, that
the relationship between the doctor and patient is regulated by
agreement between the two parties. This is unsatisfactory for a
number of reasons. First, in England there is not as a matter of
law a contract between doctor and patient in about 99% of all relationships as health care is made available through the National
Health Service. Secondly, the traditional notion of contract or
agreement contemplates two parties in equal bargaining position
possessed of all relevant information (or capable of acquiring it).
This is plainly not so in the case of the vast majority of patients
who must rely on the doctor's knowledge and who are therefore in no
position to do otherwise than agree. Third, the notion of a contract carries the implication that medical care is a commodity to
be bargained for in the market place, a notion specifically rejected
in England. Another unifying principle is said to be the concept of
trust. This, it is said, is the key factor governing the doctor-
patient relationship. This analysis is equally flawed. First, to
argue that each party must trust the other does not demonstrate
that each in fact does so. Indeed, oftentimes a doctor may expect
trust without himself reciprocating, in that, for example, he will
choose not to tell his patient certain facts, on the paternalistic
premise that the patient is better off not knowing. Secondly,
trust presupposes a conscious and reasoned decision by the patient
which in fact may be beyond many patients who, through pain, the
effect of drugs or unconsciousness, cannot make such a decision.
The unifying premise which, in my submission, informs the law is
the concept of duty. A doctor has expertise. A patient seeks help
and is therefore vulnerable. He can only rely on the doctor's skill
and good faith. Given this reality, the law imposes duties upon the
doctor which exist independently of agreement. The patient may expect and ultimately demand that these duties be observed.

THE GENERAL DUTY OF THE DOCTOR

So, what is the doctor's duty in the case of caring for the terminally ill? The classification of a patient as terminally ill is
a decision for the doctor to make based upon wholly medical criteria.
Since, however, the decision carries with it certain significant
implications it is one which must be reached in good faith and on
the basis of the exercise of proper medical skill. If arrived at
otherwise, clearly legal redress will be available to any patient
who suffers harm as a consequence. Terminally ill, in my submission, means that the patient has an illness which has been
accurately diagnosed, and which seems certain to bring about his
death within a relatively short period of time since the illness is
beyond both cure and palliation. The duty of the doctor in such a
circumstance is, stated generally, to use all appropriate medical
skills to make the time remaining for the patient as comfortable as
possible. This is both his professional, ethical duty and his legal

duty. The primary significance is in the form of caring or treatment
the doctor provides. He is no longer under a duty to adopt forms of
treatment intended to cure the patient since by definition the patient is beyond cure. Nor need the doctor adopt palliative measures,
if palliation is taken to mean the use of measures aimed at modifying pathological processes or their consequences so as to delay or
prevent the otherwise inevitable results of such processes or their
consequences. The doctor's duty is limited to the control, to the
extent it is possible, of discomforting symptoms. But even this
apparently simple principle requires some clarification before going
further. It is important to notice that while usually the symptoms
displayed by the patient relate to the terminal illness, there may
be times when they arise from some separate, independent condition.
When this happens, the doctor's first duty is to identify this fact
correctly. Then, he must decide on the appropriate response, which
is a legal as well as a medical decision. There are, perhaps, three
principles which must be followed. First, if the new condition has
discomforting symptoms these should be controlled. Secondly, if it
does not, it can be ignored. Third, both of these principles are
subject to the question whether the new condition may be cured or
palliated. If it can be and if by so doing the patient would be
able to enjoy a further period of life without increased discomfort
then the cure or palliative measure should be adopted.

This general duty of the doctor, to control symptoms as much as
possible and otherwise make the patient as comfortable as possible
has implicit in it two propositions worth noticing. First, medical
treatment other than symptom control or management is uncalled for
as a matter of law and, indeed, is inappropriate; not only is it
unethical conduct but the doctor may also attract legal sanction.
As a matter of law the doctor could be restrained by a court from
continuing such treatment and could be held liable to pay damages
for any distress or increased discomfort the patient suffered as a
consequence, in that his conduct would amount to negligence. Although this is undoubtedly the law, it seems oftentimes to be ignored
particularly in the United States where pointless efforts are made
by doctors, albeit often with the best of intentions. For example,
the doctor may fear that if he does not use every technique in his
armoury he will be accused of neglecting his patient, or the doctor
may simply not understand the real nature of his obligations. The
second implicit proposition is that the diagnosis of a terminal illness does not mean that the doctor's obligations to his patient
cease. There is some fear among lay people that this is so, that
the doctor gives up and hands the patient over to those nursing him.
Furthermore, to the extent that doctors, especially those recently
trained, see themselves as medical scientists solving problems and
curing people rather than fundamentally caring for people, this
attitude of to some extent abandoning the patient may affect some
doctors. But a dying patient is still a living patient. The law recognises this and demands that care must continue even if its nature
changes. This is an example of the english law's affirmation of its

fundamental respect for life.

SPECIFIC DUTIES

Having stated the general duty of a doctor towards his terminally ill
patient, it is necessary to examine how this general duty is made
more specific and applied in the myriad real-life situations which
arise. Analytically the process is one of deriving more specific
principles from more general ones. It is in the nature of law, however, to be couched in abstract terms. There is not one particular
legal rule for each situation which arises or may arise. This would
be a system of ad hoc law which would suggest each novel situation
warrants the creation of a new rule. Rather, the law works dynamic-
ally through the process of analogical reasoning. A principle is
enunciated which is intended and designed to regulate a certain real
situation-X. Another principle regulates another real situation-Y.
When situation-Z arises which is novel and for which no principle
has apparently been specifically designed, the law is determined by
examining the extent to which Z is closer to X or to Y. If it is
more analogous to X than the legal principle regulating X will ordinarily be invoked. Occasionally situation Z may inspire the creation
of a wholly new principle which then serves as a possible precedent
for the future. Thus, what is outlined here represents both the
existing law and the basis for determining the law in as yet un-
tested or unfamiliar circumstances.

Respect For The Patient's Right to Self-Determination

First, perhaps the most fundamental precept of the common law is the
liberty of the individual. In a medical-legal context this means
that a person's right to self-determination, to deal with his body
as he sees fit, is protected by law. The doctor's first duty is to
respect this right. Thus, if a patient who is aware of the nature
of his condition and competent to make the decision, refuses further
treatment from his doctor, continued treatment is unlawful. This is
so notwithstanding the fact that the doctor may regard the patient's
decision as wrong or ill-advised. In practice, this situation will
arise only very rarely if a regime of symptomatic control and no
more has been adopted. Nonetheless, the importance of the obligation to respect the wishes of the patient cannot be overstated. Of
course, the law only recognises the patient's right to self-determination in circumstances where the patient is both legally competent
(ie. not a child nor mentally ill) and is sufficiently lucid to comprehend what he is doing. It is obvious that there is some danger
that the principle may be swallowed by these exceptions, particularly
the second, since the determination of a patient's lucidity falls to
the doctor who may well disagree with the patient's expressed wish
and want to override it. Perhaps, the most appropriate mechanism
for safeguarding both the patient's and the doctor's interests is
for the hospital to document the circumstances fully in the notes
and have the patient's competence assessed by a qualified person
not otherwise concerned in his care. Thus, in summary, the first

duty of the doctor is to listen to and respect the wishes of his
patient.

The Prohibition Against Taking Life

Having established the point that it is the patient who ultimately
may set the limits to the doctor's intervention, it is now necessary
to consider the duties which arise in the usual circumstances where
treatment is consented to. The almost trite observation has already
been made that the patient though dying is still living. This cannot, however, be overemphasised in that respect for life is a cardinal principle of english law. It follows that the taking of a
patient's life by some conduct deliberately designed to bring about
his death is unlawful, whether it be at the patient's request or
without his knowledge or consent. In both cases, the doctor would
attract both criminal and civil liability. Many doctors specialising
in the care of the dying consider that the state of modern medicine
makes even the need to consider this as an option quite unnecessary,
quite apart from its moral repugnance. For, the regime of medicines
now available to the doctor allow him to avoid the pain, distress or
even agony which could prompt a consideration of active euthanasia.
While this is so, it is still the case that by no means all hospitals
or doctors are yet educated in the pharmacological and other management of the terminally ill and large members of patients outside
Hospices and centres of excellence may well, by virtue of their condition, continue to pose the problem of euthanasia. The appropriate
response, however, is not to alter the law so as to allow euthanasia
and thereby arguably undermine the respect for life enshrined both in
the law and medical training. Rather, attention must be directed
to ensuring that doctors who care for the dying understand and use
the medicines and techniques now available.

To Intervene Or Not

The question which next arises is whether the doctor, while prohi-
bited from doing anything deliberately aimed at causing the death of
his patient, may when the circumstances arise stand by and refrain
from doing anything so that the patient dies. The examples commonly
cited are whether antibiotics must be administered if the patient
contracts pneumonia or whether the patient must be resuscitated if
he suffers heart failure. The analysis which is often offered by
lawyers is one which distinguishes between omissions and commissions
and argues that doctors are not open to legal liability merely by
allowing the patient to die rather than doing something which brought
about the death. This analysis is, it is submitted, unsatisfactory.
It is better both morally and legally to analyse the problem in terms
of the doctor's duty. He owes the patient certain duties by virtue
of the relationship of doctor and patient. The duties which arise
in this situation can be set out as can those arising elsewhere.
Moreover, to claim that by allowing the patient to die the doctor
acted lawfully because he omitted to do anything rather than com-

mitted any act is to overlook the obvious point that, depending on
the particular circumstances, it may be the doctor's duty to act,
so that his failure to act by allowing death constituted a breach of
duty. The problem is best analysed in the following stages. The
doctor's duty to the terminally ill is centred on making the patient
comfortable until death. The doctor is not under a duty to take
action to avert death if such action will not aid in the comfort of
the patient. Each patient is different in terms of the progress of
his disease, his psychological response to it, his will to live or
otherwise and thus the general principle of each patient's comfort
is to be judged in the light of these particular facts. Obviously,
purely objective criteria such as the patient's age or the particular illness cannot be justified or relied upon. The patient's death
is not an evil to be avoided at all costs but is an inevitable consequence of his condition. Thus, if, in the light of the particular
facts, the patient may be discomforted by the doctor's conduct, the
doctor is under no duty to act. Applying these principles, the
pneumonia need not be treated if on the facts to do so would mean
that the patient recovered to endure a further period of discomfort,
pain or inevitable, distressing deterioration. If by treating it
the patient could be restored to a state whereby he could enjoy a
further period of life at the level of comfort he previously had,
then it should be treated. The same would be true of resuscitation
and any similar intervention. Given that the decision calls for considered judgment, it must always be appropriate to consider the matter in the case of each patient before it arises. This avoids the
possiblity of unwarranted decisions being taken in the heat of the
moment. It may also be appropriate to record the decision taken so
that all involved in the patient's case may know. This is not to
say it may not be revised. Indeed, it is appropriate to review it
periodically as the circumstances of the patient change. Clearly,
much room is left for the discretion of the doctor and this is as
it should be, since the assessment of the patient's prognosis is
one of his distinct skills. The law lays down the general principle
and the doctor who acts skillfully, reasonably and in good faith is
protected.

This analysis also helps to clarify another issue which taxes some
commentators. The realities of modern medical technology have made
it possible for doctors to extend the process of dying through the
use, for example, of what are colloquially but perhaps inaptly
called life-support machines. Questions are asked as to how long
the doctor must maintain his patient on such a machine before discontinuing its use. Such questions are inappropriate. They stem
from an inadequate analysis of the legal and ethical principles
involved. Life-support machines are merely one form of interven-
tionist therapy, no different in principle from medicines, surgery
or other treatment. In the case of the terminally ill, their use
is ordinarily uncalled for since they can readily be categorised as
heroic or extraordinary therapy imposing a further burden of discomfort on the patient with no foreseeable benefit in terms of increased

comfort in the future. The key question is not whether their use
may be discontinued once started. Rather, it is whether they should
be used in the first place, ie. it is not a matter of switching off
but whether they should be switched on either initially or again
after suitable tests have been carried out. This is, therefore, the
same question as whether to give antibiotics when pneumonia occurs
and is resolved by reference to the same principles.

The Doctrine of Double Effect

One further point ought to be mentioned here. There may arise circumstances in which a doctor may use a form of treatment for his
patient's benefit aware of the fact that, if he does so, it may have
the secondary effect of accelerating (or running the risk of accelerating) the patient's death. The english law clearly adopts the doc-
trine of double effect. The doctor is not in breach of his legal
duty to his patient if, by adopting the particular form of treatment,
his primary intention is the alleviation of symptoms presented by
the patient which are discomforting and irremediable in any less
drastic way. This proposition is not limited to the oft-cited
example of the use of increased doses of morphine, a practice which
the specialists argue is no longer necessary or appropriate, but
extends to any treatment decision.

Aiding Suicide

It may occur sometimes that the patient may wish to end his life
rather than wait for death. The specialists again argue that with
the right regime of treatment there is no need for this to happen
but in reality the right regime is not always available and even if
it were some patients may wish to retain their independence to choose
suicide. English law makes aiding and abetting the suicide of
another a serious crime. Thus, a doctor is under a duty to refrain
from any act which may aid his patient to commit suicide. It is,
however, a fine line between aiding suicide and making available,
for example, certain drugs to relieve pain which, if more than a
certain dosage is taken, will cause death. A court would, it is
submitted, be slow to find a doctor liable who merely facilitated
the self-determination of someone unable through illness to help
himself. This should be contrasted with the situation in which the
patient instructs the doctor to refrain from further treatment.
As has been seen, the doctor is under a duty to comply with this
request provided the patient is lucid and competent. This is not
aiding a suicide since the patient is not, in my submission, com-
mitting suicide, he is merely declining further medical care.

Proxy Decision-making

The final matter for consideration is the duty owed by the doctor
when the patient is unable to participate in treatment decisions,
through unconsciousness, lack of comprehension or legal incompetence,

and others purport to speak for him. Is the doctor under a duty to
respect treatment decisions proposed by relatives or next of kin?
Proxy consent, decision-making on another's behalf, is well-known to
the law. There are, however, certain risks involved in delegating to
people other than the patient the power to make what may be life or
death decisions, for example, the decision to discontinue certain
treatment to control symptoms, or not to resuscitate the patient.
This is one of the disquieting features of the otherwise excellent
decision of the New Jersey Supreme Court in the case of Karen
Quinlan.[2] For, in the case, the court was prepared to vest in Miss
Quinlan's guardians the power to refuse further treatment on her
behalf, on the anecdotal basis that she would have wished it. The
possibilities this raises for abuse make it a most undesirable legal
development. The law should remain as it now is in England. Where
the patient is incompetent, for whatever reason, only the person who
is a parent or lawfully appointed guardian may exercise any decision-
making power on the patient's behalf. And, equally important, any
decision made must be measured against what is deemed to be in the
best interests of the patient. But the arbiter of what is in the
patient's best interests is not necessarily the legal guardian. The
guardian must conform to the objective criteria laid down by the law.
Certainly, in the case of a decision whether to resuscitate or not,
such objective guidelines are essential. The mere allegation that
the patient would not have wished to be resuscitated, without the
possibility of any proof, is not enough.

CONCLUSION

From this recital of the general and specific duties of the doctor
it can be seen that the law in England, if understood and followed,
is sensitive to the needs of patient and doctor alike. It allows
the most sensitive care to be practised because it rests on an understanding of the realities of terminal illness and care. It retains
the flexibility necessary to meet changing circumstances, and allows
appropriate discretion to doctors without sacrificing its adherence
to fundamental principles. Occasionally, disquiet is expressed
that the law is not more coherently set out. There is little
evidence, however, that doctors hesitate to adopt certain courses of
action because of doubts as to their legality, probably because the
law is entirely in keeping with good medical care. Thus, the need
for a general statute is not pressing. Some guide in the form of a
Code of Practice for doctors, similar to the one suggested for the
determination of brain-stem death, may be desirable, if only to set
the minds of some doctors and patients at rest.

---

[2] re Quinlan (1976)   70 N.J. 10, 355 A.2nd 647

READINGS

Glover, J. (1977). Causing death and saving lives. Penguin Books, London.

Kennedy, I.M. (1976). The legal effect of requests by the terminally ill not to receive further treatment. Criminal Law Review, 217-232.

Kennedy, I.M. (1977). Switching off life-support machines: the legal implications. Criminal Law Review, 443-452.

Ramsey, P. (1970). The patient as person. Yale University, New Haven.

Sharpe, D.J., Fiscina, S.F., and Head, M. (1978). Law and Medicine. West Publishing Co., Minnesota.

Veatch, R.M. (1976). Death, dying and the biological revolution. Yale University, New Haven.

Williams, G. (1973). Euthanasia. Medico-Legal Journal, 41, 14-25.

Further Legal Considerations

R. POZZATO

Forensic Medicine Institute, Universita degli Studi, Milan, Italy

Medicolegal aspects of terminal cancer care differ in several respects from those of medical treatment in general. They relate to questions of lawfulness, which depends mainly on three facts:

1. the availability of a reasonable range of anti-cancer treatments;
2. the possibility of supportive measures;
3. the possibility of administering individually determined pain relieving therapy, reserving the more potentially dangerous drugs for use in patients with the most severe pain.

With the current range of surgical, radiological, chemotherapeutic and hormonal treatment, a malignancy with a known unfavourable prognosis will no longer necessarily be totally unresponsive to anti-cancer treatment. There are frequently opportunities to slow the development of a tumour even if its progress cannot be halted.

Thus, the terminal stage of a cancer may be characterized by:

1. no response to anti-cancer treatment, whether or not the patient is experiencing troublesome symptoms;

or

2. partial response to anti-cancer treatment, which is well tolerated by the patient, whether or not the patient is experiencing troublesome symptoms from the underlying disease;

or

3. partial response to anti-cancer treatment, which is poorly tolerated by the patient, whether or not the patient is experiencing troublesome symptoms from the underlying disease.

In all three situations, a treatment is advocated which will reconcile, as far as possible, the needs of "disease control" with those of "patient care", by resorting to procedures aimed partly at slowing the course of the disease (anti-cancer therapy, supportive measures) and partly at eliminating suffering (pain relieving therapy, discontinuation of poorly tolerated anti-cancer therapy), so as to make the most of the positive impact of the former and to minimize the negative impact of the latter.

In practice this involves an operational plan consisting of:

a. implementation of supportive therapy;

b. continuation of fairly effective anti-cancer therapy, if well tolerated;

c. discontinuation of poorly tolerated anti-cancer treatment, if the patient's
    pain cannot be controlled by commonly used analgesics, even if there are no
    alternatives to the discontinued treatment;

d. use of analgesics, proportionate to the patient's needs and with the least
    possible effect on the patient's psychophysical state.

In the majority of cases, prolongation of survival rather than a shortening can be
expected to result from such an approach. A hastening of the patient's death
remains a possibility, largely because of the unpredictable course of disseminated
cancer, particularly in those patients with an obviously unfavourable prognosis.
Thus, in terminal cancer, prolongation of survival as long as possible, although
still important, does not take priority over the equally basic aim of relieving
pain; and risk of shortening survival is offset by the greater likelihood of an
unabbreviated, pain-free death.

An analysis of this approach from a medicolegal viewpoint leads to the following
conclusions:

1. A medical procedure is lawful provided the damage it causes or may cause is
offset and justified by the purpose of saving the patient a greater damage.
Palliative measures in terminal cancer carried out in a technically competent way
may cause a damage. Generally, this takes the form of a *possibility* and is offset
and justified by the fact that it is expected to prevent a greater damage, either
distressing symptoms during the survival time of the patient's more rapid death.
In other words, a terminal cancer treatment is lawful provided it is planned and
implemented in accordance with modern technological practice and adheres to the
mandatory commitment to both prolongation of survival and patient care.

2. Terminal cancer treatments are at present intrinsically dangerous like other
technically exacting procedures. This means they place in jeopardy the right to
safety, the right to the preservation of one's life; a matter which only a legally
competent patient or his representative can deal with. Such treatments are therefore lawful only when undertaken after obtaining consent based on adequate information about the nature of the disease, and the nature and prospects of the planned
procedure. The difficulty caused by the family's refusal to allow the patient to
be informed about the nature of his illness and its probable prognosis does not
necessarily mean that it is impossible to obtain a valid consent. In fact, according to an authoritative catholic statement, consent is valid when the person who
requested and obtained it did not reveal the diagnosis because he believed the
truth would harm the patient, but had reason to conclude that the patient would
have accepted the treatment if he had been informed more fully of the nature of
his disease.

3. There is need for clarification about which procedures offer the best prospects
of helping the terminal cancer patient, from any point of view. Such procedures
would represent what the majority of doctors would consider appropriate when dealing with the various problems of terminal cancer, whether undertaken by themselves
or by a specialist colleague.

Different or less adequate care cannot, however, be censured when recourse to the
optimal procedure is impossible because of lack of necessary facilities and personnel. On the other hand, when a treatment based on modern clinical and therapeutic
principles can be adopted, any recourse to a different and less effective method of
care constitutes a departure from the practice that the majority of physicians would
regard as appropriate. The actions of a physician who planned and implemented less

adequate care would then be considered malpractice. This is covered by Article 43 of the Criminal Code which states that a doctor is guilty of culpable homicide if his failure to implement the appropriate treatment allows the patient to die sooner.

The Need for Guidelines

G. CAIZZI

Deputy Attorney-General, Milan, Italy

In a large hospital, as a result of the excessive scientific emphasis that exists today, there is a considerable risk of the patient becoming depersonalized. Concern about this inspired the recent European Council resolutions on the right of the ill person not to suffer in vain. The implication of the resolutions are, however, not immediately clear. It is generally agreed that in a terminal illness, when drugs are given to alleviate pain but at the same time hasten death, the doctor is not culpable. In Italy the situation is more complicated because of rigid judicial regulations. These derive from an unadequate consideration of the ethical and legal presuppositions of the relationship between the lawfully practising physician and the patient who is suffering.

An essential premise for treatment to be lawful is consent, either expressed or presumed, by the patient to those injuries that are necessarily inflicted in the course of medical intervention. Consent is the limiting factor in relation to the authorization of medical treatment. Its position as a safeguard to the person's human values reflects the exigency of protecting the patient's primary rights to life, health, freedom and dignity against the risks which are inherent in medical intervention. The consent of the patient to his own death, however, cannot remove liability from the doctor, as it goes beyond the limits of what is judicially acceptable. Even so, it is surprising how little room for manoeuvre the existing regulations allow when one considers the realities of everyday clinical practice.

Generally, when the patient is unable to give his consent, this is presumed on the indisputable basis of human experience represented by the instinct of self-preservation. But, in the terminally ill, it is necessary to consider the equally fundamental right of the patient not to suffer in vain and to die with dignity. Here, because death is inevitable in the near future, and curative treatments are futile, the physician's duty is to help the patient die in the most dignified and painless way. Though even here willingness expressed by the patient to hasten his own death does not remove the doctor's liability, as one may not dispose of one's own life even if suffering from painful, incurable and lethal illness. But it could justify the adoption of symptom control measures that are not directly intended to shorten life. The physician must, however, always take decisions exclusively in relation to the individual patient. If this principle is not borne in mind and the same human and social dignity accorded to all, solutions motivated by interests which conflict with the patient's interests might be adopted.

The Swiss National Council, referring to the directions issued by the Swiss Medical Academy, has given physicians a wide freedom of judgment when death is imminent and the patient is no longer capable of taking decisions. From a legal standpoint, the Council thought it could single out a "presumed willingness" by the patient who, if still conscious and in his right mind, would not be able to tolerate a continuation of his suffering. The physician's action is thus justified on legal grounds by appealing to a motive corresponding to "management without mandate". The formulation of such directions has, however, little value unless the concepts of life and death in relation to a terminally ill patient are made clear, and his real interest combined with the doctor's duty is sorted out.

A good example of the gap between principles and practice is represented by the initiative taken at the Triemli Civil Hospital in Zurich. The doctors decided to suspend feeding incurable patients who, although they did not have specific brain lesions, had lapsed into deep coma. The alleged justification was that loss of personality had taken place. At the end of an inquiry performed by the Public Attorney's Office of the Zurich Canton, the doctors' decision was substantially ratified. The Attorney's Office considered in particular that they had adhered, on the basis of inner conviction, to the theory that regards death as coincident with the permanent cessation of consciousness (death of the person). It was concluded that the doctors had not acted contrary to the law and were not guilty of culpable homicide. Moreover, their action had not been negligent or contrary to their professional duties.

In this case, the problem of the consent of the patient and of those who represent him is left unsolved, and the physician is privileged as an uncontrolled administrator of the final stage of the illness, and as the exclusive interpreter of the value of the life and death of the patient. The risks of covert euthanasia are considerable unless specific guidelines are laid down for doctors to work within. Without guidelines, it is possible that a patient who is certainly going to die, but who is still living, may be consigned to a new judicial category of a "living corpse", that is, an "ex-person", deprived of guardianship and therefore no longer a subject of rights.

Such a possibility makes it even more important to answer questions about "quality of life" when death is postponed, and whether obstinate insistence on further therapeutic endeavour (dysthanasia) infringes the patient's right not to suffer in vain and to die with dignity. This right is, in fact, constitutionally recognized by the norm that forbids treatments violating the limits imposed by respect of the human person. Therefore, if the doctor always takes into account the patient's real interest, when death delaying treatment is known to be futile or, at least, unable to maintain a sufficient quality of life, his obligation to strive to keep the patient alive is annulled, and his omissive behaviour becomes legally irrelevant as a cause of death.

On the other hand, it is a doctor's duty to help the patient die in the most dignified and painless way, even if his active intervention may unintentionally hasten the patient's death. In this situation, the prescription of medicines intended to relieve pain represents the only appropriate expression of professional activity, and as such, although the medicines are a possible contributory factor, the patient's death will rightly be considered a direct consequence of the progression of the disease.

It is, however, up to medical science to supply the indications for the suspension of life-prolonging treatment and for the adoption of symptom control measures alone. This means that with an adequate system of social controls concerning diagnosis of incurability and prognosis of imminent death, legal restraints can be imposed to control those initiatives and choices which, if made by the physician, would, by culpably exceeding the limits established in the patient's interest, violate the penal regulations protecting life.

II
GENERAL ASPECTS

Communication Between Doctor and Patient

E. R. HILLIER

Countess Mountbatten House, Southampton, UK

ABSTRACT

One vital ingredient of good quality terminal care is effective communication. Without it patients and families experience needless distress whilst their management by doctors and nurses becomes more difficult. To be effective communication will occur at two levels. First the problem should be explained in clear and simple language, a plan of action made and the patient told what this is. Second, the doctor needs to show in words and actions that he understands the physical and emotional problems of the patient and that he will do all he can to help, whatever happens. Doctors and patients view illness from different standpoints so that the doctor must realise that the solution of his problems may have little relevance to those of the patient.

There comes a time when curative treatment becomes inappropriate or even harmful and the Clinician must be able to change from curative treatment to palliative. Some patients will wish to know the diagnosis; others will not and each situation must be judged separately. There are four guidelines: do not tell lies; do not tell patients the diagnosis unless they ask or otherwise show they wish to talk; a direct question probably requires a direct answer but an indirect or evasive question almost certainly does not; if doubtful how much the patient wishes to know, counter each question by a question. Patients will then take the initiative.

INTRODUCTION

The word communication is becoming yet another casualty of the increasing vocabulary of jargon. This adds to its pomposity and implies that if I talk about it I am also good at it, which is far from the truth. Indeed I am interested in communication precisely because it is difficult and my aim today is to share with you some of the thoughts I have had about communication with patients and how I overcome the problems that occur in this surprisingly difficult area of patient care.

Although it is easy to define communication, to do so is of little practical help. It is far better to list the characteristics of successful communication from which can be built a successful scheme for imparting and receiving accurate

37

information. On one level it means talking, listening, simple tactful explanations
and a sensible commonsense approach to a particular person's particular problems.
At a deeper level it may mean a sharing or feeling of emotion between doctor and
patient, imparting confidence and trust - possibly the most effective placebos
which exist in medicine today. To do this well a doctor must have a good sense of
timing, a sense of proportion, a sense of humour and an ability to show patients
and relatives that he really understands what the patient is going through and
what are his hopes, his anxieties and his fears. Such deeper communication may
not require words for it is a meeting of personalities rather than a meeting of
intellects and the doctor must appear unhurried and not embarrassed or afraid
to answer the patient's questions.

On the other hand his approach must be a balanced one. He must not dwell on such
serious matters to the exclusion of all else. Even patients with cancer have
other interests which should never be forgotton. Frequently doctors and nurses
talk less to their cancer patients feeling that if they do they will have to
discuss the weighty problems of life or death. This is always a mistake: even
dying patients need to be treated as ordinary people in an ordinary way yet
frequently this does not happen. At one end of the spectrum we avoid serious
discussion when patients need to talk or, alternatively, we become far too morbid
about the patients' cancer and give them bad news in such a way as to completely
remove all hope. A number of patients say how they have been given apparently
"good news" by a registrar or intern only to find that facial expression
completely belies his words. Communication occurs in words and in actions. To
fail to understand this is disastrous.

To communicate successfully one has to mean what one says and there are no simple
rules for achieving this. To try and act seldom, if ever, rings true and once
found out one will never be trusted again. Most patients become bitter and
resentful if they believe their doctor has lied to them. There may be no need
to tell the truth, but lying is dangerous. We often do it - in my opinion
wrongly - when we need to control the situation for our own peace of mind. Yet,
surprisingly, the frank admission that one is finding management of the patient
difficult and conversation awkward may be surprisingly effective. It shows you
are human, and patients in real trouble appreciate this.

Three Problems

There are three major problems in cancer care today. The first and most obvious
is late diagnosis, a point at which many of the problems begin. Although one
hears and reads much in the media and the press about patients sueing doctors for
late or missed diagnoses, it is less commonly mentioned that patients with
symptoms of cancer may wait weeks, months, or even years before seeking medical
help. This inaction is brought about largely by fear of a disease which many
patients consider as a death sentence involving terrible pain. In England,
as in many other countries, there is an inordinate fear of death by cancer and in
a survey of the general population approximately 25 percent of those questioned
believed that a diagnosis of cancer meant certain death, whilst another 25 per
cent believed that cancer also meant indescribable, unbearable and uncontrollable
pain. It is no surprise, therefore, that patients are afraid of having the
diagnosis confirmed.

Our failure to diagnose is a complex and subtle problem and, although many
patient care groups believe that the problem can be solved by doctors being more
vigilant, this is far from the case. Patients must first be better educated
and doctors given more efficient tools for early diagnosis for, frequently, the
first failure of communication occurs at this stage.

One of the most angry patients I have seen was a woman pouring scorn on a chest hospital which was investigating a pleural effusion and failed to diagnose her small breast tumour which, in fact, was its primary cause. Later I learned that months before she complained of increasing breathlessness she had felt her tumour, yet had told no one about it.

The second problem in cancer management is the need for more effective treatment. Inadequacies in this area occur in two ways. First, better curative treatment will reduce the 130,000 cancer deaths that occur each year in England & Wales. The second problem is more subtle. During the past few years there has been an improved survival in some cancers and definite cures in others. Thirteen malignancies which were regarded as a death sentence are now potentially curable. Although this is good news the total number of cancer deaths each year continues to rise. Thus, despite dramatic advances in medical oncology, its real impact as seen by the patient is alarmingly small. The point to be made is this: the primary aim of the medical oncologists is to cure one of the most unpleasant diseases of our time. Cure may be almost as important to them as it is to the patient, the real danger being that there is a large emotional investment in cure, creating the trap of inappropriate optimism at inappropriate times. Most of you will know what I mean. On Day 1 of a malignant diagnosis there is every reason to be optimistic. However, when the patient returns and one's initial therapy has failed, it is too easy - and before I started working in terminal care I have fallen into this trap myself many times - it is too easy to become over-optimistic about the next line of treatment in an attempt to help the patient or, perhaps even more important, to help onself believe that one is really doing something worthwhile and useful. The patient listens to what is said about treatment and its likely effects, only to find that these prognostications are wrong. Nothing shakes patients' confidence more than a promise that this treatment will make them better when, in fact, it does no such thing. Indeed they often feel worse, and if they suffer nausea, vomiting, hair loss and prolonged hospitalisation, they are likely to be extremely resentful about what has been done to them.

One simple question must be asked: "What effect will this treatment have on the particular person?" The honest answer to the question is often different from the one we fondly hope for. To give an example - A 14 year old child with Acute Myeloid Leukaemia was being managed at a famous teaching hospital by doctors whom I know, and would be proud to have looking after my own children. Despite a good first year, this particular child had a number of relapses and the prognosis became increasingly hopeless. Her father was a doctor and was aware that, unless a miracle happened, his daughter was going to die in the next few weeks. Unfortunately, as so often happens with children, instead of becoming tolerant to venepunctures and intravenous therapy, she had become increasingly disturbed by these procedures and would spend the night before such a test sobbing and crying in her parents' bed. On visiting the hospital it was suggested by the Professor that she be readmitted for treatment with a new chemotherapeutic agent. Now, taken on face value, this was entirely reasonable, but what he failed to do was to ask the question "What will this treatment do to this particular child?" The father, however, asked it for him and obtained the following answer, tinged with a somewhat desperate attempt to help a young child in a tragic situation. The answer was "I hope it will make her better." To which the child's father replied "What do you mean by better?" "I hope it will make her live longer" explained the paedetrician, "results from America have been most encouraging." "What do these results show?" asked the father. "There have been some trials" said the paedetrician, "showing definite tumour regression."

The conversation continued in this way with the father gently asking pertinent questions about the treatment and what it would actually do to his daughter. It turned out that the hospital was conducting a trial into the agent to be used and that the child, because she did not live in London, would need to be admitted while the drug would be given by infusion. Daily venepunctures would be necessary to monitor treatment. The real likelihood of significant improvement in the child's condition, as opposed to tumour regression, were likely to be small and the side-effects unpleasant. In addition to this, the parents would find difficulty visiting, since they had a number of other children, and so the real picture of what was going to happen was almost total bad news for the child, for her parents and for her brothers and sisters. Following this conversation, her management was completely replanned and she returned home, without treatment, to her family, dying peacefully six weeks later with her parents looking after her and her brothers and sisters close by.

The third difficulty in cancer management is inadequate terminal care. The first two problems I have already mentioned - those of late diagnosis and the injudicious use of either ineffective or potentially harmful treatments, can make the management of the terminally ill patient, and communication with him, much more difficult than it need be.

How, therefore, can we learn to communicate better with our patients? Clearly it must occur at two different levels. First of all, adequate information must be given in clear, simple language. The physician should always make a plan and tell the patient exactly what it is, in words he can understand. Unfortunately, we doctors are not the best communicators because few of us have been taught how to do it. Like leadership, some have a flair for it but most have not. Too often we discuss our problems - namely the problems of pathology, investigation and treatment - while the patient's problems are quite different. This raises the point that, although for doctors, investigation and treatment are the prime issues, to the patient they are incidental items in the general management. They are not going to care about the serum calcium, or what leucocytes or platelets do in response to chemotherapy. Nor, in fact, are they going to be interested in statistical chances of cure. Statistically one looks at these things differently according to whether or not one has the disease. If I am treating a patient with a condition which has a 90 per cent cure rate, I would regard his chances as good. If, on the other hand, I am the patient, the statistics do little to reassure me that I will not be one of the unfortunate 10 per cent who die. As Harold Wilson said in relation to another subject: "To the man who is out of work, unemployment is 100 per cent." That is, he looks at the problem quite differently from the actuary who produces the figures.

All this emphasises that, in order to care for the terminally ill effectively. one needs to get slightly under the skin of the patient. One of the best ways to do this on a general, surgical or medical ward round, is to imagine oneself in the patient's bed, looking out and seeing what the doctors are doing and hearing what they are saying through the patient's eyes and ears. By doing this, occasionally one is reminded how easy it is for doctors to be insensitive, tactless or even rude - all qualities which render good communication impossible. If one can feel just a little of what the patient feels, then much has been learned.

Now it might be thought that the examples I give and the points that I make all show that good communication requires much time. However, the essential point of this approach is to touch the heart and the mind of the person for whom you are caring. What I mean by this is probably best expressed in the famous painting of the Creation by Michelangelo, where God is leaning forward from Heaven to touch the hand of lackadaisical man on earth. This pictures symbolizes the point of contact which is the true and essential ingredient for any successful communication.

When someone says "I can't get anywhere this this patient" it is usually this point of contact that is missing. If it is not there, then it is wise not to press the patient too hard. If it is there, you can do and talk about almost anything. Which brings me on to one of the commonest questions I am asked: "Should you tell patients their diagnosis and prognosis and, if so, when do you tell them?"

Telling patients

It is important to discuss this question amongst ourselves because if one can relax when talking to patients about their future, terminal care need have few fears, for here lies the Rubicon of the patient's management.

There is plenty of evidence to show that approximately 80 per cent of patients with advanced cancer either know, or have good reason to suspect, that they are either very ill or going to die. Unfortunately, in some hospitals there are hard and fast rules as to whether patients should be told or not. In some wards no patient is ever told, in other wards all are told.

So often, in medicine, we doctors look at the patient and wonder if he is sensible enough to be told the truth, and whether or not he is emotionally strong enough to cope with it. I believe that, as we do this, the patient is looking at us and asking himself the same sort of question, namely "Can I trust this doctor to talk to me reasonably and sensibly about my illness without him hurting me unnecessarily?" In other words, the question we ask, "Should he be told or not?" misses the point. What the patient is really asking is, "What is happening to me and what are you going to do about it?"

Frequently, however, it is the medical team who decides that the patient should be told and, once this decision has been made, there is no turning back. The person in England often chosen to do the telling is the young, newly qualified doctor. I recently met a man who, one day before leaving hospital, was told that he had cancer of the pancreas, that it had spread all over the abdomen, that it was inoperable, that there was no other treatment available and that he was terminal. No attempt whatever was made to find our what cancer meant to him, and no help, hope nor solace of any kind was given to gim. Ironically, in their anxiety, the staff even forgot to treat his pain. Most of us would feel devastated if given such information in this way and, although it is done with the best of intentions, it is totally misguided. Words are unnecessary until the patient himself decides that he wishes to discuss, with a person he trusts, questions of the greatest importance to him.

One word of warning, however. Cancer means different things to different people. Therefore, I urge you to choose your words with the utmost care - always think what they mean to the patient and the family, not what they mean to you.

Those reading this book, probably have a similar idea of what the word cancer means but, only last week, I saw a woman who thought that cancer happened to people who had been dirty or immoral and was a punishment from God. She also believed that patients with cancer went mad and that the disease itself was infectious. Many people think that cancer can be sexually transmitted and so, frequently, in such families all intercourse has ceased with all the stresses and strains that that is likely to induce in a young couple. This patient also believed that cancer was like a huge spider inside her, gnawing its way from the abdomen to the heart and thence to the brain. If that is what people think of when they know they have cancer, it is not surprising that they become acutely distressed on learning the diagnosis.

C.C.T.C.—C

How should one tell a patient that he has cancer? The rule is that there are no
rules, but it is generally better to wait until asked and, even then, be absolutely
certain that the patient really wants to know before you answer the question. The
directness of the question should dictate the directness of the answer. A frank,
sensible and honest, "Have I got cancer, Doctor?" should be answered in an equally
honest way. A hesitant, tentative, "I haven't got cancer, have I Doctor?" usually
means that the patient is seeking reassurance and should be answered quite
differently. If one is not sure how to proceed, each question should be answered
by a question, thus allowing the patient to direct the extent of the revelations.

"Have I got cancer, Doctor?"
"Why on earth do you ask me that?"
"Because I don't seem to be getting better."
"Why don't you think you are getting better?"
"I am losing weight, feel more tired, and the pain is worse."
"Why do you think that is?"
"I think I am getting more ill."
"Is that why you asked the original question?"
"Yes."
"If you did have cancer, are you sure you would really want to know?"

And so it goes on. By feeling one's way very carefully one can, as it were, hit
the golden moment - the point at which the time is right and the information needs
to be shared. Once shared, however, one should always return the next day so that
the patient can ask questions which will have occurred to him during the previous
night. What I call brutal telling is for a doctor to tell a pateint that he has
cancer without explanation, and then never to return to see him again. This is
not what telling the patient is all about, and is the antithesis of good
communication.

Emotional Aspects of Death
and Dying

C. A. GARFIELD

Professor, Cancer Research Instiute, University of California, San Francisco, USA
and Founder and Chairman of the SHANTI Project, Berkeley, California, USA
106 Evergreen Lane, Berkeley, California 94705, USA

INTRODUCTION

In an interesting and informative book entitled When Doctors are
Patients, physicians Max Pinner and Benjamin Miller compiled an impressive array of firsthand accounts of the experiences of physicians
who were compelled to cope with serious illness. They conclude that
no matter what the nature of the disease, a sick person often has
strong emotional reactions to illness that may be a greater source of
torment for the patient (and therefore a serious challenge to the
treating physician) than the obvious somatic symptoms. Although the
authors' use of the term symptoms inaccurately implies psychopathology when, in fact, such strong emotional responses are clearly
appropriate to the extreme stress of a life-threatening illness,
their following point is vital.

> It remains a fact that even many physicians, both in the per-
> formance of their professional work and as patients (just like
> any other patients), have the impression that the distance
> between somatic symptoms and a lie is far greater than that
> between psychogenic symptoms and a lie; that psychogenic symp-
> toms are less "real" than somatic ones--and that, in conse-
> quence, psychogenic symptoms need not be treated. All wise
> physicians, and many experienced physicians, throughout re-
> corded history have known better, but the majority of physicians
> still need to be reminded (Pinner and Miller, 1952).

One intent of this paper is to assist the physician, nurse and allied
personnel in identifying the emotional needs of the dying patient and
his family and to suggest helpful ways of providing some of the
necessary support. Another and admittedly more ambitious intent is
to identify the entire area of basic emotional support for patients
and families as a legitimate and vital concern for any fully competent health professional. An important, but often overlooked,
corollary of this proposition is that doctors, nurses, and other
health care workers who spend many hours each day with patients engaged in a life-and-death struggle against disease, and who must constantly make decisions that affect the resolution of that struggle,
need emotional support themselves. The archaic notion that emotional

43

expression and support are inappropriate or unprofessional derives
from a model of professional comportment devised by those who have
learned to view emotion as a weakness and intellect as a weapon. It
is based on an inaccurate conception of the way human beings function
under stress. Physicians, nurses and others who follow this model
inevitably treat only diseases, not people, which undermines their
competence and effectiveness.

IDENTIFYING THE PROBLEM

It does seem symptomatic that few words if any are directed to
medical students about how to help a patient die. House staff
members may be criticized for failing to carry out some
relatively minor test or procedure, but seldom is there any
evaluation of the care accorded to terminal patients' psyches
during the last days. We all believe in treating the whole
person and work hard at enhancing his physical and psychic
comfort in small ways, which may have no influence on the
final outcome of his illness, and yet it is not always noticed
that a dying person very often seems to have less attention
paid to him than to the patency of the multiplicity of tubes
that are entering him from every direction and which will enable us to study his last, hopefully balanced, chemistries.
Occasionally, it seems that more real effort is expended to
get autopsy permission than to see to it that the patient does
not die alone. It is as though, as doctors, we sometimes express our denial of death by focusing our attention upon the
tubes, the chemistries, and the autopsy (Bulger, 1963).

In identifying the basic problems associated with the care of the
terminally ill, it is necessary to examine at least two points of
view: the professionals' and the patients'. Kastenbaum and Aisenberg (1972) consider the following sociomedical issues to be the
major ones: (1) the imposition of emotional isolation upon the dying
person; (2) the routinization of treatment; (3) the condescension of
professionals who treat the patient as though he were an irrespon-
sible child, unable to cope with his situation like an adult; (4) a-
mong those responsible for the patient's well-being, the inadequate
and unreliable patterns of communication ranging from the choice of
what is communicated to the patient and how it is stated, to all the
little ways significant information is withheld or misinterpreted;
and (5) the failure of all persons engaged in caring for the patient
to recognize and fulfill their share of the total responsibility.

The major issues identified by patients are (1) that the dying person
will become quietly isolated because of a decrease in communication
resulting from the unwillingness of those responsible for his care to
maintain the openness and emotional support essential for him to live
out his life with some hope and participation in meaningful relationships; (2) that the patient will be subjected to painful, uncomfortable, and demanding procedures that might prolong existence
without prolonging a desirable quality of life, and that the disease
will force the patient to endure intense, chronic pain seemingly
without end; and (3) that the terminally ill person will lose control
of bodily, interpersonal, and cognitive functions, that will compel
him or her to confront a terrifying and alien set of experiences,
stripped of all decision-making powers.

The global problem encompassing both professional and patient ident-
ifications of the dilemma is epitomized by the question, "How do we
know when we are treating a dying patient?" More specifically, "How
do we decide when cure or prolonged life are still possibilities requiring aggressive treatment?" "When do we acknowledge that a
patient is dying and that palliation and emotional support are the
optimal strategies?" Having observed this dilemma many times, I am
quite sure that a useful approach is to communicate the medical realities to the patient as skillfully, honestly, and clearly as
possible and to allow the patient (with the help of his or her family
or advocate) to decide upon the preferred treatment. To allow the
patient to retain the basic right to choose comfort care and to ac-
cord him the opportunity to relate to his impending death in a mean-
inful way, health professionals must have the courage and willingness
to acknowledge that the patient's wishes may take priority over their
own.

PATIENT-DOCTOR COMMUNICATIONS

Fundamental to the evolution of effective doctor-patient communications is the notion that physicians answer all questions honestly,
giving as much information as is asked for by the patient. For many
people in extraordinarily high-stress situations, ambiguity produces
more emotional distress than even the most negative reality. I
occasionally hear colleagues in medicine and nursing suggest that
"the patient knows anyway." If this is true, then any reluctance to
communicate honestly and openly merely compels the patient, his
family, and the staff to collude in a lie that may severely increase
the patient's anxiety. Situations similar to the one facing Tolstoy's Ivan Ilych are all too common.

> What tormented Ivan Ilych most was the deception, the lie,
> which for some reason they all accepted. That he was not
> dying but simply ill, and that he only need keep quiet and
> undergo a treatment and then something very good would result.
> He, however, knew that, do what they would, nothing would
> come of it only still more agonizing suffering and death.
> This deception tortured him--their not wishing to admit what
> they all knew and what he knew....Those lies enacted over him
> on the eve of his death and destined to degrade this awful,
> solemn act to the level of their visiting, their curtains,
> their sturgeon for dinner--were terrible agony for Ivan Ilych.

Ambiguous or dishonest communication imposes needless emotional pain
on patients and families facing life-threatening illness. The deleterious impact of the deliberate choice to withhold information
without first accurately assessing the awareness of the patient is
illustrated by the tragic case of an elderly couple.

While the husband was dying of lung cancer, the physician and family
firmly stood by their decision not to inform him that his illness was
terminal. The wife, whom her husband described as his "bride of 50
years," tried valiantly not to leak the information to him. Given
the fact that the latest research in nonverbal communication indicates that between 70 percent and 90 percent of what we communicate
to one another is transmitted through nonverbal channels, how long
could the wife maintain this facade without nonverbally communicating
signs of her obvious distress? In minutes the tension resulting from

her emotional stress was clearly perceived by her terminally ill husband who only hours before had confided to me that he had known he was dying for several weeks. He had long since noticed his wife's distress and had chosen not to talk with her about his illness in an attempt to spare her the emotional pain of confronting his death. The inaccurate assessment of the patient's awareness of his prognosis resulted in a restricted system of communication that inflicted considerable distress on both husband and wife. Since they defined their relationship of 50 years as a "marriage made in heaven" what value existed in reducing their last set of interactions to a lie? The misguided conclusions that such withholding of information more frequently prevents (rather than causes) emotional pain results from a desire for mutual protection frequently observed among patients, families, and staff. A professional or volunteer who has been trained in communication skills, has more time, and is able to understand personal metaphor and symbolic communication is in a better position to assess the level of patient and family understanding. Without such assistance, a conspiracy of silence (in which everyone knows and yet no one is willing to share the fact that he knows) can overwhelm and alienate the patient, his family, and all health professionals.

A decade or two ago we frequently wondered: Should we tell the patient he is dying or keep it a secret? As Pattison (1978), Garfield (1978) and others have observed, the question is false. Care of the dying patient clearly does not center on verbally communicating the truth or not but rather on the gamut of human communications surrounding the dying person.

Kalish (1970) has listed a variety of information inputs that come to the patient:
1.   direct statements from the physician
2.   overheard comments of the physician to others
3.   direct statements from other personnel, including aides, nurses, technologists
4.   overheard comments by staff to each other
5.   direct statements from family, friends, clergy, lawyer
6.   changes in the behavior of others toward the patient
7.   changes in the medical care routines, procedures, medications
8.   changes in physical location
9.   self-diagnosis, including reading of medical books, records, and charts
10. signals from the body and changes in physical status
11. altered responses by others toward the future

"It is evident that the dying person is engaged in multiple communications with many people. If the messages are clear the dying person can make sense out of his experience. But if the messages are confused, ambiguous, or contradictory, the result is needless apprehension, anxiety, and the blockage of appropriate actions on the part of both the dying person and those around him...We should not expect at all times to be able to look at ourselves and others in the stark cold light of reality. There is an interplay between levels of denial and levels of awareness. Human communication is full of nuances. Thus, it seems absurd to me that patterns of human communication should change. If we are able to talk with people about their lives in many ways that are comfortable

and acceptable to both them and us, then we should be able
to talk about dying in many ways that are acceptable and
comfortable. Thus I am not concerned with the issue of how
much denial or openness there is. But I am concerned that
there be <u>opportunity</u>, <u>availability</u>, and <u>possibility</u> for
open communication with the dying." (Pattison, 1978)

UNDERSTANDING PATIENT DENIAL

The subjective experience of cancer is nearly unfathomable from the
perspective of the observer. Whereas disease-related cellular and
systemic metamorphoses have many identifiable and predictable characteristics, the phenomenology of the patient is in some ways harder
to analyze. To help identify and meet the psychosocial needs of
cancer patients, my optimal consultants are the patients themselves.
It is only by communicating with these valuable sources of information that the possibilities for effective psychosocial support can
emerge. It takes courage; but the courage necessary for us to minimize the differences between "Us" and "Them" is one prerequisite to
really understanding the emotional impact on the patient of the words
"and I, too, shall die."

The threat of ceasing to be, personality disintegration, or ego an-
nihilation (i.e., the death of one's identity) has been identified as
the core component of our fear of death (Choron, 1964). Despite the
considerable magnitude of this fear for most of us, Annas (1974)
cites seven studies from journals such as <u>Cancer</u>, <u>JAMA</u>, etc., that
note that approximately 90 percent of all patients interviewed preferred to know their diagnosis, even if terminal, whereas 60 percent
to 90 percent of their physicians opposed telling them. In my own
research, over 85 percent of those terminal patients I have counseled
strongly suspected they were dying before being formally told by
house staff. It is very difficult to deny indefinitely as monumental
a psychobiological phenomenon as a widely metastasized cancer. At
times, we all use denial as a psychological defense to preserve our
psychic integrity in the face of potentially traumatizing realities.
What is not often recognized is that this process is both interpersonal (and selective) and most often time-bound (we all process
information of a potentially traumatizing nature at differential
rates). It is important to honor a patient's denial for as long as
it is psychologically adaptive; that is, for as long as the individual chooses to admit into consciousness only those relatively non-
traumatizing aspects of the illness--those with which he or she can
cope more or less successfully. Through being emotionally accessible
to the patient in the context of a caring, trusting relationship,
physicians and others may provide the optimal occasion for a patient
to choose to acknowledge the more traumatizing aspects of his illness
--the possibility of death and his fear of dying.

Why then has so much been written about patient denial? I have consistently encountered as much denial by staff members as by patients.
As health providers we experience ourselves as trained healers and
view the death of a patient as an unacceptable conclusion to the
health care process. As professionally skilled adversaries of illness and death, we may be less able to respond effectively to the
dying patient. Our anxiety and sense of impotence may force us to
keep our distance from a patient whose death appears inevitable,
leaving the patient psychologically abandoned and emotionally and

physically isolated. The vital question is not whether or not we
have a "denier," but denial when and with whom and under what circumstances? I hope that we all subscribe to the notion that the dying
patient has a right to know, but that this right is clearly contin-
gent upon his or her right not to know. It is imperative that we
honor a patient's denial until he chooses to admit into consciousness, frequently in symbolic form, a growing awareness of the life-
threatening nature of his illness.

A 55-year-old truck driver with seriously advanced lympho-
sarcoma discussed his feelings about driving a large truck
across country late at night. He spoke intensely of the
dark, the shortage of gas, and how lonely and frightened he
felt when it seemed as if it might not be possible to reach
the next gas stop. He spoke of the loneliness of the open
road, the trucker's lack of human contact and relationships,
and his fear of the uncertainty of the situation. I honored
his chosen metaphor and we spoke "truck language" for approximately one-half hour, after which time he made intense eye
contact and said "I hope you realize that I'm not talking
about trucks and the highway." I indicated that I understood what he was referring to and thanked him for sharing
so intimate a set of feelings. (Garfield, 1978)

UNDERSTANDING PATIENT ANGER

One of the most perplexing responses for hospital staff to cope with
is patient anger. The patient may be furious at what he perceives as
a capricious universe unjustly inflicting cruelty in the form of his
cancer. The emotional stress may cause the patient to search inces-
santly for some psychological and/or spiritual explanation for the
cruel fate that has befallen him. In counseling cancer patients, it
is important to realize that no definitive research has indicated a
clear etiological equation specifying the relations between causes
and effect (malignancy); hence, to the lay public (as well as many
health professionals) the selection of those who get cancer often
appears chaotic. The possibility of a random and meaningless universe, or worse, a tyrannical and capricious god, operating without
plan or with malevolent intent can be powerfully unsettling. Some
people attempt to explain cancer as a form of severe retribution;
such an "explanation" may evoke considerable fear and guilt in many
cancer patients. It is not rare for terminally ill patients to
direct their anger against the infuriating whimsy of their illness.
The services instituted by many hospitals simply do not meet the
psychosocial needs of patients, families, and staff under considerable emotional stress. Overburdened medical and nursing personnel
and anxious family members may be too preoccupied with their own
needs and demands to provide adequate support to the patient. At
minimum, it is important for us to recognize the difference between
anger directed against a seemingly random and whimsical "death-
sentence" and anger directed against (1) a physician who may have
been slow at making a diagnosis or who had inaccurately diagnosed the
illness until it was too late to treat effectively; (2) nursing staff
who seem too busy to attend to the emotional needs of the patient;
and (3) family members who choose to withdraw in fear rather than engage in meaningful dialogue with the patient.

Anger is frequently a defense against terror and severe loss of con-

trol. An effective approach is to help the patient understand his
response by actively listening as he vents his anger and then dis-
tinguishing with him the issues that are realistically subject to
variation from those that are not. Anger can be a psychologically
adaptive and important reaction to severe emotional stress. It is
vital that we not assume that anger is an immature response directed
at an inappropriate target. We have much to learn about the emotional realities of people facing life-threatening illness and must
always guard against stereotyping their responses and rendering them
invalid.

UNDERSTANDING PATIENT DEPRESSION

Another frequently observed patient response to life-threatening
illness is depression, both reactive and preparatory. When a patient
experiences the tremendous loss of self-esteem that often results
from
  (1) prolonged and painful hospitalization and treatment,
  (2) emotional abandonment by family and friends,
  (3) the real or imagined insensitivity of hospital per-
      sonnel, and
  (4) the depletion of finances due to expensive medical care,
he may understandably become severely depressed. Those who take the
time to listen will frequently find that this depressions is trace-
able to concrete life circumstances. Furthermore, some of the circumstances may be subject to modification, and all available supports
should be mobilized to this end. Facilitating communication with
family members, helping to minimize financial burdens, diminishing
the impact of severe body-image changes, and sensitizing staff to the
emotional needs of patients can all be explored in an effort to
alleviate depression of a reactive nature.

Preparatory depression is primarily an anticipatory reaction to the
threatened "loss of oneself," that is, a grief reaction to the impending cessation of embodiment. The patient is threatened "not
only" with the loss of life, but also with the loss of self-esteem,
physical potency, and personal relationships. Typical reactions include frightening dreams, irritability, extreme sadness, anorexia,
and apathy. Intense and prolonged suffering can exacerbate preparatory depression to the point where it incorporates elements of
suicidal preoccupation. It is not helpful to interrupt this preparatory response with false promises of cure or positive response
to treatment. This is a classic mourning period that offers a true
test of the professional's (or family members') ability to provide
emotional support to the patient. One can be extremely supportive
by sitting with the patient, often in silence, in an attempt to
convey a willingness to share this emotionally demanding period. A
health professional or volunteer can help a patient cope successfully
with reactive depression by assisting in the development of a sense
of closure (i.e., a sense of completing life's "unfinished business"
--personal, interpersonal, spiritual, and financial). To offer ongoing support during the preparatory period we must stay attuned to
the emotional realities of each dying patient and the personal significance of his imminent death.

UNDERSTANDING PATIENT RESIGNATION/ACCEPTANCE

Considerable confusion centers on the issue of whether or not ter-

minal patients are able to accept their impending death. I have
found that 5 to 10 percent of those cancer patients who die in the
hospital maintain a predominately consistent death-accepting attitude.
However, 15 to 20 percent of those terminal patients who choose to
die at home achieve a similar level of acceptance (Garfield, 1978).
In caring and supportive families capable of substantially meeting
the needs of the terminally ill member, the acceptance of death may
resemble not so much the resignation of a beleaguered soldier accepting defeat, but rather an emotionally and cognitively integrated
sense of "alrightness" about the termination of one's life. The degree of this acceptance often fluctuates depending on shifts in mood
due to pain, drug side-effects, and assorted emotional conflicts. In
some instances, a major difference between the hospital and home context may be the willingness of family members and health professionals to accept the patient's chosen attitude toward death. The influence of a powerful antideath institutional belief (the basic
attitude toward life-threatening illness of many medical and nursing
staff) frequently precludes a patient's acceptance of death. Understanding the impact of a death-accepting or death-denying environment
on the dying person is crucial. It is unreasonable to expect a terminal patient to accept death when he or she is embedded in a hospital social system that views disease as an evil adversary and death
as unacceptable. It may be extremely difficult for a dying patient
who is dependent upon a fiercely death-denying family or hospital
staff to ever accept his own death. It is a rare individual (usually someone with a profound spiritual or philosophic commitment) who
can counteract the pervasive death-denying institutional bias mil-
itating against death-acceptance. The heroic measures sometimes used
to prolong the lives of patients who have peacefully and clearly indicated their preference for letting nature take its course bears
witness to the institutional abhorrence of death under any conditions.
Many patients are not physically capable of sufficient impact on the
decision-making process to prevent these aggressive measures. The
point is certainly not that death-acceptance is always the preferable
response, but rather that patient input and the right of self-determination are fundamental. As health professionals, we must avoid
those absurdly macabre scenarios wherein medical heroics are directed
at the prolongation of the life of a patient who has clearly and
nonhysterically expressed an aversion to such measures.

For many people, particularly the elderly, the completion of unfinished business-economic and work-related, psychological and
related to self-esteem, interpersonal, religious--may enhance a
sense of appropriateness of their own death. The ability to derive
a sense of purpose and meaning from life and perhaps death, to have,
in Weisman's (1972) terms, "an appropriate rather than an appro-
priated death," appears integral to any self-accepting experience of
terminality. This is not to suggest that the acceptance of death is
the equivalent of an emotionally or physically painless death, but
rather that such acceptance may enhance a person's opportunity of
relating to death in a more meaningful fashion. Few people realize
that personal change and maturation often appear more possible on
one's deathbed than perhaps at any other time in the life cycle. The
fluidity of ego boundaries and the suspension of stereotypic modes of
social interaction, of "the games people play," may allow for such
maturation. The culturally dominant notion that death, the Grim
Reaper, is nothing but tragic prevents us from realizing that even in
the midst of painful chaos and parting, the possibility of positive

change exists. However, such change can occur only with the patient's willing support and can often be facilitated by a person
trained to develop these subtle but important possibilities.

THE PHYSICIAN'S EXPERIENCE

It is clear that the physician and allied professionals are powerful
figures for most patients facing life-threatening illness. We must,
therefore, continually earn our positions of influence by earning
respect and by showing we are worthy of this power. When the professional boxer commits violence against a person outside the ring,
he is properly castigated, for his hands are registered lethal wea-
pons; but at least he is conscious of his power. For the overworked
and overburdened psychologist, nurse, or physician to commit emotional violence, even inadvertently, because he or she is unconscious of
his or her personal power, is most unfortunate. The capriciousness
of cancer is such that we can rarely outline a definitive time
schedule or map out an accurate sequence of symptomatology for a
given patient. Both physician and patient are often forced to confront considerable uncertainty. Prolonged and heightened ambiguity
may result in the physicians' rejection of the largely untenable role
as healer, psychological confidant, companion, and spiritual coun-
selor. They may reluctantly, albeit correctly, conclude that they
are unable to fulfill all the needs of the dying patient. Several
medical colleagues have communicated observations similar to the
following:
> When there's nothing more I can do medically my tools are
> gone. There's nothing I can do for the patient and that's
> upsetting for me. I would rather fulfill my promises and
> expectations or at least be able to make some headway.
> When I think of other people who have time for relationships,
> time to relate to my patient, to sit and talk, I sometimes
> become jealous. I don't have that time and it's annoying to
> think that I may lose the affection of my patient. This is
> something physicians don't talk about very often.

A more distressing attitude is revealed in the following:
> I've recently realized that for the past 25 years when a
> patient of mine has been terminally ill, I'd walk into the
> room talking constantly, approach the bed, and back out of
> the room talking. I do this because I have nothing to
> offer medically and I'm not willing to deal with the patient's
> emotional stress. That's not my training so it's probably
> better if I handle the situation that way. The psychologist
> or social worker or psychiatric nurse spends time with the
> patient and opens up a whole emotional can of worms and then
> who gets the brunt of it, I do, the physician. I don't have
> time to deal with these issues. It's better if physicians
> give brief general reassurance and don't dig too deeply.

Although the quality of the growing body of research on the psychosocial aspects of dying has improved markedly in recent years,
relatively few studies have focused on the physician's reaction to
the dying patient. Working for extended periods with dying patients
is an emotionally charged experience, and physicians frequently sustain great stress when they must relate intimately to patients and
families facing a protracted life-threatening illness. The psychological defenses and coping strategies elicited by this stressful

contact are legion. Physicians and allied professionals may view
close relationships with patients as perplexing dilemmas to be avoided at all costs. Many regard the patient's basic emotional needs as
relatively insignificant compared to the primary task of biomedical
treatment. Other professionals consider long discussions about
feelings and emotional stress a waste of invaluable time.

When Freud observed that "the ego cannot comprehend its own dis-
solution," he shared with a leukemic man named Ted Rosenthal (1971)
an appreciation for that emotionally incomprehensible question: "How
could I not be among you?" (Garfield, 1977). Physicians who acknowledge the preeminence of the ultimate contest between the possibilities of "ceasing to be" and survival become involved in supramedical
issues that affect physician and patient alike. Physicians and
others may view this as a dangerous commitment and seek to protect
their own personal and professional integrity by indicating an unwillingness to entertain any questions that elicit feelings of vulnerability. As Artiss and Levine (1973) have noted, a physician's
manner of coping with the anxiety aroused by a patient's imminent
death becomes the crucial element in considering the relationship
between patient and physician. However, physicians rarely discuss
their feelings about specific patients except in the company of other
physicians and then only seldom. It is a major drawback in medical
practice that no professional context exists in which physicians can
share their feelings about their patients, the demands of professional work, and especially the death of a patient with whom one has
worked for months or years. There are virtually no available
emotional support systems for physicians. Because a majority of
practitioners manage to continue despite the severe emotional stress
inherent in those medical specialties requiring frequent life-and-
death decisions, the medical profession participates in society's
perpetuation of the "superhuman doctor" myth that has unnecessarily
limited and isolated physicians.

At some point in a patient's terminal illness the physician must
confront the eventuality that all efforts to prevent death will likely fail (Artiss and Levine, 1973). When this point is reached,
various aspects of the doctor-patient relationship become evident.
If the concerned parties do not understand and adequately deal with
all facets of this interaction, the physician's effectiveness may be
severely hampered. Just as it is essential to understand the
emotional realities of dying from the patient's perspective, it is
equally important to comprehend its emotional impact on the physician
and other health personnel. Anger, denial, and depression/resig-
nation are the three most frequent physician reactions to the probable death of a patient. These are precisely the three most common
reactions of patients themselves. Physicians and patients alike experience basic human reactions to loss. The prospect of losing one's
own life or the loss of a patient, the end of a relationship with a
dying person or the sad conclusion to a battle with an illness all
may generate similar psychological repercussions.

Anger

Physicians may employ anger as a defense against anxiety, particularly if such anger proves effective in establishing its possessor as
the adversary of a shared "enemy" (Artiss and Levine, 1973). This
phenomenon, known as displacement, allows the physician to trace the

patient's death to external circumstances, overwhelming disease process, patient and family tardiness in seeking help, bureaucratic
complications, etc. Given the superhuman qualities imputed to
physicians and the high degree of physician-acceptance of these cultural projections, it may become necessary for physicians to explain
death in a way that allows them to escape relating to it as a personal failure. For oncologists, for example, to relate to each death
as a personal failure would result in an enormous blow to their self-
esteem. Therefore, they may direct the anger mobilized after a
patient's death toward a human, situational, or disease-related adversary that serves to "explain away the failure." The problem lies
in equating death with the failure of the physician. This equation
is most often erroneous and unfair to both physician and patient.

Denial

Physicians may deny that a patient's death appears imminent, claiming
"heavy patient load or home and social obligations" to explain their
reluctance to accept and confront the reality of impending death
(Artiss and Levine, 1973). Physician denial sometimes reaches extreme proportions as in the case of one oncologist who told me that
he had never had a patient who died. Surprised at the claim, I discussed it with him further and found that he took one of two precautions when a patient seemed near death; he either transferred the
patient to another facility in order to avoid being the physician of
record at the time of death, or he transferred the case to a younger
colleague for similar reasons. Therefore, he was able to somewhat
pathetically make the claim that he had never had a patient who died.
A more common form of denial is the disavowal of a close relationship between physician and patient. No physician would deny the
existence of the conventional, professional-client, doctor-patient
relationship. However, when treatment toward maintenance, remission,
or cure is no longer possible and emotional/physical comfort as well
as the reduction of pain become the major issues, some physicians
may deny that they have a responsibility to continue this relationship. This circumscribed definition of the doctor-patient relationship, as limited to the resolution of biomedical problems, is another
way of avoiding or denying the emotional aspects of terminal illness.

Depression/Resignation

One of the most poorly understood physician reactions to prolonged
contact with terminal patients is depression. Whereas denial and
anger allow the physician to continue functioning, albeit sometimes
at a fever pitch or in a somewhat disorganized fashion, depression
can debilitate the physician and severely impair his or her efficiency. I have known physicians who, for years, via a sheer act of will,
fought off incipient depression only to succumb finally to the cum-
ulative emotional impact of patient deaths. Depression and its real
or imagined emotional engulfment are extremely threatening to physicians whose heavy work schedule and personal expectations do not
allow them the "luxury" of more modulated and frequent emotional
expression. In the past several years, I have seen an increasing
number of physicians in psychotherapy with presenting complaints related to a variety of emotional disorders. The majority have been
highly productive in their careers but had not adequately attended to
the emotional impact of their work. Most frequently, they suffered
from one of a variety of psychosomatic disorders or depressions that

had culminated in the impairment of work efficiency and severe
emotional stress. For an individual, no matter how emotionally adaptive, to select as demanding a profession as clinical oncology without recognizing its emotional impact can only be detrimental to both
physician and patient.

Wheelis offers a vivid and literate picture of the professional man's final but necessary disillusionment. He
writes of what happens when a man travels a long road to
salvation and, until he is too far along to go back,
doesn't realize that he is headed for the abyss. Nor could
anyone have told him ealier. His hope then lies in finding
that it would have been the same no matter which route he
had chosen, and that he can help himself and others along
the way. A mature resolution, but a poor one when compared
with early dreams of ultimate conquest. For the man who
cannot mature in his profession, every subsequent day of
his life challenges his magic and with it, his identity.
He has staked his life, like Faust, on learning the secret
and he cannot turn back admitting failure. He knows well
enough that he cannot win--that he will die, as will all his
patients. He knows this not with equanimity but with the
cynicism of the frustrated idealist. He less than other
men is suited to face the dying; they are a personal affront,
a symbol of his human helplessness, and an end to his life.
He whose marriage is shaken because he cannot bear his wife's
small complaints, whose children cry in their nights of
illness for a father who has to be at an induced delivery--
this man must often help a stranger die, and what can he do?
He can be tough about it, maybe breezy, or maudlin--or maybe
he can get an intern or nurse to drink the dregs of his
heady wine while he is called to more positive and hopeful
cases (Kasper, 1959).

REFERENCES

Annas, G.: "Rights of the Terminally Ill Patient," Journal of Nursing
    Administration, 4:40-43, 1974.
Artiss, K. and A. Levine: "Doctor-Patient Relations in Severe Ill-
    ness," New England Jouranl of Medicine, 288:1210-1214, 1973.
Bulger, R.: "Doctors and Dying," Archives of Internal Medicine,
    70(3):327-332, 1963.
Choron, J.: Death and Modern Man, Collier, New York, 1964.
Garfield, C.: "The Impact of Death on the Healthcare Professional,"
    in H. Feifel (ed.), New Meanings of Death, McGraw-Hill, New York,
    1977.
Garfield, C.: Psychosocial Care of the Dying Patient, New York, 1978.
Kalish, R.: "The Onset of the Dying Process," Omega, 1:57-69, 1970.
Kasper, A.: "The Doctor and Death," in H. Feifel (ed.), The Meaning
    of Death, McGraw-Hill, New York, 1959.
Kastenbaum, R. and R. Aisenberg: Psychology of Death, Springer, New
    York, 1972.
Pattison, E. Mansell; "The Living-Dying Process," in C. Garfield
    (ed.), Psychosocial Care of the Dying Patient, NcGraw-Hill,
    New York, 1978.
Pinner, M. and B. Miller: When Doctors Are Patients, Norton, New
    York, 1952.

Rosenthal, T." How Could I Not Be Among You?, Braziller, New York,
    1971.
Weisman, A.: On Dying and Denying, Behavioral Publications, New York,
    1972.

Common Psychological Problems

A. STEDEFORD

Sir Michael Sobell House and Warneford Hospital, Oxford, UK

In terminal illness, the physician will often find that his patient is anxious or depressed and may think, quite rightly, that this is a natural reaction to his predicament. As symptoms such as pain are relieved, and the patient comes to know and trust those who care for him, his anxiety level usually drops. Although he may be very sad from time to time he regains an interest in his surroundings and his morale improves. When this does not happen, and either depression or anxiety is persistent or severe, it is appropriate to look for an underlying cause. This may be an anxiety state or a clear cut depressive illness, and may require anxiolytic drugs or antidepressants for relief. But much more often, in my experience, the patient has something on his mind which is worrying him, and he has found no one in whom he feels he can confide. The anxiety or depression here are symptomatic, and identifying and working through the problem brings relief more effectively and sometimes more quickly than medication.

The commonest resons for patients to be referred to me are depression and anxiety (Table 1). Hidden psychological problems can also present as disturbed inter-personal relationships, for example, the patient who is always complaining, who antagonises his family, other patients, and the staff; or the patient whose symptoms always seem to get worse at visiting times. These people are often very much happier if their underlying problem can be identified and resolved. The fourth condition that prompts the physician to ask for psychiatric help for his patient is the failure of physical symptoms to respond to adequate treatment. This suggests that somatisation of psychological problems may be taking places.

TABLE 1   Common Reasons for Referral to Psychiatrist

1. Depression
2. Anxiety
3. Disturbed relationships
4. Failure of physical symptoms to respond to treatment

Psychological problems in terminal illness fall into 3 broad categories:

1. those due to poor communication;
2. those directly related to the effects of the disease;
3. those due to poor adaptation to the progress of the illness.

The first group is the commonest, and also the most easily remedied. The subject
has been covered in Dr Hillier's paper on communication. It is appropriate to add
that the patient's family must be included in discussions about his progress, and
in the planning of his future care. Good communication with the family contributes
greatly to the patient's peace of mind. Where husband and wife, for instance,
cannot share the knowledge that one or both has about the seriousness of an illness,
it puts a great strain on the marriage.   Practical arrangements such as the making
of a will may be delayed if communication is deficient, and this can lead to
unnecessary family problems and anxiety. Until the truth is shared, they cannot
comfort each other, plans cannot be openly made, and the resources of the family
cannot be mobilised to support the patient and those about to be bereaved.

TABLE 2   Direct Effects of Disease

1. Organic brain syndrome:

    i.   fear of insanity
    ii.   frustration due to memory loss, etc.
    iii. distress of relatives when patient is *confused*
          or has *personality change*

2. Disfigurement and deformity:

    i.   shame
    ii.   fear of rejection by relatives
    iii. guilt of relatives who cannot face patient

3. Increasing disability:

    i.   *patient* feels a burden
    ii.   *relatives* feel guilty if they can no longer care
          for the patient

4. Chronic pain and weakness, etc.

5. Fear of suffering and of death

The psychological problems most directly related to the effects of the disease are
those resulting from an organic brain syndrome (Table 2). This is discussed in
detail in the paper on Confusional States. Personality change, as sometimes occurs
in brain tumours, is perhaps the most difficult manifestation for relatives to bear.
They feel that they have already lost the person they knew so well if he becomes,
for instance, disinhibited or aggressive. They want to withdraw from this stranger
who now inhabits a familiar body, but if they do this they feel guilty. They may
be ashamed of the changed behaviour of the patient, and if he is at home, may conceal it for a long time, enduring much suffering, until someone notices the signs
of strain and asks the right questions. Trained staff can tolerate abusive out-
bursts which would be almost unbearable for close relatives, and serious personality
change is usually an indication for admission to hospital even when the patient is
otherwise capable of staying at home.

Patients are often ashamed of the disfigurement and deformity caused by malignant
disease or surgery, and may withdraw from the family because they fear that relatives may be alienated by their changed appearance. Preparing both the patient and
the close family for operations like mastectomy or colostomy helps to minimise this
distress. Patients should feel that we understand them when they mourn the loss of
a bodily part or function. They are likely to recover more quickly if they know we
take their feelings seriously.

Some patients still fear that cancer is contagious, like a woman who refrained from cuddling her grandchildren lest she contaminate them. Another thought cancer could be spread by cups or spoons, and ceased to entertain anyone in her home, with the result that she became lonely and withdrawn. Where this is just a mistaken belief, reassurance will help the patient to be sociable again. But the idea that one could contaminate others is sometimes a feature of the endogenous type of depression. Then the use of antidepressants will be more effective.

Relatives who cannot bear to spend long with a patient who has an ugly or unpleasant condition feel guilty and need support and encouragement from staff.

As disability increases, many patients get depressed and feel they are a burden, especially as they watch a caring relative become increasingly tired. Often this depression goes when more help is given in the home, or the patient comes into hospital. But the relative who has been determined to care for the patient to the end may feel a failure. Often people who have made quite heroic efforts still think they have not done enough. Sometimes they are trying to compensate for past neglect or unkindness, and they will feel better if they can talk about this and lose some of the guilt. Others need to be told repeatedly that they have done a good job; that the staff find the patient difficult too, and that it was *their* loving care that enabled him to remain at home for so long.

Chronic pain makes patients depressed: their world contracts down to their body and immediate surroundings, and they have no energy left to take an interest in anything else. A few patients assume that pain is inevitable in cancer and that there is no point in complaining because nothing can be done. Others deny the presence of pain because they fear that large doses of analgesics will make them too sleepy or shorten their lives. They may look depressed or anxious, but more effective analgesia may be the best treatment, even though they have not complained of pain.

It is too often assumed that nothing can be done about the fear of suffering and of death. Just accepting and sharing it helps; and some patients who are ashamed of their fear need to be told that they are not expected to be brave all the time. Most people fear death itself less than they fear the prospect of intolerable pain and especially loss of control and dignity. They often want to ask what will be done for them as they get worse, and what dying will be like. Their anxieties are greatly relieved when they can be told that they will never be called upon to bear the impossible, or left to cope alone with their fears.

The third group of problems are those arising from poor psychological adaptation to the progress of the illness (Table 3). A failure to alter lifestyle in accordance with disability places unnecessary stress on the patient and those around him. The person who stubbornly tries to remain independent, perhaps living alone, struggling to do things for which they no longer have the strength, presents a well known problem. They feel frustrated and angry with themselves, and their repeated refusal of help distresses their family. Sometimes this refusal is rooted in long-standing family problems for which little can be done at this late stage. Rugged independence is an admirable part of some personalities, and here too it may not be appropriate to interfere. But there are patients who are excessively independent because they feel that this is the best way to fight the progress of the disease. Others think that there is something shameful about being ill and needing help. They may have been care-givers for most of their lives, unable to recognise that it is now their turn to receive. They need someone in loving authority to "give them permission" to stop struggling now; to lie back and let others wait on them. They are amazed at the peace that comes when they can accept this.

At the other extreme, there are those who give up too soon, taking to their beds and expecting to be waited on long before the illness makes this necessary. This self-imposed restriction on their lives leads to boredom and loss of self-esteem.

TABLE 3   Poor Psychological Adaptation to Progress of the Illness

	Result	
	For patient	For family
Attitudes to Self-Care		
1. Too independent	Frustration and suffering	Anger and distress
2. Premature helplessness and dependency	Boredom and loss of self-esteem	Resentment
Role in Family and Society		
1. Inappropriate rejection of sick role by patient and/or family	Exhaustion and guilt	Shock when family realizes. Guilt and regret after patient dies.
2. Premature loss of role	Isolation and depression	Patient treated as if already useless or dead.

They may complain of being a useless invalid and a burden, not recognising that there is still much that they can do for themselves. Sometimes this arises from false assumptions in their own minds about how someone with a terminal illness should be feeling and acting. They will respond to explanation and encouragement. They need help to discover that a day which involves short periods of activity to the point of fatigue, alternating with periods of rest, will leave them with much more sense of accomplishment than a day spent idly conserving their strength.

Some patients use the sick role as a way of getting attention from those around them. This causes much resentment in the family, and they are unpopular patients in hospital too. It should be recognised that there often lies behind this a life history singularly devoid of love. Where nursing staff have enough time and patience to win such a person's trust and to convince him that they really do care for him, this kind of behaviour may become less and the more pleasant parts of the patient's personality may emerge. Often such patients complain that almost every-one is against them. This may not be paranoia — it may be true — and the cause may be their own selfish or jealous attitudes. Once a few people have gained their confidence, it may be right to confront them with the fact that their behaviour is provoking the hostility that they sense around them. During such an interview, the patient often reveals suppressed anger about his illness or the way he has been treated in the past. Acceptance of this may also contribute to the improvement that usually occurs as a result of such confrontations.

Being ill involves losing many roles — such as those of breadwinner, housewife, and care giver. Sometimes patients relinquish their roles prematurely, or are deprived of them, and this leads to loss of self-esteem. A young mother with breast cancer, quite early in her illness refused further chemotherapy and asked to be left to die. It transpired that when her husband learned that she had cancer, he assumed that she had a short prognosis and that the kindest thing he could do for her was to spare her from all household chores and take them on himself so that she could rest. She then felt redundant and useless at home, and guilty that he was getting so tired. It took time to convince him that this was not the best way to help his wife, but gradually we worked out together a better way for them to share the tasks at home. He learned to accept that she needed to feel useful even if she got very tired. Her depression improved, she accepted treatment, and is still doing well a year later.

A person needs to maintain his role in the family for as long as he is able. Although he cannot do very much, especially if he has to be admitted to hospital, he may still want to know what is going on, bad news as well as good, so that he can still feel involves. Relatives sometimes assume that they should spare a sick person from hearing about their own anxieties, or some mishap which has occurred in the family. They need to be told something like "All he has left to give you now is his interest, his concern, and his advice — don't take that opportunity away from him too". We tend to underestimate the capacity of the dying patient to go on giving, and it is very moving to witness the person who is dying comforting the one who is about to be bereaved and helping him or her to make plans for the lonely times ahead.

Sometimes denial of the seriousness of the illness leads to inappropriate rejection of the sick role by patient or family. Then the patient, most often a housewife or mother, gets exhausted in her struggle to maintain standards, and the family complains when she does not do as much for them as she has always done. Unless someone recognises what is happening and intervenes, such a family experiences terrible guilt when she does eventually give in, realising that if only they had known, they could have made her last days or weeks so much easier. Sometimes they blame themselves unduly for being unperceptive about her illness. She may have been one of those who believe it is their duty to keep on for as long as they can, and deliberately conceal their feelings from the family in order to spare them suffering.

During bereavement, the husband of a patient like this experienced much anger that she had denied him the opportunity to love her and look after her in her last months.

When an illness is causing more depression, anxiety, or general emotional distress than one would expect, it is always helpful to ask whether the patient and his family are failing to adapt appropriately to the situation. Sometimes this happens because inadequate or inaccurate information has been given about the likely course of the illness and the prognosis, as happened to the young couple described earlier. When a prognosis cannot be given, it is particularly hard, and patients have to be helped to live with uncertainty.

Another reason for maladaptive responses to illness is the persistent use of neurotic defences either by the patient or the family. It is normal to use denial, rejection, and displacement sometimes as a temporary measure to cope with anxiety, but if the defence persists, it blocks progress in the acceptance of the situation, as the following case illustrates. A very anxious man denied that he was worried about himself, saying that his only concern was for his wife. He became distressed if she was late at visiting time, and questioned her in minute detail about what she had been doing since he saw her last. She fou d this so difficult that she made her visits shorter. This made him more upset, and she felt guilty. He was using denial to avoid experiencing anxiety about his coming death, and he was displacing his anxiety on to his wife. When confronted with this he was at first more anxious about himself, but he became more relaxed with her. She could then stay longer, offering him the companionship and comfort he needed as he came to terms with his short prognosis, and within a few days both of them were much more content.

As I have described more fully elsewhere (Stedeford, 1979), it is often worthwhile to ascertain which defence mechanisms are being used and to employ simple, focal psychotherapy in an attempt to correct the faulty adaptation. In some patients the use of neurotic defences is part of a long-standing personality disorder. Some of these will become more resistant to change at times of stress and can only be helped to cope in the ways which are familiar to them, with understanding and support for them and their relatives. But I am impressed with the resilience of human nature, and have found that many are still able to grow even when they have very little time left to live. More active psychotherapy enables them to discover inner resources of which they were previously unaware.

REFERENCES

Stedeford, A. and Bloch, S. (1979) The psychiatrist in the terminal care unit. *Brit. J. Psychiat.* 135, 1-6.

Stedeford, A. (1979) Psychotherapy of the dying patient. *Brit. J. Psychiat.* 135, 7-14.

III
PAIN RELIEF

Incidence and Assessment of Pain in Terminal Cancer

R. G. TWYCROSS

Sir Michael Sobell House, Churchill Hospital, Headington, Oxford OX3 7BR, UK

ABSTRACT

About 60% of patients with terminal cancer experience considerable pain, and possibly a third of these die with their pain unrelieved. Complete assessment implies the ability to make a diagnosis and also to initiate appropriate treatment. To do this a doctor needs:

1. to appreciate the influences of non-physical factors such as mood and morale;
2. to be aware of the diagnostic possibilities;
3. to be aware of the range of treatment options;
4. to establish realistic objectives with the patient;
5. to review efficacy of treatment at appropriate intervals and monitor side-effects;
6. to develop and maintain a good working relationship with the patient.

INCIDENCE OF PAIN

Data from several centres indicate that about 60% of patients with terminal cancer experience considerable pain (Table 1).

TABLE 1   Incidence of Pain in Cancer

Author	Number of patients	% with pain	Stage
Cartwright	215	87	Final year
Wilkes	300	58	Terminal
Haram	607	66	Terminal
Foley	397	38	All stages
Foley	39	60	Terminal
Pannuti	291	64	Advanced

The incidence of pain varies according to the primary site of the tumour. Pain is relatively unusual in leukaemia and lymphoma but is common in primary bone tumours and in cancers of the buccal cavity (Table 2).

Of greater importance is the incidence of *unrelieved* terminal pain. At St. Christopher's Hospice, the figure is about 1% (Haram, 1978) and in most cases the main

TABLE 2   Primary Site and the Incidence of Pain (%)*

Bone	85
Oral	80
Genito-urinary (male)	75
Genito-urinary (female)	70
Breast	52
Bronchus	45
Lymphoma	20
Leukaemia	5

*after Foley (1979).

reason for non-relief is lack of time — the patient lapses into coma and dies within a few days of admission. Data from the home care service at St. Joseph's Hospice indicates that the incidence of unrelieved pain in patients cared for at home is higher, about 10%. This higher percentage relates mainly to the reluctance of some patients to take any medication at all. These modern stoics decline offers of inpatient treatment and prefer to "soldier on" at home with their pain.

However, both St. Christopher's and St. Joseph's are centres of excellence. What of the patient population in general? If a report based on post-bereavement visits to the surviving spouse is representative of the general situation, 20% of those cared for in hospital and almost half of those cared for at home die with their pain unrelieved (Parkes, 1978). This means that each year in Britain alone some 36,000 people with cancer die in pain. The situation in other countries is certainly no better and may be worse. In the United States the National Committee on the Treatment of Intractable Pain has several hundred unsolicited letters on file which illustrate graphically the terminal distress experienced by many of those dying of cancer:-

"I have lost my mother with uncurable uterine cancer. Her pain was so horrid that she lost her mind and ate her bottom lip completely off from clenching her top teeth so tightly. My 13-year-old sister and I watched this for 6 weeks. We would enter the small hospital and hear her screams as soon as we closed the door. The nurses had no way to quieten her. She was immune to conventional pain killers."

"This July we lost our dad with hypernephroma (cancer of the kidney). He was a beautiful 65-year-old retired contractor in January. The pain that man went thru' in May and June is undescribable. They would inject morphine into his buttocks and it would run out through his constantly injected flesh and on to the bedsheet. He was stripped of all dignity, food forced into his throat by syringe."

"I'm sure I am only one of many who saw nothing routine about my husband's suffering an agony of pain when morphine wasn't effective ... The doctors assured me they could keep him ... 'reasonably free of pain'. There is *nothing* reasonable about the pain of a patient who is terminally ill with cancer ... Destroying a person before death."

"My brother just died Friday, Oct. 14th, of terminal cancer.
He had a painful death. It deeply hurt us in the immediate
family to sit alongside of his bed last week and see him in
great pain and have his request for relief, either a shot or
pill, turned down because it *wasn't* time for another shot."

Reasons for inadequate relief are many, but more fundamental than the incorrect
use of analgesia is the tendency for a doctor to cease to be systematic when confronted with a dying patient. Instead of carefully analysing the cause(s) of the
patient's pain(s), the doctor prescribes a fixed dose of a standard preparation or,
worse, underrates the intensity of a patient's discomfort and does nothing.

ASSESSMENT OF PAIN

Pain is a dual phenomenon, one part being the perception of the sensation and the
other the patient's psychological reaction to it. It follows that a person's pain
threshold will vary according to mood and morale (Fig. 1).

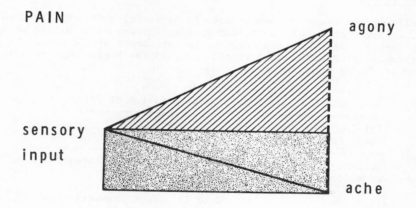

Fig. 1 For any given noxious stimulus the pain experienced
varies from ache to agony and depends on the psychological
reaction of the sufferer to his discomfort.

Attention must therefore be paid to factors that modulate pain threshold, such as
anxiety, depression, and fatigue (Table 3).

Much can be done to alleviate pain by explaining the mechanism underlying the pain
(this reduces anxiety) and by a continuing concern for the patient (this raises
morale). Ignoring mental and social factors may result in otherwise relievable
pain remaining intractable. At a weekly seminar for trainee general practitioners
(Anonymous, 1971) discussion centred on the problem of a patient with metastases in
bone from disseminated breast cancer whose pain was not relieved by narcotic analgesics. During the seminar it was suggested that the pain was intractable as the
woman was angry because her doctors and relatives would not admit that she was
dying nor discuss the problems this created. This proved to be the right explanation; a full and frank discussion resulted in a dramatic improvement in her
mental state and she no longer complained of pain.

TABLE 3 Factors Affecting Pain Threshold

Threshold lowered	Threshold raised
Discomfort	Relief of symptoms
Insomnia	Sleep
Fatigue	Rest
Anxiety	Sympathy
Fear	Understanding
Anger	Diversion
Sadness	Elevation of mood
Depression	
Mental isolation	Analgesics
Introversion	Anxiolytics
(Past experience)	Antidepressants

Description of Pain

Traditionally we are taught to assess pain by determining its PQRST characteristics (Table 4). Unfortunately a blind belief in the efficacy of so simple an approach may hinder rather than help the doctor in the assessment of the patient's pain. Determination of the PQRST characteristics is only the beginning, providing a description of the pain but no more.

TABLE 4 The PQRST Characteristics of Pain

"Tell me about your pain."
"Where is it?"

Palliative } factors	"What makes it less intense?"
Provocative } factors	"What makes it worse?"
Quality	"What's it like?"
Radiation	"Does it spread anywhere else?"
Severity	"How severe is it?"
Temporal factors	"Is it there all the time, or does it come and go?"

Complete assessment implies the ability to make a diagnosis. This demands:

   i.   a grasp of both general and neurological anatomy
  ii.   an understanding of the phenomenon of referred pain
 iii.   a knowledge of the range of pathological processes
        which are potential causes of pain.

From the history and clinical examination, supplemented if necessary by x-ray, scan, or other test, it should be possible to develop a fairly clear mental picture of the physical mechanisms underlying the pain. Then, assessment completed and diagnosis made, treatment is initiated. We are familiar with this sequence of events in relation to acute abdominal pain, for example, but often faily to apply the same relentless logic when assessing pain in far-advanced cancer. Yet assessment in this area needs to be as thorough as in any other. Cancer can cause pain in any part of the body and by a variety of mechanisms. Many patients have more than one pain. The alleviation of one pain may unmask another or a new pain may develop. To cope with what is often a complex situation, I find the use of a body chart to record pain data a great help (Fig. 2). Patients often put on a brave

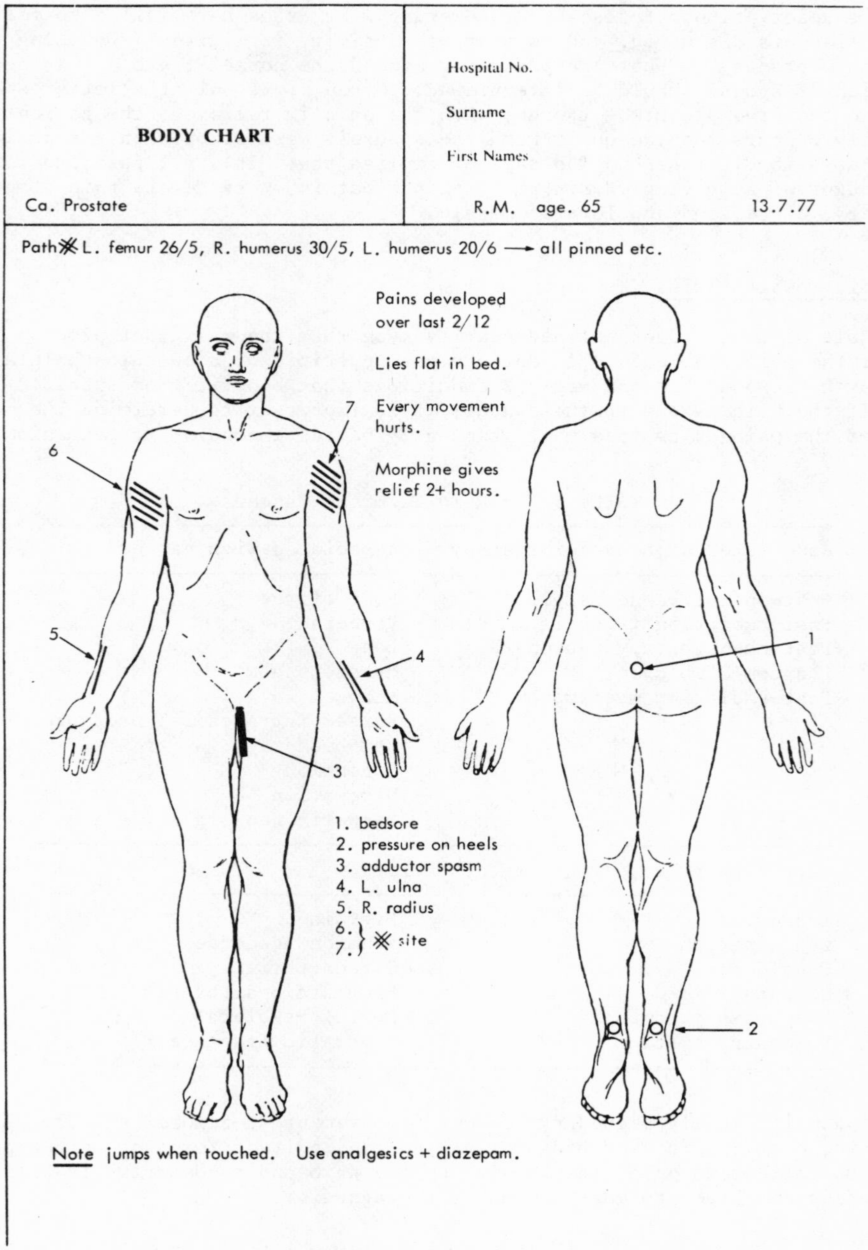

Fig. 2 Body chart used to record pain data relating to a
65-year-old man with cancer of the prostate gland

face for the doctor. This means that many patients in severe pain do not always
look distressed. Accordingly, intensity of pain is assessed not only by the
patient's description but also by discovering what drugs have failed to relieve,
whether sleep is disturbed, and in what way activity is limited ("How long is it
since you went out?", "What are you doing around the house?", etc.). In addition,
the patient's spouse should be interviewed. Often it is only the latter's comments
that give the true picture — though, when the pain is relieved, the patient
frequently concurs spontaneously with the spouse's earlier opinion. A patient who
is obviously in distress and who says or implies that "It's all pain, doctor" is
best thought of as having *overwhelming pain*, that is, very severe pain compounded
by anxiety, depression and loss of morale.

Diagnostic Possibilities

A diagnosis of cancer does not necessarily mean that the malignant process is the
cause of the pain (Table 5). A peptic ulcer, cystitis or a musculo-skeletal disorder may be responsible and are all conditions that benefit from specific treatment. If the pain is due to the cancer, it is important to determine the mechan-
ism(s) of the pain(s) as treatment frequently varies according to mechanism.

TABLE 5 Pain in Terminal Cancer

Associated with cancer therapy	Associated with cancer
Post-operative neuralgia	Soft tissue
Post-radiation fibrosis	Visceral
Post-chemotherapy neuropathy	Bone
Phantom limb pain	Muscle spasm
Post-radiation myelopathy	Nerve
	Raised intracranial pressure
	Lymphoedema
	Infection
	Ulceration
	Herpetic neuralgia

Unrelated to cancer or cancer therapy	
Bedsore	Migraine
Constipation	Tension headache
Candidosis	Osteoarthritis
Oesophagitis	Rheumatoid arthritis
Deep vein thrombosis	Musculo-skeletal
Pulmonary embolus	Traumatic fracture

Muscle spasm is usually secondary to bone involvement or deformity. Oro-pharyngeal
candidosis, constipation and bedsores are common indirect forms of cancer pain.
Asking the patient to point to the site of the pain and to describe it will usually
yield sufficient clues to make the correct diagnosis.

Case history. A four-year-old child with an inoperable
pontine glioma experienced increasing pain in the head and
occipital region. She lay flat all the time because elevation of the head caused a marked increase in pain. With
this history it was necessary to postulate a local source
of pain (possibly caused by post-radiation meningeal adhes-

ions) in addition to the diffuse headache of secondary hydrocephalus (which would have been helped by a more erect posture). The diffuse pain was relieved by small regular doses of morphine but not until she was transferred from a King's Fund to an Ellison bed (which elevates head, neck and trunk in unison) was it possible for the child to sit up without pain. Subsequently it became possible to transfer the child from bed to a high-backed reclining chair and, eventually, to lift her onto her mother's lap. This suggested that some of the pain had been caused by spasm of the neck muscles, and that the confidence engendered by the ability to sit up in bed allowed additional manoeuvres to be undertaken without pain.

TREATMENT OPTIONS

Relief of pain may be achieved by one or more of the following methods:

1. Modification of the pathological process
2. Elevation of pain threshold
3. Interruption of pain pathways
4. Immobilization.

Even in far-advanced cancer, modification of the pathological process by means of radiation, chemotherapy, or hormone treatment should always be considered. As always, it is important to ensure that the treatment is not worse than the disease. Moreover, if radiation or an oestrogen is prescribed, this does not mean that analgesics should be withheld. The best results are obtained by adopting a "broad-spectrum" approach, using two or more treatments in combination (Table 6).

The use of analgesics and other drugs is best seen as but one way — generally a powerful way — of elevating the patient's pain threshold. Interruption of pain pathways refers to chemical neurolysis (nerve blocks) and neurosurgical techniques (e.g. rhizotomy, spinothalmic tractotomy). Such procedures are of value in nerve compression pain that is inadequately relieved by the use of analgesics and a corticosteroid.

Some patients continue to experience pain on movement despite analgesics, other drugs, radiotherapy and nerve-blocks. In these, the situation may be improved by suggesting commonsense modifications to daily activity. For example, a man may continue to struggle to stand while shaving unless the doctor suggests that sitting would be a good idea. Such a suggestion is accepted more readily if accompanied by a simple explanation of why weight-bearing precipitates or exacerbates the pain. Individually designed plaster or plastic supports for patients with multiple collapsed vertebrae are occasionally necessary to overcome intolerable pain on movement in bedfast patients.

Internal fixation or the insertion of a prosthesis should be considered if a pathological fracture of a long-bone occurs, as these measures obviate the need for prolonged bedrest and pain is usually relieved. The decision whether or not to treat surgically depends on the patient's general condition; but, whereas in bronchial carcinoma or malignant melanoma pathological fracture often presages death, in breast cancer this is not generally so, particularly if the tumour is hormone sensitive. The median survival after the first or only pathological fracture associated with breast cancer is about six months ranging from two months to four years (Twycross, 1977).

R.G. Twycross

TABLE 6 Treatment of Pain in Far-Advanced Cancer

Mechanism	Analgesic	Co-analgesic	Non-drug treatment	Other measures
Soft tissue infiltration	Aspirin (mild) + laxative Codeine (moderate) + anxio-lytic? Morphine (severe) + anti-emetic?			Modification of lifestyle Diversion — heat — massage
Bone involvement		Aspirin Prednisolone	Radiotherapy	
Nerve compression		Dexamethasone	Nerve block	
Raised intracranial pressure				
Lymphoedema		Diuretic	Compression sleeve	
Abdominal visceral (a) epigastric (b) hypogastric			Coeliac axis ganglion block (Presacral block)*	
Ulceration – infection		Antibiotic		
Constipation	Specific treatment			
Second pathological process	Specific treatment			

*The use of nerve blocks for lower abdominal pain is limited by probability of causing urinary retention.

Realistic Objectives

A recent survey of patients with persistent pain suggested that patients' expectations in relation to relief are lower than they need be. Although, in some, relief
may be obtained fairly easily, it is important to bear in mind that with others,
particularly those who have pain on movement and those whose pain is compounded by
severe anxiety or depression, it may take three ro four weeks of inpatient treatment
to achieve satisfactory control. However, in all patients it should be possible to
achieve some improvement within 24 to 48 hours. Although the ultimate aim is
always complete freedom from pain, a doctor will be less disappointed but, paradox-
ically, more successful if he aims at "graded relief". Moreover, as some pains
respond more readily than others, improvement should be assessed in relation to
each pain.

REASSESSMENT

With cancer one is dealing with a progressive pathological process. This means
that new pains may develop or old pains re-emerge. It should not be assumed that a
fresh complaint of pain merely calls for an increase in a previously satisfactory
analgesic regimen; it demands reassessment, an explanation to the patient and,
only then, modification of drug therapy or other intervention. The probability of
the initial prescription being inadequate increases with the intensity of pain.
Patients should, therefore, be reassessed within hours if the pain os overwhelming,
or after one or two days if severe or moderate. If troublesome or unacceptable
side-effects result, treatment may need to be modified. In addition, the relief of
the major pain may allow a second less severe pain to become apparent.

> Case history. An 85-year-old man with carcinoma of the
> prostate and right femoral metastatic pain was treated
> with aspirin and morphine. The next day he indicated that,
> although less severe, he was still in pain. Detailed
> questioning revealed that the site of pain was now retro-
> sternal and epigastric; he had no femoral pain at all.
> The dose of morphine was left unaltered, and the prescrip-
> tion of an antacid resulted in complete relief.

In the case of the man with overwhelming pain (Fig. 2), it was necessary to review
progress in relation to each pain. On the second day he was reluctant to admit
that several of the pains were less intense but, judging by his reactions to
passive movement, they undoubtedly were. Possibly his reluctance was due to a
shifting base-line of reference. It was necessary to remind him of the difference
I observed and to encourage him to accept that the pains were beginning to ease.
It was a case of "chipping away" at his total pain experience until eventually,
after a week or so, he was considerably more comfortable and able to sit up in bed.

ACKNOWLEDGEMENTS

The author thanks the Committee for Treatment of Intractable Pain for permission
to publish the letters from their files.

Figure 1 and Table 3 are published by kind permission of Pitman Medical, Tunbridge
Wells, England; Figure 2 and Table 2 by permission of the Journal of Medical
Ethics.

REFERENCES

Anonymous (1971) Vocational training for general practice. *Brit. Med. J.* <u>2</u>, 704-706.

Cartwright, A., Hockey, L. and Anderson, A.B.M. (1973) *Life Before Death*. Routledge & Kegan Paul, London.

Foley, K.M. (1979) Pain syndromes in patients with cancer. In: *Advances in Pain Research and Therapy, Vol. 2* (Eds. J.J. Bonica and V. Ventafridda), pp. 59-75. Raven Press, New York.

Haram, J. (1978) Facts and figures. In: *The Management of Terminal Disease* (Ed. C.M. Saunders), pp. 12-18. Edward Arnold, London.

Pannuti, F., Martoni, A., Rossi, A.P. and Piana, E. (1979) The role of endocrine therapy for relief of pain due to advanced cancer. In: *Advances in Pain Research and Therapy, Vol. 2* (Eds. J.J. Bonica and V. Ventafridda), pp. 145-165. Raven Press, New York.

Parkes, C.M. (1978) Home or hospital? Terminal care as seen by surviving spouses. *J. Roy. Coll. Gen. Pract.* <u>28</u>, 19-30.

Twycross, R.G. (1977) Care of the terminal patient. In: *Breast Cancer Management — Early and Late* (Ed. B.A. Stoll), pp. 157-163. Heinemann Medical Books Ltd., London.

Wilkes, E. (1974) Some problems in cancer management. *Proc. Roy. Soc. Med.* <u>67</u>, 23-27.

The Natural History of Cancer Pain

F. PANNUTI, A. P. ROSSI, D. MARRARO, E. STROCCHI,
A. CRICCA, E. PIANA and E. POLLUTRI

Divisione di Oncologia, Ospedale Specializato M. Malpighi, Bologna, Italy

Of 324 patients with advanced cancer, who were treated and who died in our Department between January 1976 and June 1979, inclusive, 284 (87%) had tumour related pain for more than 15 days at some stage of their disease (Table 1).

TABLE 1   Patients with Pain for more than 15 Days

Primary sites	Patients	Pain for >15 days	%
Ovary	19	19	100
Cervix uteri	16	16	100
Rectum	19	18	95
Breast	63	56	94
Lung	84	71	85
Colon	19	16	84
Stomach	24	18	75
All sites	324	284	88

As pain generally appeared after the diagnosis of relapse, i.e. the pain free interval is longer than the cancer free interval (Table 2) pain may be considered as a signal-symptom of far-advanced neoplastic disease. With identical pain indices (breast 0.21; colon 0.21) it is possible to have different residual survival times without pain (5.7 months for breast and 0 for colon). This means that while the ratio between survival time with pain and total survival is identical, after the initial onset of cancer related pain, the two groups of patients tend to have different periods free from pain. The data also demonstrate that some patients from groups with long residual survival times without pain die without recurrence of pain.

Table 3 records the incidence of pain in relation to the dominant metastatic site in all patients on first examination and 15 days before death, together with separate figures for patients with lung and breast cancers. It shows that the greatest incidence of pain is associated with osseous metastases. Apart from patients with ovarian cancer, there was a consistent tendency for the incidence of pain to decrease after the first visit (Table 4). This is presumably connected with the treatments carried out.

76

F. Pannuti *et al.*

TABLE 2 Natural History of Pain in 324 Cancer Patients

	324 Patients			284 Patients with Pain			
	Total Survival[1] (months)	Cancer Free Interval[2] (months)	Pain Free Interval[3] (months)	Survival Time with Pain (months)	Pain Index[4]	Residual Pain Free Survival Time[5] (months)	
Breast	32.7	13	20	7	0.21	5.7	
Lung	10	0	2	2.5	0.25	5.5	
Stomach	22	9	14.2	2.5	0.11	5.3	
Colon	8.3	0	6.6	1.8	0.21	0	
Rectum	10.3	4.1	7.7	2.7	0.26	0	
Ovary	13.6	0	5.4	1.3	0.09	6.9	
Cervix	20.3	6.6	15.2	2.7	0.13	2.4	
Total	12.5	1	8.1	3	0.24	1.4	

[1] Median time from diagnosis to death
[2] Median time from diagnosis and initial treatment to recurrence
[3] Median time from diagnosis to the onset of pain
[4] Pain Index = Survival time with pain divided by total survival time
[5] Median time free from pain, from the first onset of pain to death.

TABLE 3   Pain and Dominant Metastatic Site

Soft Tissue	First visit	2/9	(22%)	8/11	(73%)	25/40	(63%)
	15 days before death	4/8	(50%)	2/3	(67%)	22/30	(73%)
Bone	First visit	15/19	(79%)	18/21	(86%)	41/48	(85%)
	15 days before death	12/18	(67%)	16/20	(80%)	36/47	(77%)
Visceral	First visit	33/55	(60%)	17/30	(57%)	145/230	(63%)
	15 days before death	32/57	(56%)	20/40	(50%)	145/247	(59%)

TABLE 4   Incidence of Pain at First Visit and 15 Days before Death

Primary sites	No. of patients	First visit %	15 days before death %
Lung	83	60	53
Breast	63	71	60
Colorectal	38	68	63
Stomach	25	64	52
Cervix uteri	22	82	64
Ovary	19	47	74
All sites	324	67	61

TABLE 5   Pain Remission and Chemotherapy

Treatment	Course I		Course II	Course III
Adria	11/28	(39%)	8/23	0/8
CF	7/13	(54%)	1/8	1/7
CMF	6/12	(50%)	0/2	0/2
P14	14/40	(35%)	7/17	1/10
CTX	1/8	(13%)	1/7	0/3
CHVV	2/15	(13%)	1/3	0/1
Total	41/116	(35%)	10/60 (17%)	2/31 (6%)

Adria = adriamycin
CF   = cyclophosphamide, fluorouracil
CMF   = cyclophosphamide, methotrexate, fluorouracil
P14   = cyclophosphamide, vincristine, vinblastine,
          adriamycin, methotrexate, fluorouracil
CTX   = cyclophosphamide in high dosage
CHVV = cyclophosphamide, hydroxyurea, vincristine, vinblastine

Finally, we analysed pain remission in relation to antiblastic therapy. Table 5 records the pain remission rate after the more commonly used antiblastic chemotherapies. All together, out of 259 courses, 59 induced pain remission (23%). By comparison, hormone therapy with medroxyprogesterone acetate (MAP) at high doses (500–2000 mg/day for at least 30 days) induced pain remission in 23 out of 34 cases (68%). The age and sex of patients did not seem to be significant as far as the incidence of pain is concerned (Table 6).

TABLE 6   Pain Related to Sex and Age

	First visit	15 days before death
Male	91/140 (65%)	88/140 (62%)
Female	120/184 (68%)	112/184 (61%)
≤ 50 years	44/57 (77%)	40/57 (70%)
> 50 years	173/267 (65%)	163/267 (61%)

Hormonal Treatment

F. PANNUTI, A. P. ROSSI, D. MARRARO, E. STROCCHI, A. CRICCA, E. PIANA and E. POLLUTRI

Divisione di Oncologia, Ospedale Specializzato M. Malpighi, Bologna, Italy

ABSTRACT

The literature relating to hormone therapy for relief of pain is reviewed. The
authors report their experience with medroxyprogesterone acetate (MAP) in high
doses (500-1500-2000 mg/day for at least 30 days). In a series of 212 patients
with advanced breast cancer, remission of pain was obtained in 135/154 cases (88%)
and objective remission in 94/212 (44%). Pain remission occurred as early as one
week in some patients and lasted for a median duration of 6 months. MAP is an
anti-cancer agent which, when given in high doses, results in remission of pain in
hormone-sensitive tumours to an extent not observed before.

INTRODUCTION

Table 1 summarizes the published results of additive and ablative hormone therapy
in hormone-sensitive tumours. As far as endometrial carcinoma is concerned, data
on pain remission are not available; subjective remission obtained by means of
progestins was 71%. Our own data for clear cell carcinoma of the kidney are
related to a group of patients who were treated with high doses of medroxyprogesterone acetate (MAP), that is, 1500 mg/day intramuscularly for 30 days. We
obtained 5/12 (42%) pain remissions and 2/20 (10%) objective remissions. In view
of the low rate of objective remissions that were obtained, at present we currently
combine MAP and poly-chemotherapy.

For prostatic carcinoma ablation hormone therapy induced pain remission in about
70%. Additive hormone therapy was most effective when using oestrogens (in particular diethylstilboestrol diphosphate, DES-P) or MAP at high doses. In both cases,
pain relief was obtained in more than 80%. Our own experience related to a pilot
study in which we used MAP at high doses, 1500 mg/day intramuscularly for 30 days,
and obtained pain relief in all 10 patients.

In breast cancer ablation treatments, hypophysectomy induced the highest rate of
pain relief (82%). The result varied according to the method used: varying from
72% in the case of cryodestruction to 100% after Moricca's alcoholic neuroadenolysis. Additive therapy results in pain relief in 44% of patients treated with
androgens, 33% with anti-oestrogens and 44% with non-MAP progestins. MAP at low
doses (<500 mg/day) induced pain relief in 21%; MAP at high doses (>500 mg/day)
resulted in pain relief in 83%, a similar figure to that obtained by hypophysectomy.

F. Pannuti *et al.*

TABLE 1   Chemotherapy and Advanced Cancer

	Author	Date	Pain Remission	Subjective Remission	Objective Remission
Endometrial					
MAP low doses (<500 mg/day)	Smith Serment	1966 } 1970	–	41/55 (75%)	19/55 (35%)
17-Hydroxy-progesterone	Kistner	1965	–	123/176 (70%)	58/176 (33%)
Clear-cell kidney					
Androgens	Talley	1961	–	11/11 (100%)	–
Corticosteroids	Talley	1969	–	38/38 (100%)	–
Progestins (not MAP)	Talley Vanderwermessing	1969 } 1971	–	26/49 (53%)	4/49 (8%)
MAP low doses (<500 mg/day)	Talley Vanderwermessing	1969 } 1971	–	11/17 (65%)	2/17 (12%)
MAP high doses (>500 mg/day)	Pannuti	1978b	5/12 (42%)	6/14 (43%)	2/20 (10%)
Prostate — additive therapy					
Oestrogens (DES-P)	Colapinto Band Susan	1961 1973 } 1976	34/42 (81%)	19/25 (76%)	8/19 (42%)
Cyproterone acetate	Smith Scott	1971 } 1973	12/25 (48%)	–	8/10 (80%)
MAP low doses (<500 mg/day)	Rafla	1974	9/12 (75%)	–	–
MAP high doses (>500 mg/day)	Pannuti Bouffioux	1977c } 1976	19/22 (86%)	10/10 (100%)	–
Prostate — ablative therapy					
Hypophysectomy	Straffon Fergusson Murphy	1968 1971 } 1971	62/87 (71%)	12/34 (35%)	–
Adrenalectomy	Huggins West Archimbaud	1945 1952 } 1973	15/21 (71%)	–	2/10 (20%)
Orchidectomy	Huggins	1941	–	15/21 (71%)	
Breast — ablative therapy					
Hypophysectomy	Notter Denoix Abbes Moricca Hardy Martino	1966 1979 1972 } 1974 1975 1976	454/554 (82%)	42/100 (42%)	152/508 (30%)
Adrenalectomy*	Dao Fracchia	1961 } 1967	8/18 (44%)	210/518 (41%)	186/518 (36%)

TABLE 1   (cont'd.)

	Author	Date	Pain Remission	Subjective Remission	Objective Remission
Breast — additive therapy					
Androgens	Brennan	1960			
	Lewison	1963			
	Wolk	1962			
	Wolk	1964	16/36 (44%)	77/209 (37%)	43/316 (14%)
	Wolk	1965			
	Nevinny	1964			
	Aslam	1977			
Antioestrogens	Cole	1971	8/24 (33%)	41/96 (43%)	5/144 (24%)
	Bloom	1974			
Corticosteroids	Dao	1961	5/43 (12%)	7/43 (16%)	1/23 (4%)
	Colsky	1963			
L–Dopa	Minton	1974	10/30 (33%)	10/30 (33%)	10/30 (33%)
Progestins (not MAP	Colsky	1963			
	Curwen	1963	24/54 (44%)	39/78 (50%)	35/109 (32%)
	Sonkin	1969			
MAP low doses (<500 mg/day)	Bucalossi	1963			
	Dogliotti	1968	14/67 (21%)	31/61 (51%)	37/131 (28%)
	Muggia	1968			
	Klaassen	1976			
MAP high doses (>500 mg/day)	Pannuti	1974			
	Amadori	1976	176/211 (83%)	–	125/276 (45%)
	Martino	1976			
	Pannuti	1977			

* 255 patients also had oophorectomy

HIGH DOSE MEDROXYPROGESTERONE ACETATE

In 1973 Pannuti (1976b) showed it was possible to use daily doses of medroxyprogesterone acetate (MAP) that were larger than those previously used (usually
less than 500 mg intramuscularly per day): the maximum tolerable dose (MTD) of
MAP given intramuscularly was found to be 1500 mg/day for 30 days. Subsequently
we treated 54 patients suffering from advanced breast cancer with MAP at the MTD
and obtained 44% objective remissions (Pannuti, 1976a). Even before objective
remission became apparent, treatment with high doses of MAP was shown to be capable
of inducing prompt subjective remission and producing an impressive antalgic effect
During a study aimed at identifying the maximum therapeutic dose, it was
found that MAP was able to induce pain remission in 90% of the patients treated
(Pannuti, 1976b).

In the group of 54 patients treated with a dose of 1500 mg intramuscularly per day
for 30 days the subjective remission rate was 86% (38/44) and partial or complete
relief of pain occurred in 95% (35/37) of the patients (Pannuti, 1976a). Table 2
shows that the remission of pain became apparent as early as one week after
commencement of treatment, and became proportionally greater during subsequent
weeks, while the treatment continued. After 5 weeks, all 26 patients who had had
severe pain before treatment were totally or partially pain free. The antalgic
effect was especially noticeable in patients with far-advanced breast cancer with

F. Pannuti *et al.*

TABLE 2 Pain Remission Related to Time and Total Doses of MAP

	Pain Intensity			Total MAP (gm)
	Grade 2	Grade 1	Grade 0	
Before treatment	26	11	8	0
After 1 week	7	25	13	10.5
After 2 weeks	2	24	19	21
After 3 weeks	1	18	26	31.5
After 4 weeks	1	15	29	42
After 5 weeks	0	11	34	50
After 6 weeks	0	11	34	–

multiple osseous metastases who were totally incapacitated by pain and thought to be no longer susceptaible to chemotherapy. In addition to the antalgic effect, we noted an improvement in the ability to walk in 63% (15/24). For the purpose of assessing mobility, we considered impairment in walking as a signal-symptom and, therefore, probably correlated to the presence of neoplastic foci capable of inducing motor impairment. We used the following rating scale:

Grade 0 — no or slight impairment
Grade 1 — the patient spends less than 50% of the day in bed
Grade 2 — the patient is forced to spend more than 50% of the day in bed.

In the same group of patients, the incidence of objective remission — complete remission (CR) or partial remission (PR) — was 44% (20/45) with an average duration of 7 months (Pannuti, 1976a). Prior to therapy 79% of this group of patients had pain and nearly one-half of these had severe pain. After 1 month of treatment only 15% had pain and none had severe pain. After six months pain recurred in 48% of the patients and, of these, nearly a third had severe pain. In 23 patients, following recurrence of pain, treatment with MAP was repeated employing even higher doses, 2000 mg intramuscularly daily for 30 days, using a more concentrated preparation (Farlutal 500-1500, F.I. 7401, 200 mg/ml vials). As a result of this repeated therapy, we noted remission once again in 21 patients (91%). In this second group of patients the incidence of objective remission (CR+PR) was 18% (Pannuti, 1978c). Subsequently, we treated another group of 25 patients with the same type of advanced disease with daily doses of 2000 mg intramuscularly per day for 30 days. We noted an objective remission rate of 45% and subjective remission rate of 70% (Pannuti, 1976a).

A new group of 92 patients with the same type of disease was studied as part of a prospective, randomized, multi-centre trial with the aim of assessing the effectiveness of two different dose-levels of MAP. Forty-six patients received 500 mg/day for 30 days and 46 patients received 1500 mg/day for 30 days. The drug was administered intramuscularly (Pannuti, 1979d). Analysis of objective results showed that a higher precentage of the patients who received 1500 mg had complete or partial remission, though the differences were not statistically significant. However, the remission rates in all the signal-symptoms considered were consistently higher for MAP at the 1500 mg dose level (p < 0.05; Table 3). Moreover, remission of pain was more rapid and greater for the higher dose than for the lower dose level (Table 4). The results we obtained using high doses of MAP were subsequently confirmed by other authors (see Table 1).

TABLE 3   Reduction or Disappearance of Signal-Symptoms with Two Doses of MAP

Symptoms	Patients treated with MAP 1500 mg			Patients treated with MAP 500 mg		
	Before therapy	After therapy	Remission rate	Before therapy	After therapy	Remission rate
Pain	26	4	85%	28	7	75%
Dyspneoa	9	3	67%	6	3	50%
Asthenia	25	7	72%	24	8	67%
Anorexia	10	0	100%	16	3	81%
Walking impairment	10	3	70%	12	7	42%

TABLE 4   Rate of Pain Remission During MAP Treatment

Dose (mg)	Patients with pain before therapy	% of patients without pain after			
		1 week	2 weeks	3 weeks	4 weeks
MAP 1500	20	40%	60%	70%	80%
MAP 500	21	29%	38%	48%	71%

Administration of 1500 mg of MAP intramuscularly is associated with a 15% incidence of abscess (Table 5). All the side-effects clear within 3 weeks of the end of treatment and do not delay or prevent further treatment.

TABLE 5   Side Effects of MAP 500, 1500, 2000 mg daily for 30 days

Infiltration	12/166	(7%)
Abscess	31/166	(18%)
Facies lunaris	28/166	(16%)
Fine tremor	27/166	(16%)
Sweating	25/166	(15%)
Vaginal bleeding	18/166	(10%)
Thrombophlebitis	2/166	(1%)
Cramps	15/166	(9%)

In 1977 (Pannuti, 1977b), we began a series of studies concerning the oral administration of high doses of MAP (2000 mg/day for 30 days) with the aim of assessing:

1) the effect on appetite and body weight
2) the anticancer effect on hormone-sensitive tumours
3) the effect on pain.

142 patients (40 males and 102 females) were treated orally with MAP 2000 mg daily for 30 days (Pannuti, 1979a). 77 patients had hormone-sensitive tumours; 26 had early tumours (Table 6).

F. Pannuti *et al.*

TABLE 6   High Dose Oral MAP (2000 mg daily for 30 days)

Remission of	Number of patients	%
Pain	36/68	53
Asthenia	27/73	37
Anorexia	77/141	55
Performance status	41/119	34
Body weight*	73/122	60

* Average increase: 2.5 kg after 30 days of treatment

CONCLUSIONS

Although anti-cancer activity (direct or mediated by pituitary blocking) may be the prime factor behind the antalgic effect of MAP, it is possible that there may also be a more direct anti-inflammatory or analgesic mechanism involved. Even so, it should be stressed that MAP is an anti-cancer agent which, when given in high doses, is able to induce pain relief in hormone-sensitive tumours to an extent not observed before. The value of this form of treatment becomes even more important when one considers that it is associated with a considerable objective remission rate, at least in breast cancer, and also with a strong anabolic effect which may contribute significantly to the patient's quality of life.

REFERENCES

Abbes, M. M., Bourgeon, G., Paillaud, F., Juillard, G., Kermarec, J.,
Cambon, P.,and Namer, M.(1972). A propose de 111 destruction hy-
pophysaires pér yttrium 90 on cryothérapie pour cancer du sein a-
vancé. Ann. Chir.,26, 521-531.

Amadori, D., Ravaioli, A., and Barbanti, F.(1976). L'impiego del medrossiprogesterone acetato ad alte dosi nella terapia palliativa
del carcinoma mammario in fase avanzata. Min. Med.,67, 1-14.

Archimbaud, J. P., Dex Roseax, M., and Picq, P.(1973). Le traitement
des douleurs des métastases osseuses de l'épithélioma prostatique
par la surrénalectomie unilatéralle gauche. J. Urol. Nefrol.,79,
415-419.

Aslam, J.,and Maxwell, J.(1977). Calusterone therapy for advanced bre
ast cancer. Cancer Treat. Rep.,61, 371-373.

Band, P. R., Banergee, T. K., Patwardhan, V. C., and Eid, T. C.(1973)
High dose diethylstilbestrol diphosphate therapy of prostatic cancer after failure of standard doses of estrogens. CMA J., 109,
697-699.

Bloom, H. J. G., and Boesen, E.(1974). Antioestrogens in treatment of
breast cancer. Value of nafoxidine in 52 advanced cases. Br. Med.
J., 2, 7-10.

Bouffioux, C.(1976). Traitement du cancer de la prostate par les agents progestatifs. Acta Urol. Bel., 44, 336-353.

Brennan, H. J., Beckett, V. L., Kelley, J.E., and Betanzos, G.(1960).
Treatment of advanced mammary cancer with 3-β-17-β-androstanediol
Cancer, 13. 1195-1200.

Bucalossi, P., Di Pietro, S.,and Gennari, L.(1963). Trattamento ormo-
nico del carcinoma mammario diffuso con un progestativo sintetico
il 6-α-methil-17-α-acetossiprogesterone. Min. Chir., 9, 358-366.

Colapinto, V., and Aberhart, C.(1961). Clinical trial of massive stil
bestrol diphosphate therapy in advanced carcinoma of the prostate
Br. J. Urol., 33, 171-177.

Cole, M. P., Jones, C. T. A., and Todd, D. H.,(1971). A new anti-oe-
strogenic agent in late breast cancer in early clinical appraisal
of ICI 46474. Br. J. Cancer, 25, 270-275.

Colsky, J., Shnider, B., Jones, R., Jr., Nevinny-Stickel, H. B., Hall
T., Regelson, W., Selawry, D. S., Owens, A., Brindley, C. D., Fre
i, E., III, and Uzer, Y.(1963). A comparative study of 9α-bromo,
11β-ketoprogesterone and prednisolone in the treatment of advanced carcinoma of the female breast. Cancer, 4, 502-505.

Curwen, S.,(1963).The value of norethisterone acetate in the treatme
nt of advanced carcinoma of the breast. Clin. Rad., 14, 445-446.

Dao, T. L.(1961). In:" Progress report: results of studies by the co
operative breast cancer group 1956-1960". Cancer Chemother. Rep.,
11, 109-141.

Denoix, P.(1970). Breast Cancer: Treatment of Malignant Breast Tumours. pp. 1-92. Springer Verlag, Berlin.

Di Carlo, F., Pacilio, G., and Conti, G.(1975). Sul meccanismo d' azione dei progestinici nella terapia dei tumori mammari ormono-dipendenti. Tumori, 61, 501-508.

Dogliotti, G.C., Gavosto, F., and Molinatti,G. M.(1968). Trattamento del cancro avanzato della mammella con progestatici di sintesi. Min. Med., 81, 42-83.

Fergusson, J. D.(1971). Life Sciences Monographs,1,International Symposium on the Treatment of Cancer of the Prostate. Pergamon Press Vieweg.

Fracchia, A. A., Randall, H. J., and Farrow, J. H.(1967). The results of adrenalectomy in advanced breast cancer in 500 consecutive patients. Surg. Gynecol. Obstet., 125-747.

Hardy, J., Grisoli, F., Leclercq, T. A., and Somma, M.(1975). Hypophysectomie transphenoidale dans le cancers du sein metastatiques (160 cas.). Nuov. Presse Med., 4, 2387-2390.

Huggins, C., and Scott, W. W.(1945). Bilateral adrenalectomy in prostatic cancer. Ann. Surg., 122, 1031-1045.

Huggins, C., Stevens, R., and Hodges, C. V.(1941). Studies on prostatic cancer. II. The effect of castration on advanced carcinoma of the prostate gland. Arch. Surg., 43, 209.

Juret, P., and Hayem, M.(1974). Pituitary ablation in the treatment of breast cancer. In: Mammary Cancer and Neuroendocrine Therapy, edited by B. A. Stoll, pp. 283-311. Butterworths, London.

Kistner, R. W., Griffiths, C. T., and Craig, J. M.(1965). Use of progestational agents in the management of endometrial cancer. Cancer, 12, 1563-1579.

Klaassen, D. J., Rapp, E. F., and Hirte, W. E.(1976). Response to medroxyprogesterone acetate (NSC-26386)as secondary hormone therapy for metastatic breast cancer in postmenopausal women. Cancer Treat. Rep., 60, 251-253.

Lewison, E. F., Trimble, F. H., Grow, G. L.,.and Masukawa, T.(1963). Results of combined hormone therapy in advanced breast cancer. Cancer, 16, 1243-1245.

Martino, G., and Ventafridda, V.(1976). Effetto antalgico dell'alcolizzazione ipofisaria,del medrossiprogesterone acetato ad alte dosi e della loro associazione nel carcinoma mammario in fase avanzata. Tumori, 62, 93-98.

Minton, J. P.(1974). The response of breast cancer patients with bone pain to L-DOPA. Cancer,33, 358-363.

Moricca, G.(1974). Chemical hypophysectomy for cancer pain. Adv. Neurol. 4, 470-714.

Muggia, F. M., Cassileth, M. O., Ochoa, M., Jr., Flatow, F. A., Gellhorn, A., and Hyman, G. A.(1968). Treatment of breast cancer with medroxyprogesterone acetate. Ann. Intern. Med., 68, 328-337.

Murphy, G. P., Reynoso, G., Schoonees, R., Gailani, S., Bourke, R., Kenny, G. M., Mirand, E. A., and Schalck, D. S.(1971). Hypophysectomy and adrenalectomy for disseminated prostatic carcinoma. J. Urol. 105, 817-825.

Nevinny-Stickel, H. B., Dederick, M. M., Haines, C. R., and Hall, T.

(1964). Comparative study of 6-dehydro-17α-methyltestosterone and
  testosterone propionate in human breast cancer. Cancer, 17, 95-99.
Notter,G., and Melander, O.(1966). Pituitary implantation with 90yt-
  trium in the treatment of advanced breast cancer. Coll. Int.(Ly-
  ons), pp. 113-121.
Pannuti, F., Martoni, A., Pollutri, E., Camera, P., and Lenaz, G. R.
  (1974).Ormonointerferenza da medrossiprogesterone acetato: Risul
  tati relativi a 50 pazienti affetti da carcinoma mammario in fase
  avanzata.Proposta di una nuova metodologia di caratterizzazione
  e di valutazione. Bull. Sci. Med., 144, 1-43.
Pannuti, F., Martoni, A., Lenaz, G. R., Piana, E., and Nanni, P.
  (1976a). Management of advanced breast cancer with medroxyprogesterone acetate(MAP, F.I. 5837, F.I. 7401, NSC-26386)in high do-
  ses.In: Functional Explorations in Senology,pp.253-265. European
  Press, Ghent, Belgium.
Pannuti, F., Martoni, A., Pollutri, E., Camera, P., Losinno, F.,and
  Giusti, H.(1976b). Massive dose progestational therapy in oncolo
  gy(medroxyprogesterone). Preliminary results. Acts of the IV sym
  posium on the locoregional treatment of tumours, St. Vincent 1973
  Pan. Min. Med., 18, 129-136;
Pannuti, F., Castellari, S., Camera, P., Di Marco, A. R., Fruet, F.,
  Giusti, H., Lelli, G., Martoni, A., Piana, E., Pollutri, E., Ros
  si, A.P., and Strocchi, E.(1977a). I protocolli oncologici dell'
  ospedale M. Malpighi. In: La chemioterapia dei tumori solidi, edi
  ted by F. Pannuti, pp. 517-553. Editrice Universitaria Bolognese,
  Bologna.
Pannuti, F., Fruet, F., and Cricca, A.(1977b). Pilot trial of the use
  of massive doses of medroxyprogesterone acetate(MAP) orally in on
  cology. IRCS Med. Sci.,5,433.
Pannuti, F., Rossi, A. P., and Piana, E.(1977c). Massive doses of me
  droxyprogesterone acetate(MAP): Pilot study in the treatment of
  advanced prostate cancer. IRCS Med. Sci., 5,375.
Pannuti, F., Rossi, A. P., Piana, E.,and Iafelice, G.(1977d). A new
  polychemotherapy schedule in the treatment of advanced stomach
  cancer: pilot study. IRCS Med. Sci., 5, 439.
Pannuti, F., Rossi, A. P., Piana, E., Palenzona, D., and Rocchetta,
  G.(1977e). Combination chemotherapy of advanced gastrointestinal
  cancer with injection of cyclophosphamide plus 5-fluorouracil.
  IRCS Med. Sci., 5,578.
Pannuti, F., Lelli, G., Giusti, H., Camera, P., Piana, E., and Casadio, M.(1978a). Combination chemotherapy of lung cancer with cyclophosphamide, methotrexate, and hydroxyurea(CMFH). IRCS Med.
  Sci., 6, 33.
Pannuti, F., Martoni, A.,and Cricca, A.(1978b). Treatment of renal
  clear cell carcinoma by high doses of medroxyprogesterone aceta-
  te(MAP): Pilot study . IRCS Med. Sci., 6, 177.
Pannuti, F., Martoni, A., Lenaz, G. R., Piana, E., and Nanni, P.(1978
  c). A possible new approach to the treatment of metastatic breast
  cancer: massive doses of medroxyprogesterone acetate. Cancer Tre-

at. Rep., 62,499–504.

Pannuti, F., Martoni, A., Strocchi, E., and Piana, E.(1978d). Clinical comparison of two polichemotherapy regimens in advanced bre
ast cancer: cyclophosphamide, methotrexate and 5-fluorouracil in
combination with and without hydroxyurea. IRCS Med. Sci., 6, 40.

Pannuti, F., Burroni, P., Fruet, F., and Piana, E.(1979a).Il medrossi
progesterone acetato ad alte dosi come anabolizzante in oncologia. In: La chemioterapia dei tumori solidi, edited by Pannuti
F. vol.2 pp. 805–815. Editrice Universitaria Bolognese,Bologna.

Pannuti, F., Cricca, A., Fruet, F., Burroni, P.,and Rossi, A. P.(1979
b).New polychemotherapy regimen for head and neck tumours: Pilot
study. Cancer Treat. Rep., 63,' 805.

Pannuti, F., Lelli, G., Casadio, M., Giusti,H., Busutti, L., Di Marco
A. R., and Gentili, M. R.(1979c).Ciclofosfamide ad alte dosi ver
sus ciclofosfamide+methotrexate+5fluorouracile+idrossiurea (CM
FH)nel trattamento del carcinoma non a piccole cellule del pol-
mone (studio fase III). In: La chemioterapia dei tumori solidi,
edited by Pannuti F. vol.2 pp. 599–611. Editrice Universitaria
Bolognese ,Bologna.

Pannuti, F., Martoni, A., Di Marco, A.R., Piana, E., Saccani, F.,Bec
chi,G., Mattioli, G., Barbanti, F., Marra, G. A., Persiani, W.,
Cacciari, L., Spagnolo, F., Palenzona, D.,and Rocchetta, G.(1979
d). Prospective, randomized clinical trial of two different high
dosages of medroxyprogesterone acetate(MAP) in the treatment of
metastatic breast cancer . Europ. J. Cancer, 15,539–601.

Rafla, S., and Johnson, R.(1974). The treatment of advanced prostate
carcinoma with medroxyprogesterone. Curr. Ther. Res., 16, 261–
267.

Rifkind, A. B., Kulin,H. E., Cargille, C. M., Rayford, P. C., and Ross
G. T.(1969). Suppression of urinary axcretion of luteinizing hor
mone(LH)and follicle stimulating hormone(FSH)by MAP. J. Clin.En-
docrinol. Metab.,29, 506.

Scott, W. W.(1973). Rationale and results of primary endocrine therapy in patients with prostatic cancer. Cancer, 32, 1119–1125.

Serment, H., Spitalier, J. M., Ayme, E., De Giovanni, E., and Bardin,
J. P.(1970). Médroxyprogestérone et adénocarcinomes de l'endomé
tre. Bull. Fed. Gynecol. Obstet., 22, 93–97.

Smith, J. P., Rutledge, F., and Soffar, S. W.(1966). Progestins in
the treatment of patients with endometrial adenocarcinoma. Ann.
J. Obstet. Gynecol., 94, 977–984.

Smith, R. B., (1971). Cyproterone therapy in stage IV. In : Life Scien
ce Monographs, 1,International Symposium on the Treatment of Cancer of the Prostate. Pergamon Press, Vieweg.

Sonkin, R., Coudeyras, M., and Thévenet, M.(1969). L' utilisation de
la noréthindrone à doses fortes dans le traitement de certains
cancers génitaux hormonodépendants. Obstet. Gynecol., 68, 355–
372.

Straffon, R. A., Kiser, W. S., Robitaille, D. F., and Dohn, D. F.
(1968). ^{90}yttrium hypophysectomy in the management of metastatic

carcinoma of the prostatic gland in 13 patients. <u>J. Urol</u>., 90, 102-108.

Susan, L. P., Roth, B. R., and Adkins, W. C.(1976). Regression of pro static cancer metastases by high doses of diethylstilbestrol di- phosphate. <u>Urology</u>, 7, 598-601.

Talley, R. W., Moorhead, E. L., Tucker, W. G., San Diego, E. L., and Brennan, M. J.(1969).Treatment of metastatic hypernephroma.<u>JAMA</u> 207, 322-328.

Twycross, R. G.(1979). The Brompton Cocktail. In:<u>Advances in Pain Re- search and Therapy</u>. Edited by Bonica, J. J.,and Ventafridda, V. vol. 2 pp. 291-300. Raven Press.

Van der Werfmessing, B., and Van Gilse, H. A.(1971). Hormonal treat- ment of metastases of renal carcinoma. <u>Br. J. Cancer</u>, 25, 423- 427.

Volk, H., Ciprut, S., and Escher, G.(1962). Hormonal therapy in advan ced breast cancer. II: Effect of oral 11β-hydroxy-17α-methyl- testosterone compared with fluoxymesterone on clinical course and its effects on metabolism of nitrogen and selected electro- lytes. <u>Cancer</u>, 15, 726-732.

Volk, H., Foley, C.J., Sanfilippo, L.J., and Escher, G. C.(1964).Hor monal therapy in advanced breast cancer. III : Effect of 6-β-di bromomethilene-testosterone propionate compared with that of 2α- A-methyl-dihydrotestosterone propionate on clinical course and metabolism of selected serum electrolytes. <u>Cancer</u>, 17, 1073-1078

Volk, H., Wilde, R. C., Carabasi, R., and Bisel,H.(1965). Anti-tumor efficacy of norandrolone propionate compared with testosterone propionate in advanced breast cancer . <u>Cancer</u>, 18, 651-655.

West, C. D., Hollander, V. P., Whithore, W. F., Jr., Randall, H. T. and Pearson, O. H.(1952). The effect of bilateral adrenalectomy upon neoplastic disease in man. <u>Cancer</u>, 5, 1009-1018,

Radiation Therapy

S. BASSO-RICCI

Department of Radiology, Istituto Nazionale per lo Studio e la Cura dei Tumori,
Milan, Italy

It is well known that radiotherapy can relieve pain in a number of situations in terminal cancer. The results of radiotherapy can be attributed to the following effects of the ionizing radiation:

a) reduction of pressure on and infiltration of organs and nerves;
b) promotion of healing of malignant ulcers;
c) resolution of inflammatory processes in and around the tumour;
d) capillary haemostasis within the tumour.

These effects are sufficient to explain the results obtained in relation to cough, dysphagia, dyspnoea, oedema, haematic seepage, and motor disturbances. On the other hand, they do not completely explain the results obtained in relation to pain, perhaps because of the influence of psychological factors in this area.

TUMOURS OF THE HEAD AND NECK

We include here cases of recurrence that involve the nerves at the base of the skull, particularly the trigeminal, and metastatic lymph nodes involving the nerves of the neck or base of the skull. Good results can be expected from radiotherapy with respect to pain, though improvement of motor function is generally negligible (Felci, 1964).

Among the tumours of the oral cavity we should consider chronic recurrences, some of which are predominantly soft tissue infiltrations while others are predominantly ulcerations. The former are not very radiosensitive and it is consequently generally advisable to use other therapies. Radiotherapy is indicated more in those cases of recurrence in which radiation has not previously been used. Even in these, a decreased palliative effect may be expected if previous surgery, such as ligation of the carotid, has reduced the blood supply to the area. For tumours of the paranasal sinuses, which when very advanced are inevitably accompanied by pain, radiotherapy is indicated even for recurrences. As some of the pain may be caused by inflammation secondary to infection, antibiotics should ·be used as well.

For tumours of the hypopharynx which, after combination radiotherapy and surgery, are frequently complicated by fistulas and necrosis of the carotid, one should be extremely cautious and avoid further radiotherapy. For tumours of the thyroid, radiotherapy is indicated if there is compression or infiltration of the cervical plexus.

TUMOURS OF THE CHEST

This group includes primary tumours of the lung, primary and secondary tumours of the thoracic wall, and carcinoma of the breast. A tumour of the lung accompanied by pain is already in a far-advanced stage. It is in these cases that radiotherapy is particularly indicated whether the pain is attributable to infiltration of the brachial plexus or intercostal nerves, or to secondary costal lesions. Often pain occurs some time after initial treatment with radiotherapy or surgery and before radiology can confirm recurrence. In these cases, examination with radioisotopes, such as bleomycin labelled with radioactive iridium — used in our Institute in more than 30 patients — has allowed the irradiation of a more specific limited field (Kahn and co-workers, 1977). Radiotherapy often results in improvement of dysphagia and cough as well as pain. Radiotherapy may also be used, often with good effect, to relieve similar symptoms caused by mediastinal and lung metastases from distant tumours. It is also useful in the relief of pain caused by metastatic or primary lesions of the chest wall, ulcerated breast cancer, lymph node metastases that compress or infiltrate the brachial nerve plexus, and large axillary lymph node metastases causing lymphoedema of the arm.

TUMOURS OF THE ABDOMEN

Especially included in this group are tumours of the large intestine, which may cause pain by nerve compression as a result of retroperitoneal lymph node metastases. Treatment of these metastases with labelled bleomycin is useful, above all when the metastases are pre-sacral. In our Institute in the last seven years we have treated more than 60 cases of recurrent carcinoma of the large intestine with radiotherapy and achieved good pain relief. There are reports of good results obtained from radiotherapy given purely to achieve pain relief in cases of advanced cancer of the pancreas (Green and co-workers, 1973) and in inoperable cancer of the biliary tract (Smoron, 1977).

TUMOURS OF THE FEMALE GENITAL SYSTEM

The effect of radiotherapy on pain from uterine cancer caused by infiltration of neighbouring structures, lymph node metastases, or involvement of the pelvic bones can be marked, but less than with other tumours (Basso-Ricci and Bianchi, 1966). Even less effective is radiotherapy to the inguino-iliac and common iliac lymph node chains with the intention of reducing oedema of the lower limbs. Recanalization of the ureter in the presence of malignant obstruction is almost never obtained (Basso-Ricci and Bianchi, 1966).

TUMOURS OF THE MALE GENITAL SYSTEM

These include tumours of the testicle and the prostate. Massive retroperitoneal lymph node metastases from testicular tumours can cause intense pain. That caused by metastases of seminoma regresses with radiotherapy more quickly than that caused by metastatic carcinoma, and relates to differences in radiosensitivity. This observation is based on a study of about 40 cases treated in the Institute. In the cases of tumours of the prostate with endopelvic spread, radiotherapy can bring about complete remission of pain and disorders of bladder function (Hazra, 1974; Rodriguez and co-workers, 1973).

TUMOURS OF THE URINARY SYSTEM

Patients with local recurrences or lymph node metastases from renal tumours, bladder tumours with infiltration of the bladder wall and endopelvic tissues, or with lymph node metastases and endopelvic recurrences after total cystectomy benefit considerably from radiation therapy when there is associated pain.

TUMOURS OF THE NERVOUS SYSTEM

Primary tumours of the brain whether multiple, inoperable or recurrent, are often accompanied by cephalalgia. Although palliative surgical procedures can be a great help, particularly when there is hydrocephalus, radiotherapy may be beneficial when surgical procedures are not feasible. In cases of cerebral metastases that are associated with headache or neurological disorders of another type, radiotherapy and cortisone have been found useful in 85% of cases (Hendrikson, 1975). In our Institute we have treated at least 100 patients with these lesions in the last seven years with similar results. It is important to remember that when cerebral oedema is related to compression of the venous sinuses, as can happen in the presence of extracerebral, epidural and arachnoidal metastases, cortisone has little effect, and only radiation therapy is effective. In the presence of thrombosis of the venous sinuses, no therapy is effective (Posner, 1971). The pain from epidural or vertebral metastases (which may precede other neurological symptoms, particularly motor, by several months) regresses with radiotherapy. In the presence of compression of the spinal cord, pain regresses after laminectomy and radiotherapy. Even pain from involvement of the cauda equina, which may be accompanied by alterations in functions of the bladder and large intestine, can be effectively resolved with radiotherapy (Posner, 1971). In the Institute from 1965 to 1975, about 40 patients with epidural metastases without radiological evidence of bony involvement, have been treated with radiation therapy. Radiotherapy has consolidated, in at least one-third of the cases, the success of the laminectomy, not only with regard to pain and motor dysfunction, but it has also prevented local recurrences from metastases incompletely removed by the surgeon. As a result the patient has permanently regained the use of the lower limbs, death occurring after several years from dissemination of the cancer to other sites.

TUMOURS OF THE BONES

Amongst the most important results of radiotherapy are those obtained in relation to osseous metastases, which are commonly accompanied by pain. No other therapy has the same effectiveness as radiotherapy, though the same positive results can be obtained with chemotherapy and hormone therapy in a smaller number of cases. With radiotherapy, in addition to the analgesic effect, re-calcification of the affected bone is also obtained. Radiotherapy is generally used externally, but it is also possible to recalcify affected areas by destruction of the pituitary gland with radioisotopes and the administration of radiophosphorus, P32, particularly in the presence of sclerotic prostatic metastases after preliminary sensitization with parathormone.

SYSTEMIC TUMOURS

This group includes all those cases in which lymph node metastases involve paravertebral nerves, the meninges or bones. The response to radiotherapy in these cases is generally good.

CONCLUSIONS

Response to radiotherapy is influenced by the histological type of the tumour, by its macroscopic characteristics and, possibly, by previous treatment. Radiotherapy is especially indicated in cases of osseous metastases, even if diffuse, with the purpose of allowing the patient to remain mobile and to prevent fractures, particularly of the lower limbs. It is also indicated for epidural metastases, even if laminectomy has already been carried out. Although the aim is purely palliative, radiotherapy is also indicated especially in cases of relapse of cancer of the lung and large intestine which, even in those with a very poor prognosis, are generally limited to local recurrences or regional metastases. In fact, in these cases it is possible to achieve with radiotherapy, especially if not previously treated, the double goal of relieving symptoms and slowing tumour progression. Better results can, of course, be obtained when the tumour is not so far advanced.

Among the contra-indications to radiotherapy, the most important are previous or repeated radiation treatments, especially if the latter concerned the dorsal region of the thorax and the lumbar area of the back, because of the particular radio-sensitivity of the cutaneous tissues of these regions and the possibility of bed sores. In very debilitated patients extensive radiation of the abdomen is contra-indicated, as it rarely achieves any positive benefit but almost always causes considerable worsening of the patient's general condition. Finally, radiotherapy is absolutely contra-indicated in those cases where the pain has resulted from fibrosis after previous radiotherapy, especially when the brachial plexus is involved (Basso-Rissi and co-workers, 1976).

The method of treatment deserves some mention. A small number of sessions of relatively high doses are recommended, because the patients are usually suffering and move with difficulty. However, in the majority of cases there is no benefit in exceeding an overall dose of 3000 rad.

REFERENCES

Basso-Ricci, S. and Bianchi, F. (1966) Terapia delle recidive pelviche del carcinoma del collo dell'utero. *Minerva Ginecol.* 18, 603-609.

Basso-Ricci, S., Ventafridda, V., Zanolla, R., Cassani, L. and Spreafico, R. (1976) Presentazione di 25 casi di lesioni postirradiatorie del plesso brachiale e loro trattamento. *Tumori*, 62, 365-372.

Felci, U. (1964) La radioterapia dei tumori della rinofaringe. In: *Corso Superiore sulla Terapia dei Tumori della Testa e del Collo*, Milano, 6-11 April, pp. 181-215. CEA, Milan.

Green, N., Beron, E., Melbye, R.W. and George, F.W. (1973) Carcinoma of the pancreas: palliative radiotherapy. *Am. J. Roentgenol. Radium Ther. Nucl. Med.*, 117, 620-622.

Hazra, T.A. (1974) The role of radiotherapy in management of carcinoma of the prostate. *Maryland Med. J.* 23, 48-49.

Hendrikson, F.R. (1975) Radiation therapy of metastatic tumors in the brain. *Semin. Oncol.*, 2, 43-46.

Kahn, P.C., Milunsky, C., Dewanjee, M.K. and Rudders, R.A. (1977) The place of ^{57}Co-bleomycin scanning in the evaluation of tumors. *Am. J. Roentgenol. Radium Ther. Nucl. Med.*, 129, 267-273.

Posner, J.B. (1971) Neurological complications of systemic cancer. *Med. Clin. North Am.*, <u>55</u>, 625-646.

Rodriguez, A., Cook, S.A., Jelden, G.L., Hunter, A.T.W., Sraffon, R.A. and Stewart, B.H. (1973) Management of primary and metastatic carcinoma of the prostate. *Am. J. Roentgenol. Radium Ther. Nucl. Med.*, <u>118</u>, 876-880.

Smoron, G.L. (1977) Radiation therapy of carcinoma of gallbladder and biliary tract. *Cancer*, <u>40</u>, 1422-1424.

Narcotic Analgesics

B. M. MOUNT

Director, Palliative Care Service, Royal Victoria Hospital, Montreal,
Quebec, Canada

ABSTRACT

Recent experience suggests that the chronic pain of advanced malignant
disease can be controlled with very few exceptions using an oral morphine elixir in doses carefully titrated to analgesia and given regularly at intervals based on the serum half-life of the narcotic being
used. Pain is continuously just prevented rather than being repeatedly treated. Significant dependance, tolerance, and attendant dose
escalation are not a problem even when narcotics are administered in
this fashion for several years. The patient remains alert, pain free,
with an unclouded sensorium and an unaltered affect. The oral and
parenteral use of morphine, heroin, methadone, anileridine and other
commonly employed narcotics is reviewed as is the role of adjuvant
therapy. While further studies are needed, a new standard of pain
control has been established in this clinical setting.

INTRODUCTION

The last decade has seen significant changes in our understanding of
chronic pain and the use of oral narcotics for its control. Most physicians gain experience in the use of narcotic analgesics while treating acute pain. Too frequently the prescribing practices appropriate
to that setting have been utilized in the treatment of chronic pain.
The significant differences between acute and chronic pain and the
host of factors which modulate all perception of pain, acute and chronic,
are now more clearly appreciated (Lipman 1975, Melzack 1973).

Acute pain warns of a problem that needs attention; thus it has a
meaning. It can be viewed as linear, with a beginning and an end.
In directing attention to the offending organ the noxious stimulus is
seen as "helpful", "useful" or "justifiable", however else it is perceived. How different is the experience of chronic pain. Early in its
course, the perception of the physical stimulus is modified by psycho-

logical considerations (Leshan, 1964, Lipman 1975). Anxiety and depression develop and lead to insomnia. A vicious cycle is established. The very chronicity of the pain underscores the hopelessness of
the situation and the inadequacy of therapeutic intervention. The
pain is thus meaningless in that it does not lead to a corrective
therapeutic response. Nietzsche has said (Allport 1959), "He who has
a why to live can bear with almost any how." Deprived of helpful
therapy that would give the pain an acceptable "why" the patient is
to a large degree stripped of his defences.

Saunders (1967) has coined the term "total pain" to describe the all-
consuming nature of chronic pain and our need to attack all of its
components - physical, psychological, social and spiritual. For the
patient with advanced malignant disease, chronic pain is a forceful
reminder of his prognosis and a potent factor accentuating his total
agony.

An important factor influencing our use of narcotics in the past has
been the fear of producing dependance (addiction), tolerance and resultant dose escalation. The physician has been faced with further
problems:

- the fear of running out of effective agents before the patient's
  death;
- the belief that morphine taken orally is sufficiently poorly absorbed to render it useless by that route;
- the dilemma of having to choose between a patient in pain and one
  sedated by narcotics;
- the difficulty in evaluating a subjective and highly personal experience such as pain;
- the problem of interpreting the scattered, often anecdotal and
  frequently conflicting data relating to narcotics in the literature.

All these factors have led to an endemic inadequacy in pain control
(Bonica 1979), and the conclusion that the use of narcotics implies
poor medical care (Black 1974). Much of this has changed.

Many comprehensive reviews of the pharmacology, toxicology and therapeutic uses of narcotic analgesics are available (for example,
Lasagna, 1964: Catalano, 1975: Jaffe and Martin, 1975: Evens and
Koda-Kimble, 1978). The purpose of this paper is not to reproduce
these reviews but to focus specifically on the use of narcotic analgesics in the treatment of cancer patients with chronic pain. Recently, in reviewing 10 years experience with 3,362 such patients, Saunders (1978B) reported that pain was "difficult to control" in only
34 (1%) using oral narcotics as the mainstay of therapy, complemented
by a variety of other drug and non-drug treatments. Although the
assessment of relief in these patients was clinical and lacked rigorous objective quantification, the writing on the wall is now clear.
It is possible to relieve the pain of terminal cancer with the improved use of narcotics and other drugs now available. Furthermore,

iatrogenic sedation, clouding of consciousness and the spectre of
addiction are avoidable in virtually all patients.

The roles of non-pharmacologic approaches including ablative neurosurgical procedures, the use of P32, or whole-body irradiation, must
now be reassessed taking into consideration their attendant morbidity
and mortality risks and the quality of life they provide, as compared
to those associated with the skilled use of a simple solution or elixir
of morphine taken orally. The use of narcotic analgesics for patients
with advanced malignant disease will be reviewed, therefore, from this
perspective.

AIMS OF TREATMENT

The therapeutic aims against which the efficacy of narcotics must be
measured in treating the intractable pain of advanced malignant disease, including the following:

(1) Identifying the Etiology: Clarification of the cause of pain is
    the first step in its control and may lead to specific forms of
    therapy. The patient with pain related to metastatic breast or
    prostate cancer, for example, may respond dramatically to estro-
    gen therapy. It should not be assumed, however, that the patient's
    pain is invariably due to the malignant process. Rather than anal-
    gesics, the patient with severe abdominal pain in the presence of
    constipation may require purgatives. Rather than irradiation for
    metastatic disease, a carious molar may need dental extraction,
    while osteitis pubis will require curettage of the synchondrosis.
    Careful assessment is essential.

(2) Pain Prevention; Not Treatment: The aim is to anticipate and con-
    tinuously to prevent the resurgence of pain, rather than to re-
    peatedly treat it, thus breaking the vicious cycle of pain-despair-
    more pain with resultant dose escalation. This requires the regu-
    lar administration of individually optimized doses of an appro-
    priate analgesic. Waiting for pain to reappear, as with "as re-
    quired" narcotic orders or self-administered "demand" analgesia
    only perpetuates the fear of pain and the need for higher anal-
    gesic doses for its control.

(3) Erasing Pain Memory: Consistent pain prevention will lead to a
    lessening of the anxious anticipation and memory of pain and a
    frequent diminution in the narcotic dose required for pain control.

(4) An Unclouded Sensorium: Many patients feel trapped between per-
    petual pain on the one hand and perpetual somnolence on the other.
    The balance, a pain-free state without sedation, requires careful
    regulation of analgesic dose according to the individual patient's
    needs.

(5) <u>An Unaltered Affect</u>: The ability of a patient to relate to his
    family, friends, and environment with an affect that is neither
    euphoric or depressed is an important goal. The practice of using
    intravenous alcohol and psychotropic drugs that lead to a state of
    euphoria or altered consciousness is, therefore, questionable.

(6) <u>Ease of Administration</u>: Oral administration of analgesics can
    allow a patient to retain a degree of independence and mobility
    that he cannot have when analgesics are given parenterally. Cac-
    hexia may also make the regular administration of parenteral medi-
    cation difficult and painful.

                THE USE OF DIAMORPHINE AND MORPHINE

Although for many years British physicians have used a number of oral
narcotic mixtures, often bearing the name of the Brompton Chest Hospital, London, it was not until 1973 that such a formulation was included in the British Pharmaceutical Codex (1973).

The important experience of Saunders (1967) and her co-workers at St.
Christopher's Hospice, London, a medical foundation for patients mainly with advanced malignant disease, has led to a refinement of approach
associated with greatly increased effectiveness in achieving the six
aims of therapy listed above. In a retrospective review of 500 patients Twycross (1974) described their experience with the use of diamorphine (heroin). More than 80% of the patients admitted to St.
Christopher's Hospice received diamorphine at some time. About 15%
of patients on diamorphine received it either predominantly or exclusively by injection, the remainder took it by mouth in an elixir containing both diamorphine and cocaine (Table 1, A). The dose was adjusted to produce analgesia and the elixir given regularly so as to
produce a continuous pain-free state. Twycross concluded:

    1. Although, on account of increasing debility, most patients re-
        ceived parenteral treatment during the last 12-48 hours, the
        majority can be maintained on orally administered diamorphine
        prior to this time.
    2. There is no single optimal dose or maximum effective dose of
        diamorphine.
    3. The prescription of diamorphine does not, by itself, lead to
        impairment of mental faculties.
    4. Tolerance is not a practical problem.
    5. Psychological dependance does not occur.
    6. Physical dependance may develop, but appears not to prevent
        the downward adjustment of the dose of diamorphine when con-
        sidered clinically feasible.

In a further study of the long-term use of diamorphine Twycross and
Wald (1976) analyzed the course of 115 patients with advanced cancer
who received individually optimized doses of diamorphine hydro-

chloride regularly for 12 weeks or longer. Dose reductions were common and the median final dose was _less_ than the median maximum dose.
The data supported the hypothesis that in general, increases in dose
reflect a change in pathophysiology as with new metastases or collapse
of a vertebral body,rather than tolerance.

Oral Morphine

How effective is morphine taken orally? Following a pilot trial that
demonstrated a diamorphine to morphine oral analgesic potency ratio
of 1.5:1, Twycross (1977) carried out a controlled cross-over trial
to compare the effectiveness of these two narcotics taken orally. He
concluded that provided allowance is made for the difference in potency, morphine is a satisfactory substitute for orally administered
diamorphine. The lack of clear cut superiority of heroin, as compared
to morphine, noted by Twycross, agreed with the earlier conclusions of
Lasagna (1964) who reviewed the literature relating to the testing of
narcotics in human subjects and concluded that there was little evidence to suggest that heroin was the better drug. In light of these
findings St. Christopher's Hospice started using orally administered
morphine instead of heroin in April 1977.

The findings supporting the effectiveness of oral morphine also cor-
roborated the earlier observations of Melzack and his colleagues
(1976) who had for the first time attempted to quantify the response
to oral morphine, prescribed according to Saunders and Twycross, in
a population of cancer patients with advanced disease, in a general
hospital. The study used the McGill Melzack Pain Questionnaire, a
pain rating tool offering three indices of pain measurement, (the
present pain intensity, the pain rating index and the number of words
chosen). A morphine elixir similar to the diamorphine elixir in Table
1A was employed. The effectiveness of pain control was assessed in
cancer patients in the palliative care unit, ward and private hospital
accommodations. Results were also compared with the pain relief obtained with a variety of traditional approaches to pain control other
than oral morphine in an unmatched group of cancer patients seen in
the hospital pain clinic. Eight (9%) of the 90 patients entered in
the study could not be controlled using oral morphine as the basis
for analgesia. Of these, one had severe bladder spasm, two had sharp
nerve root pain radiating into the legs and five complained of severe
pain, a major component of which was the despair and anguish associated with their impending death. (Several years subsequent experience
has confirmed that these problems are consistently the most refractory
to control by oral morphine). The study showed that oral morphine was
strikingly effective in controlling the pain of advanced cancer in all
hospital settings but significantly more effective in the therapeutic
milieu of the hospital palliative care ward (PCU) than on other wards.
In the PCU 92-96% of patients taking the morphine elixir had no pain
or mild pain and none had severe pain, while 65-81% of patients elsewhere in the hospital had mild or no pain and 10-16% had severe pain.
Pain control using other agents in the unmatched group of pain clinic

patients was significantly poorer than that obtained with oral morphine.

TABLE 1   Formulation for: A) Diamorphine Elixir
                             B) Aquous Morphine Elixir

A. Diamorphine Hydrocloride   2.5 mg or more
    Cocaine Hydrochloride   10 mg
    Ethyl Alcohol 95% BP   2.5 ml
    Syrup (66% sucrose in water (W/V)   5.0 ml
    Chloroform water ad   20.0 ml

B. Morphine Sulphate   2.5 mg or more
    Syrup BP   5.0 ml
    Ethyl Alcohol 94%   1.5 ml
    Water ad   20 ml

To what extent does the documented effectiveness of a "Brompton Mixture" depend on the narcotic ingredient? In a further study a traditional Brompton mixture formulation containing morphine was compared in a double-blind, cross-over trial to an aqueous solution of
morphine sulphate (Melzack, Mount and Gordon, 1979) (Table 1B).
There was no significant difference in mean morphine dose used, effectiveness of pain control attained, or incidence of side effects
encountered (confusion, nausea, drowsiness) using morphine alone or
the Brompton mixture. It is concluded that a simple elixir of morphine is as effective as the traditional elixirs containing cocaine
and alcohol in higher concentrations.

The series of studies cited suggest that oral morphine may be tolerated in approximately 85-90% of those patients with advanced cancer
who require narcotic analgesics, and that as many as 95% of patients
given oral narcotics will attain excellent pain control with this
basic approach in conjunction with adjuvant therapy. The studies relate, however, to a highly selected group of patients — those with
advanced cancer, particularly those in specialized care centres spe-
cially designed to meet the needs of the terminally ill. Their relevance to other clinical settings has not been well established.

Administration: Clinical and Pharmacologic Considerations

For most patients the chronic pain of advanced malignant disease can
be controlled with less than 30 mg of morphine per oral dose (Melzack, 1976, 1979). In reviewing the administration of diamorphine
to 2,000 patients admitted to St. Christopher's Hospice, Twycross
(1978) reported that approximately 80 percent received 20 mg diamorphine or less as a maximum 4-hourly dose.

Small or elderly patients with easily controlled pain may require as little as 2.5 mg morphine per dose. There is insufficient data concerning dose response curved when these very low oral doses have been clinically effective to firmly establish pharmacokinetic explanations for these results. There is a similar paucity of data at higher dose ranges. Furthermore, Berkowitz and colleagues (1975) remind us that to date there are no studies showing any direct evidence in man suggesting that serum levels of morphine or metabolics may be a useful indicator of pharmacologic activity. Further study is clearly needed.

In studying the disposition of parenterally administered morphine in anesthetized surgical patients using radioimmunioassay (Berkowitz, 1975) found that initial serum levels of morphine correlated with the age of the patient. The degree to which this accounts for the greater sensitivity of older patients to morphine (Belleville 1971) is uncertain. The half-life of its analgesic effect was found to be independent of age and averaged from 2-4 hours after either parenteral or oral administration, an interval which parallels the plasma morphine concentration quite closely.

Because the therapeutic ratio for morphine is not large some important conclusions follow about both the peak plasma concentration and the frequency of dosing. The aim is to keep the plasma concentration within the zone of efficacy, but below the zone of toxicity (Vere 1978). This is achieved in a given patient by careful titration of narcotic dose to the point of pain relief using a regular schedule of oral doses at intervals based on the duration of clinical effect of the narcotic in that patient (for morphine this is usually 4 hours). The night time dose is omitted only when the patient can sleep through the night free of pain. Careful individualization and attention to exact dosage and timing will pay dividends in improved results. Careful observation of the patient's condition over a complete 24 hour period may suggest augmentation of one or two specific doses at periods of peak activity.

Oral doses reach peak plasma concentrations more slowly and also diminish more slowly than those given parenterally and are thus safer. Although the area under the curve when plotting plasma drug concentration against time is similar following parenteral and oral administration, there is a higher initial peak in plasma concentration following parenteral administration. This may reach toxic levels at a dose which is safe when given orally. Vere (1978) has presented a helpful review of these issues.

For most patients, a pain free state can be achieved by titrating to the point of relief with sequential increments in narcotic dose. (Fig. 1). In the treatment of excruciating pain one may, however, elect to start with a higher dose then use sequential decrements with successive doses until analgesia without sedation is achieved. During titration of dose to the patient's need, dose alterations may be made at intervals of 24 to 48 hours and even more frequently if the patient

is not experiencing significant relief. While dose titration is in
process, further relief can be achieved with the use of supplemental
oral or parenteral morphine as necessary. Sequential increases in
oral dose are usually in the increments shown.

INCREMENT	DOSE RANGE
5 mg	2.5-20 mg
10 mg	20-60 mg
20-30 mg	over 60 mg

The maximum effective oral dose of morphine is ill-defined. Recent
experience suggests that continuing effectiveness may be obtained
with oral doses of 150 mg or more. Such doses are rarely needed.
As already noted, the majority of patients have excellent pain relief at 30 mg or less morphine every four hours by mouth. Where pain
control is inadequate the role of the non-physical components of the
patient's "total pain" such as anxiety, depression, social stress or
unresolved spiritual concerns should be examined. Alterations in tumour status are looked for and a careful repeat history and physical
examination performed. Hyperaesthesia and dysaesthesia in an area of
acute sensory loss, and spasms of acute pain present special management problems not responsive to simple augmentation of a routine narcotic dose.

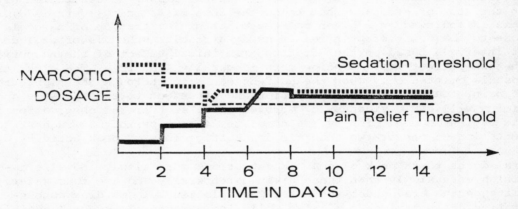

Fig. 1

Tolerance with resultant escalation of dose requirements in not encountered (Mount 1976, Twycross 1974, Vere 1978) when attention to
detail is observed in analgesic dose titration as described, even
after narcotics have been used for periods of several years.

If parenteral medication becomes necessary one half the previous oral
dose is given (Twycross 1974). The experience of others has varied
in this regard (Houde 1965, Evens 1978), with the parenteral to oral
dose ratio in terms of total relief being reported by Evens as 1 to
6. Our clinical experience confirms the observations of Twycross that
such major differences between oral and parenteral doses are not called

for and that the 1:2 ratio is clinically effective (Mount 1976).

Concurrent Use of Phenothiazines

In many of the studies reported above (Melzack 1976, 1979, Mount 1976, Saunders 1967, Twycross 1974) phenothiazines were routinely given with the oral narcotic elixir. Prochlorperazine 5 mg may be used for its antiemetic effects. If restlessness or agitation is a feature, chlorpromazine 10 to 25 mg may be substituted. After the first 48-72 hours on narcotics the nausea associated with their initiation passes and the phenothiazine can usually be discontinued. In general it is wise to increase the dose of one variable, the narcotic or the phenothiazine, at a time. Since the phenothiazines and narcotics are additive in producing CNS and respiratory depression, small changes in either variable may produce profound changes in analgesia and sedation. Prolongation of narcotic analgesic effect on addition of a phenothiazine appears to occur in some cases but has not been objectively quantified in any of the studies cited.

When phenothiazines are being used, dispensing the morphine mixture and the phenothiazine syrup separately allows greater flexibility in adjusting dosage. Once a continuous pain-free state is achieved, they may be combined in dispensing for greater ease of administration, or the phenothiazine may be discontinued.

Adverse effects: The oral regimen described affords a safe and reliable means of controlling pain in these very sick patients. Problems are uncommon and rarely serious. They are the adverse effects common to all narcotics and include the following:

Sedation: Writing in Goodman and Gilman's textbook The Pharmacological Basis of Therapeutics, Jaffe (1975) states, "In man, morphine produces analgesia, drowsiness, changes in mood and mental clouding." It is important to emphasize that of these effects ONLY the analgesia need be encountered when oral morphine is used as described.

When narcotic therapy is first introduced transient sedation frequently occurs. Both patient and family should be reassured that this will clear within 48-72 hours and that complete pain control with a clear sensorium can be expected. The potential of the phenothiazines to act additively with narcotics in producing CNS and respiratory depression has been referred to. This is avoided by care in titrating the doses of both variables. It should be remembered that analgesia is encountered at a lower dose than toxicity. One may therefore rely on the analgesic response as a safe and pragmatic indicator of appropriate dose for a given patient. When somnolence is encountered in the presence of residual pain one should re-examine the possibility that previously unsuspected anxiety, depression or other unresolved psychosocial distress is augmenting the patient's total pain and that the present narcotic dose is excessive relative to the physical component of the pain. A lowering of the narcotic dose, the judicious pursuit

of the non-physical factors in the patient's anguish and the control
of other symptoms is required. Excellence of pain control requires,
in effect, excellence in the control of all other symptoms as well.
Reviews of effective approaches to the control of symptoms other than
pain in these patients have recently been published (Baines 1978,
Mount 1978).

Should the above factors be ruled out as the cause of uncontrolled
pain in the presence of somnolence, other factors unrelated to the
use of morphine should be sought. These include hepatic and renal
insufficiency, brain metastases and the complete list of differential
diagnoses for somnolence common to general medical practice.

Sedation may be encountered also as a terminal event. Frequently it
is noted that patients require less narcotic in the final days or hours
of life. Terminal somnolence, then may simply reflect a relative
over-dose of narcotic in the dying patient at dose levels that were
required for effective pain control a few days earlier. The physician
or nurse alert to this phenomenon may carefully titrate down the narcotic dose being careful to maintain effective analgesia yet avoiding
sedation thus providing patient comfort while enabling him to relate
to family and friends until the end.

Respiratory depression: It is extremely rare for the respiratory depression to be clinically significant when morphine is given as described. Individual variation in the disposition of morphine is seen
at any age but is particularly marked in the very young and old. As
with sedation, respiratory depression is caused by narcotics at doses
above the analgesic doses except in patients with poor respiratory re-
serve. Even so, the margin of safety is not wide (particularly when
given intravenously). It follows that with patients who represent a
particular risk one should begin with small doses and work up quickly
until the pain is controlled, watching ventilation at each dose increase. This requires some experience and attention to detail on the
part of both doctor and nurse (Vere 1978).

In treating several hundred patients over the past five and one half
years we have administered narcotic antagonists on only three occasions when morphine was used as described: In one case following an
error in the dose of narcotic given by a nurse, in the second case,
probably unnecessarily, to a somnolent terminally ill cancer patient
who had longstanding chronic respiratory insufficiency and in the
third instance following respiratory arrest that occurred as part of
an idiosyncratic response to a low dose of morphine.

Nausea and vomiting: Routine use of a phenothiazine with the narcotic elixir counters this common side effect of all narcotics. If
a patient is vomiting before therapy is instituted, control should
first be achieved with parenteral medication and subsequently maintained with oral medication. In addition to stimulating the chemoreceptor trigger zone in the medulla, narcotics induce nausea by

increasing vestibular sensitivty. (Gutner, L.B., 1952). This may
account for the heightened incidence of nausea in morphine treated
patients when ambulatory as compared to recumbant. Antihistimines may
be helpful in controlling this problem (Jaffe, J.H., 1975).

A separate problem is the nausea and vomiting simulating small bowel
obstruction occasionally seen in patients maintained on morphine as
described. Radiologic assessment fails to demonstrate evidence of
bowel obstruction. The phenothiazines and antihistamines are of little
help. The presumed etiologic factor is the narcotic induced delay in
gastric emptying. The increase in resting tone and associated marked
decrease in propulsive contractions in the small bowel play a further
role. Metoclopramide is useful in this setting. In several refractory
cases dramatic relief has been afforded by discontinuing morphine and
substituting methadone. The mechanism of this response is unclear
since the effect of methadone on gut is similar to morphine and controlled clinical studies usually demonstrate that in equianalgesic
dosage the incidence of nausea and vomiting is similar with all
clinically useful narcotics (Jaffe, J.H., 1975).

Constipation: Constipation is the most important and consistently encountered side effect of morphine used in this context. The combined
effects of poor dietary intake, dehydration, inactivity and narcotic
therapy almost invariably lead to constipation. This should be anticipated and preventative measures instituted when narcotics are initiated. These very sick patients are frequently unable to tolerate
the fluid volumes required with bulk forming laxatives and bran is not
only often unpalatable to the very sick but may be of little help if
colonic propulsion is reduced by the narcotic. A combination of a stool
softener and a bowel stimulant, such as dioctyl sodium sulfosuccinate
and senna concentrate, is effective. Either agent may be increased as
required. As in pain control itself, the aim is dose titration to prevent, rather than treat, the problem.

Tolerance: Tolerance occurs with all narcotics. The term implies that
with time it is necessary to give larger doses to achieve the same
therapeutic effect. Progressive tolerance with escalating dosage requirements and the danger of respiratory depression with large doses
of narcotic are often given as reasons for delaying the onset of narcotic therapy. Fortunately this does not pose a problem when morphine
is given as described since:

- the dose needed to produce respiratory depression is always higher
  than the dose producing analgesia;
- the impact of tolerance on dosage requirements, if it does occur,
  is negligible;
- tolerance levels off in most cases and usually ceases to operate
  after a few weeks (Twycross, 1974, 1976). Tolerance is not an
  issue even when narcotics used as described are required for several
  years.

Cumulation: Because of the brief half-life this is not a practical
problem with morphine or heroin used as described. It is, however,
a potential problem with methadone (see below).

Dependence: The term "drug addiction" has been replaced by "drug dependence", which is defined by the World Health Organisation (1969)
as "A state, psychic and sometimes also physical, resulting from the
interaction between a living organism and a drug, characterized by
behavioural and other responses that always include a compulsion to
take the drug on a continuous or periodic basis in order to experience
its psychic effects, and sometimes avoid the discomfort of its absence.
Tolerance may or may not be present."

While undertreatment with analgesic medication may encourage craving
and psychological dependence, this does not occur when narcotics are
used regularly in analgesic doses as described.

Eddy (1959) found that physical dependence develops in the majority
of patients within four weeks when narcotics are given by injection.
Lee (1942) noted, however, that dependence develops less rapidly and
possibly to a lesser degree following oral administration. It is possible but not certain that physical dependence regularly occurs when
oral morphine is used as described. If it occurs it does not prevent
the downward adjustment of narcotic dose and even cessation of therapy
when that is clinically feasible. Indeed withdrawal reactions do not
occur if the dose is tapered in stopping the narcotic, even after periods of regular administration extending to years.

Allergy: A true allergic reaction to morphine is uncommon but may
present with a rash, puritis, dyspnoea or, after injection, an itchy
wheal and flare response at the injection site. These are due to his-
tamine release and antihistamines should be administered and the narcotic changed to an agent of substantially different structure such
as methadone. Codeine (methylmorphine) should be avoided because of
its similar structure.

            OTHER AGENTS

With severe pain, only the narcotic analgesics provide adequate control. Milder analgesics should always be tried for less severe pain
and may be helpful in combination with more potent drugs. A wide
variety of agents is available. Catalano (1975) presents a good recent review.

Weak Analgesics were tested in cancer patients with advanced disease
in a double-blind cross-over study by Moertel and colleagues (1974).
None of the newer agents tested, including several weak narcotics,
displaced aspirin as the agent of choice. Aspirin 650 mg was superior
to pentazocine (Talwin) 50 mg and codeine 65 mg, which were both significantly superior to placebo (p < 0.05). Propoxyphene (Darvon) 65 mg,

gave no significant evidence of therapeutic activity. Young (1972)
has reported nine deaths due to propoxyphene overdose.

In a further study of various analgesic combinations aspirin 650 mg
plus either codeine 65 mg, oxycodone 9 mg or pentazocine 25 mg produced significantly greater pain relief than aspirin alone (Beaver
1966, Moertel 1974).

Initial claims that pentazocine was non-addicting have proven incorrect (Lewis 1974). Catalano (1975) has summarized its other disadvantages. These include: weak antagonism to morphine; local irritation
at the site of injection with parenteral use and lack of dependability
taken orally; high incidence of side effects including sedation, drowsiness, nausea, vomiting, blurred vision, visual and auditory hallucinations and other psychic reactions.

Parenteral Diamorphine

The reports by Lasagna (1964), Twycross (1977) and the Interagency
Committee on New Therapies for Pain and Discomfort (1979) all suggest
that with adjustment in dose according to the difference in oral potency there is little difference in the effectiveness of morphine and
diamorphine (heroin) taken by mouth. It is clear from the studies
cited earlier that an oral morphine solution will, when used with a
variety of adjunct approaches (Mount 1978, Saunders 1978A) as required,
control the intractable pain due to advanced malignant disease in more
than 80% of all cases with pain. It is in the remaining patients that
there may be a potential place for diamorphine. When injections are
necessary the greater solubility of diamorphine hydrochloride (1g in
1.6 ml) gives diamorphine an important practical advantage over morphine sulphate or hydrochloride (1g in more than 20 ml) (Martindale
1972), especially when large doses are required. It is important to
note, however, that in the experience of the Royal Victoria Hospital
the mean dose of orally administered morphine has varied from 10.5 to
27 mg (Melzack 1976, 1979). This is equivalent to approximately 5-10
mg given parenterally. Since concentrations of 15 mg morphine per ml
are available for parenteral injection, these doses may be well tolerated by even the most cachectic patient. A small portion of the highly
selected group of patients requiring parenterally administered narcotics may, however, require higher morphine doses in volumes as large
as 4-8 ml per injection. Such volumes are poorly tolerated in cachectic patients with depleted muscle mass. In this uncommon situation a
more soluble narcotic would be desirable. While diamorphine would be
useful if available, methadone has been a satisfactory alternative in
our hands. Its safe use requires, however, an appreciation of the potential dangers involved (see below).

While a small but vocal group is actively lobbying for the legalization
of diamorphine in both Canada and the United States it must be recognized that the availability of diamorphine would not correct the tragic
inadequacy of pain control that is endemic in North American hospitals.

What is required is not new legislation but new attention to detail
and improved use of available agents.

Methadone

As noted above, methadone is a highly soluble narcotic which may be
given orally or parenterally. Its attractive features include the
fact that it is effective parenterally and is well absorbed orally
with little gastrointestinal intolerance. Furthermore, it has a prolonged half-life permitting less frequent administration than morphine
or heroin.

With its great solubility relatively large doses may be conveniently
given in a small volume (80 mg per ml). When oral doses are poorly
tolerated because of taste, even large doses may be injected into an
empty gelatin capsule to mask the bitter narcotic taste when taken by
mouth. This should be done immediately pre-administration at the bedside so that the gelatin capsules remain intact until swallowed.

Unfortunately the fate and excretion of methadone are rather more complex than with morphine. Life threatening accumulation may occur when
the drug is administered according to manufacturer's recommended doses
(Ettinger 1979). Relevant pharmacokinetics must be appreciated in order for methadone to be used safely and effectively.

Clinical studies show that the average plasma half-life of methadone
is 25 hours with a range from 13 to 47 hours (Verebely 1975). The
problem arises in how methadone is handled. Following initial administration there is a biexponential plasma decay with an average primary phase half-life or 14.3 hours and a slower secondary phase half-
life averaging 54.8 hours. With repeated administration there seems
to be a monoexponential plasma half-life of approximately 22.4 hours
(Verebely 1975) suggesting the presence of a depot compartment in
which methadone is tightly bound and released at a slower rate than
that from the compartment represented by the primary-phase half-life
(Verebely 1975). As a result, with an increase in methadone dose
there is a gradual increase in plasma concentration which finally
reaches equilibrium and "steady-state" levels after 4-5 days on the
new dose. Seriously complicating the picture is the fact that there
is no correlation between these slowly equilibrating plasma levels
and the duration of methadone analgesic effect. In spite of the prolonged serum half-life, the analgesia produced by methadone may last
only 3 hours (Berkowitz, B.A., 1976), though generally lasting 6-8
hours. Residual pain in the face of regular methadone administration
may lead the unwary physician to use frequent dose escalations and
short dose intervals. Life threatening accumulation may result.
Several additional factors add further uncertainty to the use of
methadone (Ettinger 1979):
(a) Methadone is known to interact with other drugs which may alter
    its protein binding, metabolism and excretion.

(b) Hepatic and renal dysfunction will tend to increase the half-life of methadone.

(c) The influence of advanced patient age on methadone metabolism is uncertain (Symonds 1977).

(d) The response to initial exposure to methadone may be exaggerated in those not previously on narcotics.

For safe use methadone should be given at initially low doses with time allowed for a steady (plateau) state to develop. Our pratice has been to vary the frequency of administration using intervals varying from 12 to 6 hours between doses, as required. While titrating to analgesia morphine may be used parenterally as required to obtain supplementary short term pain relief. It should be kept in mind that plasma levels will continue to rise for about 4 days before reaching a plateau following an increase in dose. Should respiratory depression occur, Nalaxone 0.4-0.8 mg may be given sc, IM, or IV. Response is prompt but its antagonistic effect lasts only 1-4 hours (Jaffe 1975) and repeated doses may be needed.

Other Narcotics

A wide variety of other narcotics is available. Lasagna (1964), Catalano (1974), Jaffe (1975), and Evens (1978) among others have extensively reviewed comparative features of these agents including data related to equianalgesic dosage by various routes of administration, duration of action and variations in pharmacologic activity. The wealth of tabular data presented in these and other similar articles is often difficult to interpret since they have been derived from many disparate clinical settings encompassing both acute and chronic pain. Experience suggests that when regularly administered oral morphine is used as the narcotic therapy of choice in the setting of advanced cancer there will only infrequently be the need to broaden the armamentarium to include other agents. Observations related to the use of other narcotics in this fashion include:

Meperidine (Pethidine): Jaffe (1975) lists the duration of action for meperidine at 2-4 hours making it unsatisfactory for the treatment of chronic pain.

Anileridine: While the duration of action of parenterally administered anileridine is also only 2-4 hours (Jaffe 1975), Houde and Wallenstein (1959) reported that in their patients with advanced cancer it produced more prolonged pain relief when given orally than parenterally and noted that it was more consistent in its effect than meperidine.

Extensive experience at the Smythe Pain Clinic, Toronto has led Evans (1977) to use anileridine with methotrimeprazine (levomepromazine) as the analgesic combination of choice in patients with severe pain due to head and neck carcinomas. The effectiveness of this combination has been substantiated in cases of head and neck carcinoma responding poorly to oral morphine in the Royal Victoria Hospital experience.

These observations have not been based, however, on controlled trials.

Levorphanol: The long duration of action (4-8 hours: Evens 1978), its
effectiveness when taken orally and its relative freedom from side effects (less nausea and vomiting than morphine: Jaffe 1975) make levorphanol an attractive alternative for the ambulatory, non-hospitalized
patient. When pain is relatively easily controlled such patients may
find the 2 mg tablet taken 8-hourly effective and more convenient than
the regular 4-hourly dispensing of oral morphine. As pain increases,
however, and precise titration of narcotic dose is required, morphine
is better tolerated and provides greater flexibility.

Among the other agents, those available in suppository form, including
hydromorphone, oxymorphone and oxycodone may be particularly useful in
avoiding injections when patients are transiently unable to take narcotics by mouth.   In Great Britain, morphine is available in 10, 15,
20, 30 and 60 mg suppositories (BNF)

COMMENT

To be effective against the "total pain" of advanced malignant disease,
narcotics must be used in combination with other therapies. Pain control may require additional measures such as radiation therapy, peripheral or intrathecal nerve blocks, ablative neurosurgical procedures
or physical measures such as splinting and passive exercises. Benzo-
diazepines, phenothiazines, tricyclic antidepressants, glucocortico-
steroids, anti-inflammatory agents, and hypnotics can all be useful
in attacking the vicious cycle of chronic pain. Environmental mani-
pulations may also influence pain perception. The experience of spe-
cially designed services for the terminally ill have suggested the
importance of creating a pleasant, supportive environment in which a
patient is able to communicate his concerns and where the resources of
a skilled interdisciplinary team are available to help in areas of
interpersonal, psychosocial and philosophical need. Bonica (1979B)
has commented, "It is important to emphasize that, regardless of which
of the major approaches is used, physiologic and psychologic support
of the patient and his family is an essential, if not the most essential, part of the management of patients with cancer pain."

REFERENCES

Allport, G.W., (1959) Preface in Frankl, V.E., Man's Search for Meaning, Beacon Press, Boston, p. xi

Baines, M.J., (1978), Control of Other Symptoms in Saunders, C.M. (ed.) The Management of Terminal Disease, Edward Arnold, London, pp. 99-118

Beaver, W.T., (1966) Mild Analgesics: A Review of Their Clinical Pharmacology, Part II, Am. J. Med. Sci. 251: pp. 576-599

Bellville, J.W., Forrest, W.H., Tr. Elashoff et al. (1968) Evaluating Side Effects of Analgesics in a Cooperative Clinical Study, Clin. Pharmacol. Ther. 9: pp. 303-313

Bellville, J.W., Forrest, W.H., Miller, E. Brown, B.W., (1971): Influence of Age on Pain Relief from Analgesics, JAMA, 217: pp. 1835-1839

Berkowitz, B.A. (1976) Research Review: The Relationship of Pharmacokinetics to Pharmacologic Activity: Morphine, Methadone and Naloxone, Clin. Pharmacokinet. 1: pp. 219-230

Berkowitz, B.A., Nagi, S.H., Yang, J.C., Hampstead, J., Spector, S. (1975) The Disposition of Morphine in Surgical Patient, Clin. Pharmacol. Ther. 17, pp. 629-635

Black, Leinbach, G., Eisendorfer, C., Videotapes (1974) University of Washington, Learning Resources Center

Bonica, J.J. (1979A) Cancer Pain: Importance of the Problem, in Bonica, J.J. and Ventafridda, V. (ed.) Advances in Pain Research and Therapy, Vol. 2, Raven Press, New York, pp. 1-12

Bonica, J.J. (1979B) Introduction to Management of Pain of Advanced Cancer, Bonica, J.J., Ventafridda, V. (ed.) Advances in Pain Research and Therapy, Vol. 2, New York, pp. 115-130

British Pharmaceutical Codex (1973), London Pharmaceutical Pr.,p. 669

Catalano, R.B. (1975) The Medical Approach to Management of Pain Caused by Cancer, Seminars in Oncol., 2, pp. 379-392

Dundee, J.W., Love, W.T., Moore, T. (1963) Alterations in Response to Somatic Pain Associated with Anaesthesia, XV., Further Studies with Phenothiazines Derivatives and Similar Drugs, Br. J. Anaesth: 35, pp. 597-610

Eddy, N.B., Lee, L.C., Harris, C.A. (1959), The Rate of Development of Physical Dependence and Tolerance to Analgesic Drugs in Patients with Chronic Pain, 1. Comparison of Morphine, Oxymorphone, and Anileridine, Bull. Narcot, 11, pp. 3-17

Ettinger, D.S., Vitale, P.J., Trump, D.L. (1979) Important Clinical Pharmacologic Considerations in the Use of Methadone in Cancer Patients, Cancer Treat. Rep., 63, pp. 457-459

Evans, R.J. (1977) Personal Communication

Evens, R.P., Koda-Kimble, M.A., Katcher, B.S., Young, L.Y. (ed) 1975 Applied Therapeutics Inc., San Francisco, pp. 86-101

Gutner, L.B., Gould, W.J., Butterman, R.C. (1952) The Effects of Potent Analgesics Upon Vestibular Function, J. Clin. Invest. 31, pp. 259-266

Houde, R.W., Wallenstein, S.L., (1959) Minutes of 20th Meeting Committee on Drug Addiction and Narcotics, App. B

Houde, R.W., Wallenstein, S.L., Beaver, W.T., (1965), Clinical Measurement of Pain, in, De Stevens, G., (ed.), Analgesics, Academic Press, New York, pp. 75-122

Interagency Committee on New Therapies for Pain and Discomfort (1979) Report to the White House: U.S. Department of Health Education and Welfare, Public Health Service, National Institutes of Health, May

Jaffe, J.H., Martin, W.R., Narcotic Analgesics, Ch. 15, in Goodman L.S., Gilman, A. (ed.) (1975), The Pharmacological Basis of Therapeutics, 5th Edition, MacMillan, New York, pp, 245-283

Lasagna, L., (1964) The Clinical Evaluation of Morphine and Its Substitutes as Analgesics, Pharmacol. Rev. 16, pp. 47-83

Lee, L.C. (1942) Studies of Morphine Codeine and Their Derivations XVI, J. Pharmacol. Exp. Ther. 75, pp. 161-173

Leshan, L. (1964) The World of the Patient in Severe Pain of Long Duration, J. Chronic Dis. 173, 119

Lewis, J.R. (1974) Misprescribing Analgesics, JAMA:228, pp. 1155-1156

Lipman, A.G. (1975), Drug Therapy in Terminally Ill Patients, Am. J. Hosp. Pharm. 32, pp. 270-276

Martindale, W., (1972), Extra Pharmacopeici, 26th ed. Pharmaceutical London

Melzack, R., (1975), The McGill Pain Questionnaire, Major Properties and Scoring Methods, Pain, 1, pp. 227-

Melzack, R., (1973), The Puzzle of Pain, Penguin, Harmondsworth, England

Melzack, R., Mount, B.M., Gordon, J.M., (1979), The Brompton Mixture Versus Morphine Solution Given Orally: Effects on Pain, CMAJ, 120, pp. 435-438

Melzack, R., Ofiesh, J.G., Mount, B.M., (1979), The Brompton Mixture: Effects on Pain in Cancer Patients, CMAJ, 115, 125-129

Moertel, C.G., Almann, D.L., Taylor, W.F., Schwartam, N., (1974) Relief of Pain by Oral Medications, A Controlled Evaluation of Analgesic Combinations, JAMA, 229, pp. 55-59

Mount, B.M., (1978), Palliative Care of the Terminally Ill, Royal College Lecture, Annals Roy. Coll. Phys. Surg. Can., July, pp. 201-208

Mount, B.M., Ajemian, I., Scott, J.F., (1976), Use of the Brompton Mixture in Treating the Chronic Pain of Malignant Disease, CMAJ, 115, pp. 122-124

Saunders, C.M., (1978A) The Management of Terminal Disease, Edward Arnold, London

Saunders, C.M., (1967) The Management of Terminal Illness, London, Hosp. Med. Publ.

Saunders, E.M., (1978B) Standards and Accreditation, presented at the First Annual National Hospice Organization Meeting, Shoreham Americana Hotel, Washington, D.C., October 5th

Symonds, P., (1977) Methadone and the Elderly, Br. Med. J., 1, p. 512

Twycross, R.G., (1977) Choice of Strong Analgesic in Terminal Cancer: Diamorphine or Morphine?, Pain, pp. 93-104

Twycross, R.G., (1974) Clinical Experience with Diamorphine in Advanced Malignant Disease, Int. J. Clin. Pharmacol. 9, p. 184, 198

Twycross, R.G., (1978) Reliefe of Pain in Saunders, C.M., (ed.) The Management of Terminal Disease, Edward Arnold, London, pp. 65-92

Twycross, R.G., Wald, S.J., (1976) Long Term Use of Diamorphine in Advanced Cancer, in Bonica, J.J., Albe-Fessara, D. (ed.) Advances in Pain Research and Therapy, Vol. 1, Raven Press, New York, pp. 653-661

B.M. Mount

Vere, D.W., (1978) Pharmacology of Morphine Drugs Used in Terminal
Care, in Vere, D.W., (ed.) Topics in Therapeutics, 4, Pitman, London,
pp. 75-83

Verebely, K., Volavka, J., Mule, S., (1975), Methadone in Man, Clin.
Pharmacol. Ther., 18, pp. 180-190

World Health Organization, (1969), Expert Committee on Drug Dependence, 16th Report, Technical Report Series, No. 407

Young, D.J., (1972), Propoxyphene Suicides, Arch., Inter. Med. 129,
pp. 62-66

Non-Narcotic, Corticosteroid and Psychotropic Drugs

R. G. TWYCROSS

Sir Michael Sobell House, Churchill Hospital, Headington, Oxford OX3 7BR, UK

ABSTRACT

Many osseous metastases produce a prostaglandin which causes osteolysis and also lowers the "peripheral pain threshold" by sensitizing free nerve endings. Aspirin (in high dosage) and other non-steroidal anti-inflammatory drugs (NSAID) inhibit the synthesis of PGs and by so doing alleviate pain. This suggests that, compared with morphine, NSAID should be relatively more efficacious in bone pain than in pain caused by soft tissue infiltration. Corticosteroids have a definite place in alleviating pain associated with extensive soft tissue infiltration in relatively circumscribed areas, e.g. head and neck cancers or pelvic malignancy and with massive hepatic metastases.

Data relating to the use of psychotropic agents in the relief of pain in terminal cancer is limited. Anxious patients benefit from the concurrent use of an anxiolytic sedative and depressed patients from the use of an antidepressant. Whether these same drugs have a general application as narcotic-sparing or potentiating drugs is not known. Clinical experience suggests that psychtropic drugs have a definite place in the treatment of a number of specific cancer pain syndromes. For example, diazepam helps to relieve muscle spasm pain; chlorpromazine is of benefit in cases of rectal and bladder tenesmus; and tricyclic antidepressants may alleviate dysaesthesiae associated with partial nerve damage or the burning pain of post-herpetic neuralgia.

NON-NARCOTIC ANALGESICS

In most countries aspirin (acetylsalicylic acid) and paracetamol (acetominophen) are the two most readily available non-narcotic (or antipyretic) analgesics. They are the drugs of choice in pain of mild or moderate intensity. Only if these fail to relieve is it necessary to use a narcotic analgesic. Paracetamol may be preferred to aspirin in view of the absence of gastro-intestinal side-effects. However, when the pain originates in bone, there are certain theoretical reasons for prescribing aspirin (vide infra). Both drugs are available in soluble and non-soluble forms, either "over the counter" or on prescription. If unsupervised, patients tend to take these preparations not more than three times a day. This generally results in a "switchback" effect. When this occurs, patients should be advised to take medication more frequently, either 6 or 4 hourly, in order to anticipate and prevent the re-emergence of pain.

Many patients can tolerate up to 1200 mg of aspirin 4-hourly, obtaining relief
denied to them with the more usual 600 mg dose. If a higher dose is recommended,
the problem of patient compliance can be overcome by using a soluble form which
converts four tablets into one drink, or by prescribing a preparation such as
glycine-aspirin (Table 1). If dyspepsia or gastrointestinal bleeding is a problem,
enteric-coated aspirin or aloxiprin may be tried. The size of the former preparation tends, however, to reduce its usefulness in advanced cancer. Benorylate, an
ester of aspirin and paracetamol, needs only to be administered two or three times
a day. It is useful in the elderly where drug compliance may be a problem, though
it cannot be recommended for routine use because of its greater cost.

TABLE 1 Useful Preparations of Aspirin

Preparation	Aspirin content per tablet (mg)	Mode of administration	Time between doses (hours)
Aspirin	300	Swallow whole	4
Soluble aspirin	300	Dissolve in water	4
Glycine-aspirin (Paynocil)	600	Dissolve on tongue	4
Enteric-coated aspirin (Nu-seals)	325, 650	Swallow whole	8
Microencapsulated aspirin (Levius)	500	Swallow whole	8
Aloxiprin (aluminium polyox-aspirin; Palaprin Forte)	500	Dissolve in water, suck, chew or swallow whole	4

When aspirin or paracetamol fail to relieve, weak narcotic analgesics, such as
codeine, dihydrocodeine (DHC) and dextropropoxyphene, should be used, either alone
or in combination with aspirin or paracetamol (Table 2). It is generally stated
that DHC is one-third, and codeine one-sixth as potent as morphine. These are

TABLE 2 Weak Narcotic Analgesic Preparations

	Narcotic	Non-narcotic	Proprietary preparation
Dextropropoxyphene	65	–	Doloxene
hydrochloride	150	–	Depronal SA
+ aspirin	(50)*	500	Napsalgesic
	(100)*	325	Dolasan
+ paracetamol	32.5	325	Distalgesic
Codeine phosphate	15, 30, 60	–	–
+ aspirin	8	500	Codis
+ paracetamol	8	500	Neurodyne Panadeine
Dihydrocodeine tartrate	30	–	DF 118
+ aspirin	10	300	Onadox-118
+ paracetamol	10	500	Paramol-118

*Weight refers to dextropropoxyphene napsylate; equivalent to 32.5 and
  65 mg of hydrochloride, respectively.

almost certainly over-optimistic estimates; in cancer pain, DHC is approximately one-sixth as potent as morphine (Seed and co-workers, 1958), and codeine one-twelfth (Houde, Wallenstein and Beaver, 1965). Although DHC is more potent that codeine, any difference between them is reduced by the constraints of tablet size. DHC is said to be less constipating than codeine.

Dextropropoxyphene continues to enjoy considerable vogue. In Great Britain, it is generally used in combination with paracetamol (Distalgesic), whereas in the United Stated it is used both alone (Darvon) and in combination (Darvon-Co). The popularity appears to result from several factors, including a widespread belief in its efficacy, not wholly supported by evidence from clinical trials (Miller, Feingold and Paxinos, 1970) and the fact that, unlike aspirin and aspirin-compound tablets, dextropropoxyphene is available only on prescription. In other words, it will not have been tried and found wanting by the patient prior to prescription by the doctor, and will therefore be taken with a higher expectancy of success than a self-prescribed remedy. Until more evidence is forthcoming to show that it is superior to aspirin or paracetamol, either alone or in combination with codeine, its true place in therapeutics will continue to be uncertain.

ASPIRIN AND BONE PAIN

Traditionally, analgesics have been graded according to afficacy; and the basic "analgesic ladder" — aspirin, codein, morphine — paralleled the clinical classification of pain as mild, moderate or severe. While this classification still holds good for pain in general, it is no longer appropriate for bone pain. The reason for this related to new information about:

1. osteolytic factors produced by osseous metastases;
2. the mechanism of action of aspirin and other non-steroidal anti-inflammatory drugs (NSAID).

The growth of an osseous metastasis appears to be linked with induced bone resorption. Initially, this is mediated via osteclastic activity but, subsequently, an osteolytic agent is produced by the tumour itself (Editorial, 1976). Most studies relating to solid tumour implicate prostaglandin E_2 (PGE_2) as the principal factor involved (Seyberth and co-workers, 1975; Bennett and co-workers, 1977). Other work has shown that prostaglandins of the E series cause pain when injected sub-dermally at high concentrations (Ferreira, 1972). In lower concentrations, the same prostaglandins exacerbate pain by sensitizing free nerve endings. Aspirin (in high dosage) and other NSAID are potent inhibitors of prostaglandin synthetase. This suggests that, compared with morphine, NSAID should be relatively more efficacious in bone pain than in pain caused by other mechanisms. Our experience in Oxford would support such a hypothesis.

Response to prostaglandin inhibitors is, however, variable; a fact which can be explained if certain cancer cell types synthesize osteolytic agents other than or in addition to PGE_2. It has been shown, for example, in patients with hypercalcaemia in association with multiple myeloma or a reticulosis, that the urinary excretion of prostaglandin metabolites is normal and that bone resorption appears to be due to secretion of "osteoclast activating factor" by tumour cells (Mundy and co-workers, 1974). Other candidates include ectopic parathyroid hormone and active vitamin D metabolites or related sterols. Although complex, as further research elucidates the relative importance of these substances, the ability to relieve bone pain by pharmacological means should steadily improve.

Meanwhile, we need to ask and attempt to answer a number of questions.

1. Is There a NSAID of Choice?

Aspirin (3-4 G or more a day), indomethacin (75-150 mg a day) and phenylbutazone
(400-600 mg a day) have all been used at difference centres. Many doctors, however,
avoid using phenylbutazone for fear that it will cause agranulocytosis or, worse,
aplastic anaemia, though this is less important in terminal cancer than in arth-
ritis. More important is its ability to cause fluid retention and so precipitate
or exacerbate dependent oedema. Concurrent use with prednisolone is, therefore,
generally contra-indicated. Although it has been claimed that indomethacin is
superior to aspirin in myeloma and other haematological neoplasia, its use is often
limited by gastro-intestinal side-effects. It also causes frontal headache in up
to 50% of chronic users. Moreover, as it is known on occasion to cause confusion,
depression or hallucinations, it should be used with caution particularly in association with narcotic analgesics in the elderly or debilitated. In the light of
these considerations, the author favours the humble aspirin. Other forms of long-
acting or modified aspirin, no doubt, also have their place (Table 3).

TABLE 3 Long-acting NSAID

Enteric-coated aspirin (Nu-Seals)
Microencapsulated aspirin (Levius)
Benorylate (Benoral)
Salsalate (Disalcid)
Diflunisal (Dolobid)
Sulindac (Clinoril)
Flurbiprofen (Froben)

2. Is Clinical Efficacy Proportional to a Drug's Ability to Inhibit PGE_2 Synthesis?

Data about relative molar potency for 50% inhibition of PGE_2 synthesis have been
obtained from in vitro studies (Table 4). The relatively poor showing of aspirin
and phenylbutazone indicates that, although of interest, such studies are not a
good guide to clinical efficacy. This means, for example, that it should not be
assumed that flurbiprofen is, by definition, superior to the well tried drugs
referred to above.

TABLE 4   Relative Molar Potency for 50% Inhibition of PGE_2 Synthesis
In Vitro. Potency of Aspirin Taken as Unity*

Drug	Potency
Paracetamol	< 0.01
Salicylic acid	< 0.02
Aspirin	1
Phenylbutazone	2.7
Ibuprofen	22
Naproxen	45
Indomethacin	257
Flurbiprofen	5610

*from Crook and co-workers (1976)

The same paper which places aspirin low in the efficacy table stresses that in other tests aspirin is unique in its superiority over other NSAID (Crook and co-workers, 1976). It would seem necessary, therefore, to postulate that in contrast to NSAID in general, aspirin acts at more than one site and possibly via more than one mechanism (Morley, 1975).

3. Are Corticosteroids as Effective as NSAID?

Corticosteroids prevent the release of prostaglandins by their "stabilising" effect on cell membranes; they do not inhibit prostaglandin synthesis. They also have an impact on other elements of the inflammatory process that are not connected with prostaglandins and are of considerable symptomatic benefit in certain patients with advanced cancer. Yet, in the absence of evidence from controlled studies, the answer to the question is probably no.

4. Should NSAID be Used Alone or with a Narcotic Analgesic?

The NSAID have been described as "40-50%" drugs, a reminder that they relieve only that proportion of the pain related to the production of prostaglandins. It is, however, possible that elevation of the peripheral pain threshold by administration of a NSAID may be enough to raise the patient's total pain threshold to a degree sufficient to relieve the pain complete.y When aspirin is used, this is more likely because of its suggested multifocal action. A decision to use aspirin alone or with a narcotic will, in practice, depend on the intensity of pain. If severe, a combination should be used, at least initially.

INJECTABLE ASPIRIN

Although it is generally possible to administer non-narcotic analgesics by mouth, it is important to note that a preparation of injectable aspirin is available in Italy. Lysine-acetylsalicylate (Flectadol) is prepared in freeze-dried ampoules, each containing 900 mg (equivalent to aspirin 500 mg). In a trial in patients undergoing major gynaegolocial surgery, 1.8 G of IM lysine-acetylsalicylate was shown to be as effective as 10 mg of IM morphine hydrochloride (Kweekel- De Vries and co-workers, 1974). No trials appear to have been undertaken in terminal cancer patients.

NEFOPAM

A new non-narcotic analgesic has recently been introduced into the British pharmaceutical market. Nefopam (Acupan) is in a novel class of analgesics, the benzoxazocines. It is chemically related to orphenadrine and diphenhydramine, but it is not an antihistamine. How nefopam acts as an analgesic is not known. It does not cause respiratory depression, does not lessen opiate withdrawal signs and its effects are not reversed by naloxone. It is neither anti-inflammatory nor does it inhibit prostaglandin synthesis. It lowers normal body temperature slightly but its action on fever has not been evaluated. It has anticholinergic and sympathomimetic activity which is not usually noticeable unless other drugs with these properties are taken at the same time.

Nefopam can be given by mouth or injected intramuscularly. The plasma concentrations and the analgesic effect reach a peak after about two hours when given by mouth and about $1\frac{1}{2}$ hours after i.m. injection. The plasma half-life is about $4\frac{1}{2}$ hours. The drug is mostly excreted as an inactive metabolite in the urine. An

oral dose of 60 mg has about the same analgesic effect as 20 mg intramuscularly.
The main unwanted effects are insomnia and dryness of the mouth. Other reported
unwanted effects include nausea, nervousness and light-headedness. Less frequent
vomiting, blurred vision, drowsiness, sweating, tachycardia and headache may occur.
These effects are dose-related and transient, becoming less troublesome with continued treatment. Because of its anticholinergic action it should be used with
caution in patients with glaucoma or urinary retention. Nefopam enhances motor
neurone activity and therefore patients with epilepsy should not take it. In dogs
high doses of nefopam increased the hepatic toxicity of high doses of paracetamol.
This effect was not observed at doses closer to those used in man, but, even so,
it would possibly be unwise to give nefopam and paracetamol concurrently to
patients.

Most clinical trials have been completed in patients with non-malignant pain.
Intramuscularly, nefopam 15 mg is approximately equivalent to 50 mg of pethidine.
There is probably a low ceiling effect.   In one study (Tigerstedt and co-workers,
1977) nefopam 30 mg was no more effect than 15 mg, though it lasted longer and was
associated with a higher frequency of adverse effects. This ceiling effect may
explain wht reports of the potency ratio of nefopam to morphine vary between 1:1
and 1:3 (Beaver & Feise, 1977; Sunshine & Laska, 1975). The place of nefopam in
the relief of cancer pain is at present uncertain. It may prove to be a satisfactory alternative to the weak narcotic analgesics. At the moment, however,
there is unsufficient evidence to recommend its use; it is also very expensive.

                    CORTICOSTEROIDS

Corticosteroids are widely used in far-advanced cancer (Table 5). Inclusion in
this list does *not* imply that their use represents the sole or most important
treatment for these indications. It simply means that the use of corticosteroid
may be of benefit and should be considered as a treatment option to be tried alone
or in association with other recognized measures. In the majority of patients
with, for example, incipient paraplegia, superior venal caval obstruction or
haemoptysis, a corticosteroid will be given in association with radiation therapy.
Similarly, a corticosteroid is not generally the treatment of choice for malignant
effusions but, where other measures have failed or seem inappropriate, may be tried
with or without a chemotherapeutic agent.

The use of a corticosteroid as a "co-analgesic" should be considered wherever there
is a large tumour mass within a relatively confined space. There is often an
oedematous area around a tumour and pressure on neighbouring veins and lymphatics
may lead to further local or regional swelling. In other words, the total tumour
mass = neoplasm + surrounding hyperaemic oedema. Corticosteroids reduce this
oedema and thereby reduce the total tumour mass.

The classical situation is that of headache caused by raised intra-cranial pressure
in association with cerebral neoplasm. There may be other central nervous symptoms
or signs and patients often show improvement lasting for weeks or months after
starting treatment. When headache is the main symptoms, analgesics, a diuretic and
elevating the head of the bed may also help to relieve the pain. Corticosteroids
are also of benefit in relieving the pain of nerve compression (Fig. 1). About
one-third of nerve compression pains respond to analgesics alone, and a further
third to the combined use of analgesics and a corticosteroid. Thus, only a minority of patients with nerve compression pain fails to respond to pharmacological
measures, and thereby become candidates for neurolytic techniques.

Metastatic arthralgia (Table 5) refers to the pain caused by metastatic involvement
of the acetabulum (relatively common) or glenoid fossa (relatively uncommon) in
patients with, in particular, cancer of the breast, bronchus or prostate. In

TABLE 5 Corticosteroids in Terminal Cancer

Non-specific uses	Other specific uses
1. To improve appetite	1. Hypercalcaemia
2. To reduce fever	2. Carcinomatous neuromyopathy
3. To enhance sense of well-being	3. Incipient paraplegia
4. To improve strength	4. Superior vena caval obstruction
	5. Airways obstruction
Co-analgesic	6. Haemoptysis
	7. Leucoerythroblastic anaemia
1. Raised intra-cranial pressure*	8. Malignant effusion*
2. Nerve compression	9. Discharge from rectal tumour**
3. Hepatomegaly	10. To minimize radiation induced reactive oedema
4. Head and neck tumour*	11. To minimize the toxic effects of radiation or chemotherapy
5. Intra-pelvic tumour	12. As an adjunct to chemotherapy
6. Abdominal tumour	
7. Retroperitoneal tumour	
8. Lymphoedema*	
9. Metastatic arthralgia	

*May benefit by concurrent use of a diuretic. **Given rectally (Predsol enema).

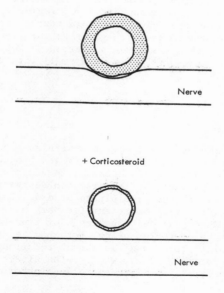

Fig. 1 Diagram illustrating action of corticosteroids in relief of nerve compression pain. Total tumour mass = neoplam + surrounding hyperaemic oedematous tissue.

addition to radiation therapy, sometimes maximum relief is obtained only by the combined use of a narcotic, a NSAID and a corticosteroid. Alternatively, injection into the joint space of a long-acting preparation of either methylprednisolone (Depo-medrone) or triamcinolone hexacetonide (Lederspan) may be considered.

Which corticosteroid?

Patients with cerebral oedema are usually given dexamethasome 4 mg 3 or 4 times a day initially. This drug is seven times more potent than prednisolone and has less mineralocorticoid activity. No controlled comparisons, however, have been made. In other situations, prednisolone is usually given in a dose of 5-10 mg three times a day. The dose needed to achieve maximum benefit varies from patient to patient. It is often advisable to commence with a higher dose to avoid missing a treatment effect; the dose can subsequently be adjusted downwards after 1-2 weeks, or sooner if unacceptable, unwanted effects occur.

Since the early 1960's a number of French physicians have used IV methylprednisolone as the corticosteroid of choice (Pierquin, Baillet & Maylin, 1978). A dose of 125 mg IV is given daily for 30 days, followed by oral maintenance therapy with prednisolone 5 mg three times a day. There is no evidence that the IV regimen is superior to the use of oral dexamethasone or prednisolone in terms of pain relief or general benefit. Consequently, the use of the IV regimen cannot be recommended.

Unwanted effects

Apart from leg oedema, unwanted effects are not often troublesome in patients receiving prednisolone. Weight gain and the development of a 'moon-face' may indeed be welcomed by the patient. Many patients receiving dexamethasone become cushingoid and this may be a limiting factor. However, it is sometimes possible to reduce the dose without the original symptoms reappearing. Autopsies on over 500 patients with terminal cancer, of whom more than half were treated with prednisone, have shown that the only real risk from glucocorticoid therapy is an increase in complicated peptic ulcer. Death due to haemorrhage or perforation occurred in only 5% compared with 1% in the patients not given a steroid (Schell, 1972). In view of the patients' already poor prognosis, this is a small risk and one which many physicians are prepared to accept.

HYPERCALCAEMIA

Hypercalcaemia occurs in 10-20% of all patients with advanced malignant disease. The figure is much higher in cancer of the breast and bronchus. It is important to reduce hypercalcaemia when it occurs because, in addition to causing or exacerbating nausea, vomiting, constipation, lethargy and depression, a high serum calcium concentration appears to be able to precipitate or exacerbate pain by modifying a patient's pain threshold (Fig. 2). No scientific work has, in fact, been done on this apparent effect but the occasional experience of improved pain relief occurring when hypercalcaemia has been corrected using, for example, calcitonin rather than prednisolone or NSAID, points to a possible causal relationship. In the absence of reliable data, it is not possible to say whether the effect is a peripheral one (as with prostaglandins) or centrally mediated (? elevation of mood).

In the majority of cases a high daily fluid intake (3 L) and prednisolone (initially 10 mg t.d.s.) will correct hypercalcaemia and decrease intensity of pain. Alimentary and other symptoms also improve. If there is no response to prednisolone after 7-10 days, intramuscular calcitonin 200 IU six-hourly for 48 hours should be

E.S. ♀ 37y   MAMMARY CARCINOMA WITH OSTEOLYTIC METASTASES

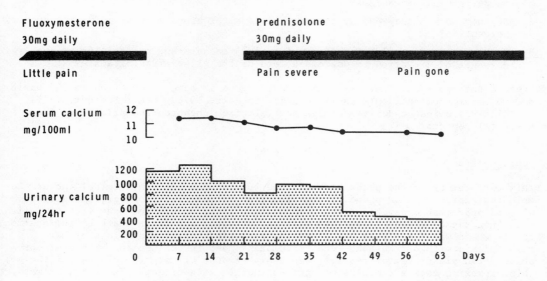

Fig. 2   Does hypercalcaemia lower pain threshold?   (from Stoll, 1963)

given. The initial effect may be maintained by using effervescent phosphate tablets   in daily divided doses of 1-3 g. It is, of course, possible initially to
give phosphate intravenously instead of calcitonin.

It is important to remember that it is the high ionized calcium concentration that
causes symptoms. Many patients with advanced cancer are hypoalbuminaemic and, on
routine estimation, may appear to have a normal, or even a low normal, serum calcium. A number of centres have recommended ways in which the serum calcium may be
corrected in relation to the serum albumin. Which method one uses is not important
and will depend largely on local custon. In the author's experience, quite small
above-normal calcium concentrations have, on occasion, caused definite hypercal-
caemic symptoms.

PSYCHOTROPIC DRUGS

Psychotropic drugs may be grouped together into five categories:

        Neuroleptics   (e.g. chlorpromazine, haloperidol)
        Anxiolytic sedatives   (e.g. diazepam)
        Antidepressants   (e.g. imipramine, amitriptyline)
        Psychostimulants   (e.g. dexamphetamine, cocaine)
        Psychodysleptics   (e.g. LSD, marihuana)

The value of certain neuroleptic drugs and antidepressants in the relief of chronic
pain states of *non-malignant* origin is well documented (Merskey and Hester, 1972;
Merskey, 1974; Kocher, 1976). The conditions in which such drugs have been found
beneficial are those which do not respond well to conventional analgesics. They
include thalamic syndrome, atypical facial pain, causalgia, phantom limb pain, post-
herpetic neuralgia and other painful neuropathies. These same drugs have a small
but definite place in the treatment of a variety of pain syndromes in cancer.

The use of psychotropic drugs in the treatment of pain raises a number of questions:

1. Do these drugs have specific analgesic activity, either by acting centrally or on peripheral mechanisms?

2. Do they work by depressing the general level of arousal or by modifying sensory perception?

3. Is the apparent analgesic effect of antidepressants and tranquillizers purely a result of elevation of depressed mood or the alleviation of anxiety?

These questions remain largely unanswered. There is some information on the basic mode of action of antidepressants in pain (Spencer, 1976; Lee & Spencer, 1977), but clinical evidence derives almost entirely from uncontrolled trials and from anecdotal reports.

Neuroleptics

This term refers to the phenothiazines and butyrophenones. In terminal cancer the main indication for a phenothiazine is as an antiemetic. However, in patients with an appreciable psychological component to their pain — for example, the patient with lung cancer experiencing both pain and dyspnoea who fears death by suffocation, or the woman who feeds that her fungating breast cancer is jeoparidizing her relationship with her husband — chlorpromazine used in conjunction with oral morphine often yields better results than a higher dose of morphine alone. If the chlorpromazine causes troublesome anticholinergic side-effects (Table 6), it may be necessary to use prochlorperazine with diazepam, though in the absence of nausea and vomiting diazepam can, of course, be used alone.

TABLE 6   Common Anti-cholinergic Side-effects

1.	Blurred vision
2.	Dry mouth
3.	Oesophageal reflux
4.	Tachycardia
5.	Urinary retention
6.	Constipation
7.	(Convulsions)

In addition, phenothiazines have a definite place in the relief of a number of less common pain states and other symptoms associated with malignant disease (Table 7). It is sometimes considered that the beneficial effect is mediated via a modification of the reactive component of pain, a sort of "dissociative" phenomenon. On the other hand, it has been demonstrated that chlorpromazine increases the intensity and duration of analgesic drugs in man (Hougs & Skouby, 1957; Boreus & Sandberg, 1959). Moore and Dundee (1961) studied the analgesic properties of nine phenothiazines (as distinct from their analgesic *potentiating* properties) in women undergoing uterine curettage. Intramuscular injections of the phenothiazines were given in the doses commonly employed in anaesthesia with atropine 0.6 mg as a premedication. Pain thresholds were measured between 60 and 90 minutes later by applying an increasing pressure to the anterior surface of the tibia. The results indicated that the nine compounds could be classified into three groups:

1. those showing some analgesic activity —
        trimeprazine
        chlorpromazine
        promazine

TABLE 7   Tranquillizers in Terminal Cancer

	Chlorpromazine	Diazepam
Nausea and Vomiting	++	–
Insomnia	+	++
Overwhelming pain	+	++
Anxiety	+	++
Tension headaches	+	++
Muscle spasm pain	+	++
Rectal tenesmus	++	+
Bladder tenesmus	++	+
Urethral spasm pain	++	+
Agitated confusional state	+	++
Coma + restlessness*	+	++
Coma + rigidity	+	++
Coma + twitching	+	++
Convulsions	–	++

This table summarizes the use of tranquillizers at Sir
Michael Sobell House, Oxford.

*May indicate unrelieved pain, full bladder or overloaded
rectum. A tranquillizer is appropriate only when these
aspects have been dealt with and the restlessness persists.

 – means not used for this indication
++ means generally regarded as drug of first choice
 + means also used but less often than drug of choice or if
     latter fails to relieve

    2.   those mildy algesic —
             prochlorperazine
             perphenazine
             trifluoperazine
             triflupromazine

    3.   those markedly algesic —
             promethazine
             pecazine.

There was no clear relationship between analgesic action and chemical structure.
Thus, while those with analgesic properties all have a dimethylaminopropyl side
chain, so does promethazine.

There is, however, no definite evidence that promethazine is algesic in cancer
patients with pathological pain when used, for example, as a night sedative. Like-
wise, in many centres both in Britain and elsewhere, prochlorperazine is used in
patients with terminal cancer concurrently with morphine as the antiemetic of choice
without any apparent loss of analgesic efficacy.

Although chlorpromazine (50 mg) and promazine (100 mg) were equally analgesic,
subsequent practice has favoured chlorpromazine when seeking analgesic potentiation.
Moreover, despite the superior showing of trimeprazine, there is a dearth of
subsequent interest in this drug. This is particularly surprising in view of the
marked analgesic properties of its congener, methotrimeprazine (levomepromazine).
By injection, methotrimeprazine 15 mg and morphine 10 mg are equipotent (Bonica &
Halpern, 1972). The oral potency ratio has not been determined, but when allowance

is made for differences between absorption and plasma half-time, it is possible
that methotrimeprazine by mouth is as potent as morphine on a weight-for-weight
basis. Its use in terminal pain is, however, limited because it is too sedative
for most patients, causing unacceptable drowsiness. Methotrimeprazine also
commonly causes marked orthostatic hypotension and, because of this effect, some
believe its use should be restricted to non-ambulant patients. However, provided
one is aware of this potential problem, this is unnecessary. Its use should be
considered in the younger, anxious patient, requiring above average amounts of a
narcotic, or in those who experience marked vestibular disturbances when given a
morphine-like drug. In those aged under 40, it would be reasonable to prescribe
25 mg 4-6 hourly with 50-100 mg at night; in older patients, a smaller dose should
be given. Generally, it is wise to reduce the dose of morphine or other narcotic
analgesic when first prescribing methotrimeprazine.

Haloperidol

This is a butyrophenone neuroleptic (Ayd, 1976). Compared with chlorpromazine, it
is a more potent anti-emetic but causes less sedation and less anticholinergic and
cardiovascular effects. On the other hand, it has a greater propensity to cause
extra-pyramidal reactions. It has been claimed that haloperidol is able to relieve
chronic cancer pain, either alone or in combination with narcotics (Cavenar &
Maltebie, 1976; Maltebie & Cavenar, 1977). The six case reports on which this
claim is made indicated that the patients treated with haloperidol were all
suffering from prolonged pain complicated by insomnia and physical and mental
exhaustion, a situation best described as *overwhelming pain*. Analgesics were
generally modifed and patients received between 10 and 30 mg of haloperidol at
night, usually starting with 10 mg and increasing rapidly if sleep had been disturbed. Benzhexol 5 mg twice a day was also given to counter the extrapyramidal
side-effects. Thus, although the reports demonstrate that haloperidol is a useful
alternative to diazepam or chlorpromazine in this situation, they do not support
the contention that haloperidol is necessarily better or has specific analgesic
properties. Our experience in Oxford suggests that overwhelming pain will respond
equally well to analgesic modification and a large bedtime dose of diazepam or
chlorpromazine. The most important step in the treatment of this syndrome is to
ensure that the patient has a good night's sleep.

Anxiolytic sedatives

From Table 7 it will be seen that, at Sir Michael Sobell House, diazepam is commonly
preferred to chlorpromazine in many situations. In relation to pain control,
diazepam is generally used as the drug of choice where there is muscle spasm or
tension, and chlorpromazine in the less well defined discomforts of rectal and
bladder tenesmus. Other centres use chlorpromazine more widely, stressing the
depressing tendency of diazepam. In our experience, neither drug is notably
depressing, possibly because of the counteracting effect of the symptomatic relief
afforded. However, it is important to be aware that patients receiving these drugs
may become depressed and that an antidepressant may need to be prescribed.

Antidepressants

The need for an antidepressant increases the longer a patient is maintained on a
narcotic analgesic (Table 8). Whether the onset of depression is precipitated by
the protracted terminal illness itself or is a side-effect of long-continued treatment with a narcotic and a phenothiazine is not clear. It is important to be aware
that depression not only can, but frequently does, supervene in patients receiving
so-called 'euphoriant' drugs, and to initiate a trial of therapy when it does.

TABLE 8   Incidence of Antidepressant Prescriptions in Terminal Cancer
Patients receiving Diamorphine for more than 12 weeks *

Group	Number of patients	Length of treatment (weeks)	% prescribed antidepressant
I	23	12–13	17
II	22	14–17	32
III	32	18–25	41
IV	19	26–41	42
V	19	42+	68

* after Twycross and Wald (1976).

Amitriptyline is the most commonly used antidepressant. Treatment should be
started with half the usual adult dose, as debilitated patients commonly become
confused and disorientated if a higher dose is given initially, particularly if
they are receiving a narcotic or another psychotropic drug.

As might be expected, not all patients respond to an antidepressant. If after a
reasonable trial of therapy no effect is noted, treatment should be stopped. In
these circumstances, alternative measures to be considered include:

1. Use of corticosteroids, e.g. prednisolone.
2. Prescription of dexamphetamine.
3. Change of environment, e.g. temporary admission to a hospice or similar unit.

Support and companionship are always necessary, particularly in cases where the
depression is more properly described as sadness at the thought of leaving behind
one's family, friends and all that is familiar.

Tricyclic antidepressants are also of benefit in terminal care in other ways
(Table 9), particularly as the main analgesic agent in the management of superficial
dysaesthesiae and post-herpetic neuralgia (Hatangdi and co-workers, 1976; Gerson
and co-workers, 1977). Either amitriptyline or clomipramine may be used, beginning
with a dose of 25 mg at night and increasing every few days until unacceptable side
effects occur (dry mouth, drowsiness, confusion) or the pain is alleviated. If
the patient is also experiencing intermittent stabbing or shooting pain, the
addition of carbamazepine or valproate may help considerably. The therapeutic
range of valproate in this condition appears to be narrower than for carbamazepine
and unwanted effects less; a dose of 200 mg two or three times a day after meals
is often sufficient (Rafferty, personal communication).

TABLE 9   Antidepressants in Terminal Cancer

1. Depression
2. Insomnia
3. Nocturnal frequency
4. Nocturnal enuresis
5. Superficial dysaesthetic pain
6. Post-herpetic neuralgia
7. (Rectal tenesmus)

Psychostimulants

Cocaine. More than 80 years ago, Snow (1896) began to prescribe cocaine with opium
or morphine for patients with advanced cancer. He maintained that cocaine helped
to 'sustain vitality', though subsequently he had to stop using it because of the
cost. Thirty years later it was re-introduced by Roberts, a surgeon at the Brompton
Hospital, London, who used a morphine-cocaine elixir as a post-thoracotomy analgesic.
The mixture subsequently became known as the Brompton Cocktail. Since 1973, the
British Pharmaceutical Codex has included a standard formulation for both morphie-
cocaine and diamorphine-cocaine elixirs.

Only recently, however, has the effect of a standard 10 mg dose of cocaine hydrochloride been evaluated (Twycross, 1979). In this study patients were stabilized
on morphine-cocaine, or diamorphine-cocaine, or morphine alone or diamorphine alone.
After 2 weeks, patients receiving cocaine stopped receiving it, and vice versa.
Stopping cocaine had no effect at all, either in relation to pain, mood or other
subjective states. On the other hand, starting cocaine resulted in a small but
definite improvement in feelings of alertness and strength though did not affect
pain ratings. This order of treatment effect suggests that when cocaine is given
in a small fixed dose tolerance develops after a few days. Cocaine would thus be
of benefit during the initial period of treatment with morphine or diamorphine, but
thereafter would be relatively ineffective. The results of a second trial comparing the traditional Brompton Cocktail with morphine hydrochloride alone also failed
to demonstrate measurable differences in relation to pain, nausea, drowsiness, or
confusion (Melzack, Mount & Gordon, 1979).

Many physicians have, however, experience of patients — usually elderly — who have
become restless, agitated, confused and hallucinated when prescribed a morphine-
cocaine mixture and whose symptoms have persisted until the cocaine was withdrawn.
In view of this, and the equivocal nature of the trial results, I no longer prescribe cocaine concomitamtly. Instead, the patient is told that he may feel drowsy
for 2 or 3 days following the start of treatment, but subsequently the drowsiness
will become less. If the drowsiness persists, dexamphetamine 5 mg may be prescribed
once or twice daily.

Amphetamine. Dexamphetamine has been shown to potentiate the action of narcotic
analgesic drugs when used post-operatively (Forrest and co-workers, 1977). Its
place in terminal cancer is probably limited as most patients appear to do better
on a milder sedative regimen. In those patients in whom there is continued troublesome drowsiness or lack of concentration, the addition of dexamphetamine 5 mg in
the morning and at midday is sometimes of considerable benefit. It is generally
necessary to increase the dose after a number of weeks on account of tolerance, when
the patient complains that "it is no longer working". Dexamphetamine antagonizes
phenothiazine induced *sedation* and is itself antagonized by phenothiazines. Whether
their analgesic potentiating properties are additive or not is not known. However,
at the present time, the concurrent use of a neuroleptic and a psychostimulant as
co-analgesics cannot be recommended.

Psychodysleptics

In recent years there has been renewed interest in psychdysleptic drugs such as
lysergic acid diethylamide (LSD) and marihuana. LSD is the most potent member of
this group. It has been used successfully in a small number of cancer patients,
but not primarily as a co-analgesis but as an aid to psychotherapy. In one study
(Richards and co-workers, 1972), the following criteria were used in patient
selection:

1. The patient must be suffering from some degree of physical pain, depression, anxiety or psychological isolation associated with his malignancy.
2. He must have a reasonable life expectancy of at least three months.
3. No evidence of brain metastases or organic brain disease must be apparent.
4. The patient must not manifest gross psychopathology or appear pre-psychotic.

The treatment procedure consisted of three phases:

1. A series of interviews over a period of 2-3 weeks in which rapport was established and the patient was prepared for the drug session. (This preparation lasted from 6-12 hours).
2. The LSD session.
3. Several subsequent drug-free interviews for the integration of the LSD session experiences.

Pain relief following LSD-assisted psychotherapy often lasted weeks or months. There was no clear dose-response relationship and the effect of LSD was not predictable. Almost certainly the relief resulted from a change in the patients' psychological outlook.

Marihuana is a much less potent psychodysleptic. Tetra-hydrocannabinol (THC), the active principle in marihuana, possessed euphoriant, analgesic, appetite stimulant and anti-emetic effects. Controlled trials have shown that in patients without prior marihuana exposure, use of THC for analgesia has no advantage over codeine, and carried with it a risk of unacceptable side-effects including sedation, thought impairment, and depersonalization (Noyes and co-workers, 1975, 1976). Nabilone is a new THC homologue with anxiolytic properties (Lemberger & Rowe, 1975). As yet studies of its use in terminal cancer are not available.

It must be stressed that the casual use of either LSD or marihuana, cannot be recommended; rather it must be condemned as likely to cause considerably psychological harm. Moreover, it must not be forgotten that much can be done to assist terminal cancer patients in their adjustment to the implications of their disease by the more down-to-earth support and companionship offered by the increasing number of hospice programmes in Britain and North America.

ACKNOWLEDGEMENTS

Tables 1 and 2 are reproduced by kind permission of Edward Arnold; Figure 1, Tables 3 and 4 by permission of Pitman Medical, Tunbridge Wells; Figure 2 by permission of the Editor of the British Medical Journal and Dr. B.A. Stoll.

REFERENCES

Ayd, F.J. (1976) Haloperidol update: 1975. *Proc. Roy. Soc. Med.* 69, 14-18.

Beaver, W.T. and Feise, G.A. (1977) A comparison of the analgesic effect of intramuscular nefopam and morphine in patients with post operative pain. *J. Clin. Pharmac.* 17, 579-591.

Bennett, A., Charlier, E.M., McDonald, A.M., Simpson, J.S., Stanford, I.F. and Zebro, T. (1977) Prostaglandins and breast cancer. *Lancet*, 2, 625-626.

Bonica, J.J. and Halpern, L.M. (1972) Analgesics. In: *Drugs of Choice 1972-1973* (Ed. W. Modell), pp. 185-217. Mosby, St. Louis.

Boreus, L.O. and Sandberg, F. (1959) The influence of three phenothiazine derivatives and of amiphenazole on the action of methadone. *J. Pharm. (Lond.)* 11, 449.

Cavenar, J.O. and Maltebie, A.A. (1976) Another indication for haloperidol.
Psychosomatics 17, 128-130.

Crook, D., Collins, A.J., Bacon, P.A. and Chan, R. (1976) Effect of "aspirin-like"
drug therapy. Prostaglandin synthetase activity from human rheumatoid synovial
microsomes. *Ann. Rheum. Dis.* 35, 327-332.

Editorial (1976). Osteolytic metastases. *Lancet* 2, 1063-1064.

Ferreira, S.H. (1972) Prostaglandins, aspirin-like drugs and analgesia. *Nature
New Biol.* 240, 200-203.

Forrest, W.H., Brown, B.W., Brown, C.R., Defalque, R., Gold, M., Gordon, H.E.,
James, K.E., Katz, J., Mahler, D.L., Shroff, P. and Teutsch, G. (1973) Dextro-
amphetamine with morphine for the treatment of postoperative pain. *N. Engl. J. Med.*
296, 712-715.

Gerson, G.R., Jones, R.B. and Luscombe, D.K. (1977) Studies on the concomitant use
of carbamazepine and clomipramine for the relief of post-herpetic neuralgia.
Postgrad. Med. J. 53 (Suppl. 4), 104-109.

Hatangdi, V.S., Boas, R.A. and Richards, E.G. (1976) Postherpetic neuralgia:
management with antiepileptic and tricyclic drugs. In: *Advances in Pain Research
and Therapy, Vol. 1* (Eds. J.J. Bonica and D. Albe-Fessard), pp. 583-587. Raven
Press, New York.

Houde, R.W., Wallenstein, S.L. and Beaver, W.T. (1965) Clinical measurement in
pain. In: *Analgesics* (Ed. G. de Stevens)., pp. 75-122. Academic Press, New York
and London.

Hougs, W. and Skouby, A.P. (1957) The analgesic actions of analgesics, antihistamines and chlorpromazine in volunteers. *Acta Pharmacol. (Kbsh.)* 13, 405.

Kocher, R. (1976) Use of psychotropic drugs for the treatment of chronic severe
pain. In: *Advances in Pain Research and Therapy, Vol. 1* (Eds. J.J. Bonica and
D. Albe-Fessard), pp. 579-582. Raven Press, New York.

Kweekel-De Vries, W.J., Spierdijk, J., Mattie, H. and Hermans, J.M.H. (1974)
A new soluble acetylsalicylic derivative in the treatment of postoperative pain.
Br. J. Anaesth. 46, 133-135.

Lee, R. and Spencer, P.S.J. (1977) Anti-depressants and pain: a review of the
pharmacological data supporting the use of certain tricyclics in chronic pain.
J. Int. Med. Res. 5 (Suppl 1), 146-156.

Lemberger, L. and Rowe, H. (1975) Clinical pharmacology of nabilone, a cannabinol
derivative. *Clin. Pharmacol. Ther.* 18, 720-726.

Maltebie, A.A. and Cavenar, J.O. (1977) Haloperidol and analgesia: Case reports.
Milit. Med. 142, 946-948.

Melzack, R., Mount, B.M. and Gordan, J.M. (1979) *Can. Med. Ass. J.* 120, 435-439.

Merskey, H. (1974) Psychological aspects of pain relief; hypnotherapy; psychotropic drugs. In: *Relief of Intractable Pain* (Ed. M. Swerdlow). Excerpta Medica,
Amsterdam.

Merskey, H. and R.A. Hester (1972) The treatment of chronic pain with psychotropic drugs. *Postgrad. Med. J.* <u>48</u>, 594-598.

Miller, R.R., Ferngold, A. and Paxinos, J. (1970) Propoxyphene hydrochloride: a critical review. *J. Amer. Med. Assoc.* <u>213</u>, 996-1006.

Moore, J. and Dundee, J.W. (1961) Alterations in response to somatic pain associated with anaesthesia. VII: The effects of nine phenothiazine derivatives. *Brit. J. Anaesth.* <u>33</u>, 422-431.

Morley, J. (1975) In: *Proceedings of the Aspirin Symposium* (Ed. T.L.C. Dale).

Mundy, G.R., Raisz, L.G., Cooper, R.A., Schechter, G.P. and Salmon, S.E. (1974). Evidence for the secretion of an osteoclast stimulating factor in myeloma. *New Eng. J. Med.* <u>291</u>, 1041-1046.

Noyes, R., Brunk, S. and Avery, D. (1975) The analgesic properties of delta-9-tetrahydrocannabinol and codeine. *Clin. Pharmacol. Ther.* <u>18</u>, 84-89.

Noyes, R., Brunk, S. and Avery, D. (1976) Psychologic effects of oral delta-9-tetrahydrocannabinol in advanced cancer patients. *Compar. Psychiatry* <u>17</u>, 641-646.

Pierquin, B., Baillet, F. and Maylin, C. (1978) In: *La Corticothérapie en cancérologie* (Ed. S.A. Malaine). Paris.

Richards, W., Grof, S., Goodman, L. and Kurland, A. (1972) LSD-assisted psychotherapy and the human encounter with death. *J. Transpers. Psych.* <u>4</u>, 121-150.

Schell, H.W. (1972) The risk of adrenal corticosteroid therapy in far-advanced cancer. *Am. J. Med. Sci.* <u>252</u>, 641-649.

Seed, J.C., Wallenstein, S.L., Houde, R.W. and Belville, J.W. (1958) A comparison of the analgesic and respiratory effects of dihydrocodeine and morphine in man. *Arch. Int. Pharmacodyn.* <u>116</u>, 293-339.

Seyberth, H.W., Segre, G.V., Morgan, J.L., Sweetman, B.J., Potts, J.T. and Oates, J.A. (1975) Prostaglandins as mediators of hypercalcaemia associated with certain types of cancer. *New Eng. J. Med.* <u>293</u>, 1278-1283.

Snow, H. (1896) Opium and cocaine in the treatment of cancerous disease. *Br. Med. J.* <u>2</u>, 718-719.

Spencer, P.S.J. (1976) Some aspects of the pharmacology of analgesia. *J. Int. Med. Res.* <u>4</u> (Suppl. 2), 1-14).

Stoll, B.A. (1963) Corticosteroids in therapy of advanced mammary cancer. *Br. Med. J.* <u>2</u>, 210-214.

Sunshine, A. and Laska, E. (1975) Nefopam and morphine in man. *Clin. Pharmacol. Ther.* <u>18</u>, 530-534.

Tigerstedt, I., Sipponen, J., Tammisto, T. and Turunen, M. (1977) Comparison of nefopam and pethidine in postoperative pain. *Br. J. Anaesth.* <u>49</u>, 1133-1138.

Twycross, R.G. (1979) Effect of cocaine in the Brompton Cocktail. In: *Advances in Pain Research and Therapy, Vol. 3* (Eds. J.J. Bonica, J.C. Liebeskind and D.G. Albe-Fessard), pp. 927-932. Raven Press, New York.

Twycross, R.G. and Wald, S. (1976) Long-term use of diamorphine in advanced
cancer. In: *Advances in Pain Research and Therapy, Vol. 1* (Eds. J.J. Bonica and
D.G. Albe-Fessard), pp. 652-661. Raven Press, New York.

Nerve Blocks

V. VENTAFRIDDA*, C. FOCHI** and F. DE CONNO***

*Division of Pain Therapy and Rehabilitation, Istituto Nazionale per lo Studio e la
Cura dei Tumori, Milan, Italy
**Department of Anesthesiology and Resuscitation, Ospedale Maggiore
Policlinico, Milan, Italy
***Ospedale L. Sacco, Milan, Italy

ABSTRACT

Peripheral nerve blocks, autonomic system blocks and neurolytic epidural and
subarachnoid blocks are the main procedures used in terminal cancer patients.
After a description of some typical pain syndromes and of the relevant nerve blocks,
the authors record their experience with 84 patients during the last five weeks of
life at the Pain Therapy Department of the Istituto Nazionale per lo Studio e la
Cura dei Tumori, Milan, Italy. Approximately 80% benefited from nerve blocking
procedures, including those who continued to need smaller doses of analgesics to
relieve residual pain.

Two cases are reported in which the neurolytic block led to almost complete relief
of pain that had not been responsive to the use of oral morphine. Nerve blocks
should not be regarded as a sole treatment of choice for terminally ill patients
but should be supplemented as necessary with systemic analgesics in order to
achieve optimal results.

INTRODUCTION

Nerve blocks should be considered in patients with pain resulting from nerve
compression. This type of pain is typically localized to a well define unilateral
or bilateral area and tends to be exacerbated by movement. The interruption of the
sensory input brings about a sudden relaxation of the reflex tension in the muscles,
and either reduces or overrides the associated neurovegetative phenomena. In this
situation, anaesthetic and neurolytic blocks have the following advantages:

1) less trauma than with neurosurgical techniques
2) low toxicity
3) a reduction in the need for analgesics
4) prolongation of the antalgic effect by repeat block
5) low cost
6) relatively easy to perform.

GENERAL PROCEDURE

To increase the chance of success, the following procedures should be adopted:

1. Evaluate the nociceptive focus on the basis of the dermatomal pattern of the
    pain. This may require the use of diagnostic techniques such as X-ray, tomo-
    graphy, scintigraphy and C.T. scan.

2. Examine the patient neurologically both as regards function (possible presence
    of paresis or paraparesis and faecal incontinence) and in relation to the
    patient's ability to perceive and discriminate pain. It is important to differ-
    entiate between pain induced by a nerve lesion and that caused by lesions of
    other tissues. Deafferentation of nervous tissue causes an imbalance of the
    afferent sensory input which results in paroxysmal pain. If the damage is more
    severe, with the loss of small and large diameter axons, a change in the impulse
    pattern occurs which results in dysaesthesiae associated with sensory deficit.
    In these cases, a nerve block is only effective for a very short time because
    neuronal activity central to the damaged region resumes almost immediately,
    and the pain become severe again (Pagni, 1979).

3. Inform the patient and his relatives about the type of treatment intended to
    reduce or suppress pain, and explain the procedure to be undertaken.

4. Precede any infiltration with adequate local cutaneous anaesthesia and, where
    possible, by the administration of a short-acting local anaesthetic.

5. Locate precisely the nerve fibre to be blocked: if possible, by electrical
    stimulation; visualization by image intensifier; the use of contrast media
    to demarcate clearly anatomical points of reference; and possibly a prelim-
    inary block with a local anaesthetic. A study using fluoroscopy showed that
    errors in needle placement may be as high as 40% (Ferrer and Brechner, 1976).
    Further, a "needle effect" exists. This refers to the phenomena of analgesia
    following the insertion of a needle into a partcicularly painful focus, whether
    or not the area is infiltrated by local anaesthetic or neurolytic agent (Lewit,
    1979).

6. Control and reduce side-effects by means of rehabilitation, physical therapy,
    bladder re-education, and so on.

LIMITATIONS

The main limitations of neurolytic blocks in terminally ill patients are:

1. Unwillingness on the part of the patient.

2. The presence of diffuse intractable pain or deafferentation pain.

3. Mental clouding in the patient due to both toxaemia and the excessive use of
    narcotic and psychotropic drugs.

4. The possibility of side-effects that may interfere with the patient's way of
    life and level of activity.

COMMONLY USED AGENTS

Local anaesthetics and neurolytic agents are the most widely used preparations.
The former are used for both diagnostic and prognostic purposes as well as thera-
peutically. Infiltration around the given nerve may result in a selective blockade
depending on the anaesthetic concentration. Consequently, a sympathetic and

sensory afferent block is obtained when both C and A-delta fibres are affected
(Bonica, 1979b).

The preliminary use of a local anaesthetic is important in predicting the effects
of an irreversible block with a neurolytic agent. Local anaesthetic should also
be used to anaesthetize the site of infiltration with a 30 gauge needle that the
patient does not feel. Sometimes local anaesthetics are given repeatedly or by
infusion through a catheter into the epidural space to obtain a prolonged analgesic
effect (Ciocatto, Moricca and Cavaliere, 1967).

The most widely used neurolytic substances are ethanol and phenol. They cause the
destruction both of sensory motor fibres accompanied by protein coagulation and
cell necrosis in surrounding tissues (Wood, 1978). A neurolytic agent may be
injected both around the peripheral nerve and in the epidural space (with great
care because of the unpredictability of its effects) or intrathecally with hypo-
baric (ethanol) or hyperbaric (phenol in glycerin) solutions.

TYPES OF BLOCKS

The types of nerve blocks that can be accomplished in a terminally ill patient are:

1. Infiltration of trigger points with a local anaesthetic to control the
    distressing myofascial pains that often occur in patients who have been bed-
    ridden for a long time and who, in addition to muscle atrophy, often have to
    contend with the sequelae of earlier radiotherapy and surgery (Brechner, Ferrer-
    Brechner and Allen, 1977).

2. Peripheral nerve blocks, that is, anaesthetic and neurolytic infiltration of
    nerves such as the trigeminal,peripheral cervical, brachial plexus and inter-
    costal.

3. Autonomic nervous system blocks such as infiltrations of the stellate, coeliac
    and lumbar ganglia; the latter two for the control of abdominal pain.

4. Epidural and subarachnoid anaesthetic and neurolytic blocks (Fig. 1). Sub-
    arachnoid infiltrations are undoubtedly the best way of controlling pain which
    affects large areas, including up to 4 or 5 dermatomes.

In order to obtain maximum neurolytic absorption by the posterior roots intrathecally, the patient must be positioned appropriately. This can only be done with
precision on an operating table. Consequently, this technique is not easy when
performed in an ordinary hospital bed.

The possibility of urinary, anal spincter and motor complications must always be
borne in mind. If such deficits pre-exist, the risks associated with a neurolytic
block are correspondingly lessened. In more than 2,500 patients with far-advanced
cancer submitted to various neurolytic blocks, improvement was obtained in 75% of
cases (Swerdlow, 1979). In a smaller series of 290 patients, it was demonstrated
the best results were generally in terminally ill patients (Papo and Visca, 1979).
The incidence of complications lasting longer than seven days ranges from less than
12% (Swerdlow, 1979) to 40% (Ventafridda and Martino, 1976), and depends on whether
pre-existing functional deficits that were made worse are considered. The mean
duration of the analgesic effect varies from a few weeks to several months, according to different investigators.

C.C.T.C.—F

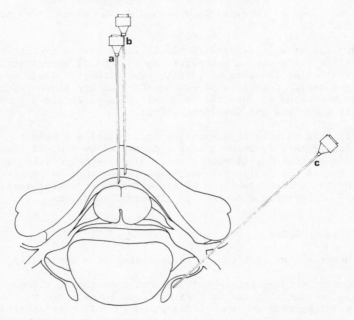

Fig.1 - a: intrathecal block.
         b: epidural block.
         c: paravertebral sympathetic block.

CHOICE OF BLOCK

To help indicate when nerve blocks may be of benefit, a number of typical cancer pain syndromes are described together with the appropriate blocks.

Head and Neck Pain

Head and neck pain (Fig. 2) is generally caused by tumours of the oral cavity and nasopharynx with trigeminal, glossopharyngeal or cervico-occipital neuralgia due to metastatic compression or concomitant radionecrosis. These patients frequency have their faces widely disfigured by vast ulcers that render social relations quite impossible because of the appearance and the odour emanating from the necrosed tissue. The survival of these patients, for whom there is no specific treatment, is more protracted than in most other terminal cancer patients. Thus blocks are just a transient or partial way to ease pain and generally need to be supplemented by systemic analgesics. The infiltration of Gasser's ganglion through foramen ovale with 0.4 ml of ethanol and 0.5 ml of phenol in 5% glycerin results in the control of pain in a vast area of the face and oral cavity. A more distal mandibular nerve block produces anaesthesia supplied by the third branch of the trigeminal nerve, which includes the lingual nerve (Madrid and Bonica, 1979). Pain in the upper part of the neck is a frequent picture; infiltration of 2-3 ml of 6% phenol in water at the transverse processes of 2nd and 3rd cervical vertebrae diminishes pain significantly in this area (Bonica and Madrid, 1979). This block can be enhanced by the infiltration of the occipital nerve.

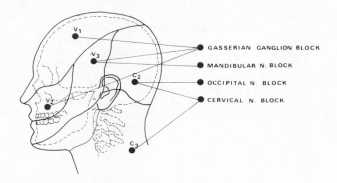

FIG.2 - Head and neck painful areas and proper nerve blocks.

Chest and Upper Limb Pain

Chest and upper limb pain (Fig. 3) represent one of the most difficult treatment problems. In fact, the terminally ill patient, generally with lung cancer with Pancoast's syndrome or brachial plexus involvement from carcinoma of the breast with vascular compression and attendant limb lymphoedema, also suffers from dysphagia, respiratory and other functional troubles. In these patients where the pain in often extremely intense, neurolytic, subarachnoid or extradural blocks have unpredictable effects both as regards the duration and the degree of pain relief; nor are they devoid of functional complications (Swerdlow, 1979). When pain is localized to the hemithorax with no evident sign of respiratory impairment percutaneous cordotomy allows more complete and prolonged relief.

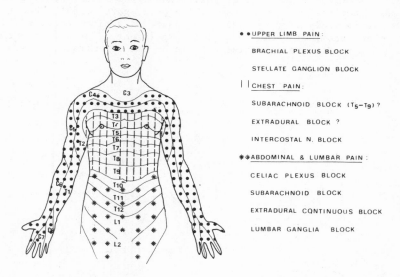

FIG. 3 - Upper limb, chest, abdominal and lumbar painful areas and proper nerve blocks.

Extradural infiltration of 10-20 mg of dexamethasone may prove beneficial in pain
caused by epidural neoplastic invasion. Intercostal nerve block with anaesthetics
or neurolytic agents (2 ml of 6% phenol in water for each space) is a useful procedure that can be done, repeatedly if necessary, at the patient's home. It relieves
most pains caused by metastatic involvement of the chest wall. The direct anaesthetic infiltration of the brachial plexus by the axillary route produces temporary
loss of limb function that can be made irreversible by using large doses of neurolytic agent. This technique has some drawbacks, notable the common early onset of
dysaesthesiae. Repeat stellate ganglion block with local anaesthetic frequently
brings about relief of pain caused by partial denervation and by vascular spasm or
compression.

Abdominal Pain

Abdominal pain (Fig. 3) is usually visceral and commonly results from the compression and invasion of the thoracic and lumbar sympathetic nerve supply by metastatic
spread. In epigastric tumours, pancreas and stomach, or with large intestinal
metastases (in the absence of intestinal obstruction) blocking the coeliac axis
ganglion with alcohol reduced or abolishes pain (Brindenbaugh, Moore and Campbell,
1964; Moore, 1979). Continuous epidural infusion of local anaesthetic brings
about pain relief for short periods (1-2 weeks), while neurolytic subarachnoid
block covers an area extending over two or three dermatomes. Pain confined to the
lower abdomen as a result of bladder or uterine compression or invasion can be
partially controlled by means of paravertebral infiltration, or infiltrations of
lumbar sympathetic ganglia from L_2 to L_4.

Perineal and Lower Limb Pain

As a rule, pain in the sacral, perineal and lower limb regions (Fig. 4) is due to
the presence of a large neoplastic mass within the pelvis or to osseous metastases
involving the sacral or lumbar spine, pelvis and lower limbs, accompanied at times
by spontaneous fractures and lymphoedema. The pain, particularly when it affects
the perineum, is commonly very intense. The patient is often bedridden and is
likely to have an abdominal stoma as well as impairment of urinary function. If
the patient has a spastic paraparesis, a large amount of intrathecal ethanol or

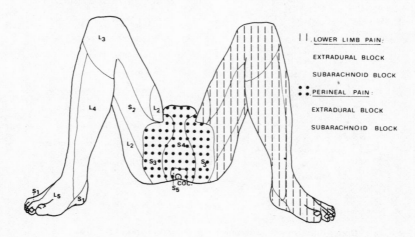

FIG.4 - Lower limb and perineal painful areas and proper nerve blocks.

phenol-in-glycerin to produce a spinal transection is particularly helpful. When
pain is confined within a small area, such as S3,4,5 perineal pain, with trigger
points, a complete remission of pain may result without any loss of lower limb
power (Ventafridda and co-workers, 1979). When pain is unilateral, affecting one
half of the pelvis and the corresponding lower limb, subarachnoid phenol in glycerin
or ethanol with several needles in different interspaces in the lumbar-sacral
region often completely relieves the pain, with muscle weakness the only common
side-effect.

CASE REPORTS

Unfortunately, many patients have a number of pains affecting different parts of
the body either simultaneously or consecutively. This limits the value of nerve
blocks and commonly makes the administration of systemic analgesics necessary. On
the other hand, a defeatist attitude about blocks, often stemming from their limited
availability, results in drug therapy being used as the only approach to pain
control.

The effectiveness of neurolytic blocks is seen in the results from 84 patients who,
during the last five weeks of life, had at least one blocking procedure at the
Department of Pain Therapy at the Istituto Nazionale per lo Studio e la Cura dei
Tumori, Milan (Table 1). All the patients were in a poor general condition, with
severe functional deficits and experiencing pain in a number of places. Some
patients were already receiving narcotic analgesics. In order to obtain satisfactory relief, a number of the patients had more than one block.

Intrathecal phenol was used most commonly, especially when the pain affected
dermatomes in the lower part of the body. Peripheral nerve blocks were used in
head and neck regions and coeliac axis ganglion block was the procedure of choice
for abdominal pain. The best results were obtained in relation to pelvic, perineal
and lower limb pain. A good result, meaning relief until death without recourse to
systemic analgesics, was obtained in only a minority. However, if fair results are
considered as well — pain relief achieved with the additional though reduced use of

**TAB. I — PAIN RELIEF OBTAINED BY NEUROLYTIC BLOCKS PERFORMED WITHIN 5 WEEKS BEFO-
RE DEATH ON 84 TERMINAL CANCER PATIENTS.**

No. of patients	Pain location	No. of blocks	Good	Fair	None	Per.	S.	C.R.
11	head and neck	27	1	4	6	22	5	—
19	chest and upper limb	32	3	11	5	18	6	8
13	abdominal	13	4	7	2	—	10	3
41	pelvic and lower limb	56	10	27	4	—	13	43
84	TOTAL	128	18(21%)	49(58%)	17(20%)	40	34	54

Results: Good = pain relief till death, no need of analgesic drugs.
     Fair = pain relief with < analgesic drugs.
     None = no pain relief and > analgesic drugs.

Type of blocks: Per. = peripheral.
     S. = simpathetic.
     C.R. = chemical rizothomy.

drugs — about 80% of the patients benefited. In patients receiving oral morphine without complete relief, the use of a nerve block resulted in both reduction of pain and a reduction in the amount of morphine required to alleviate the residual discomfort.

Two histories are recorded to illustrate the benefit of a nerve block in patients with pain only partly responsive to oral morphine. The intensity of pain was monitored on a daily basis using a visual analogue scale (Scott and Huskisson, 1979)

Case No. 1

Male patient, 51 years, with rectal carcinoma. Had had a defunctioning colostomy and currently experienced difficulty with micturition; also suffered from intract-able perineal pain associated with a large necrotic metastatic ulcer. Morphine, up to 250 mg a day by mouth, only partially controlled the pain. After two weeks, an intrathecal block was done in the L5-S1 interspace with 2 ml of phenol in 7.5% glycerin. There was an immediate marked reduction in pain and an associated loss of bladder control (Fig. 5). The dose of oral morphine was reduced to 30 mg a day in the course of one week. The analgesic effect lasted approximately four weeks, after which the patient experienced slightly more pain during the final two weeks of life.

Case No. 2

Female patient, 65 years, with lumbo-sacral compression due to a large tumour in the right half of the pelvis associated with uterine cancer. Suffered from extremely severe pain in the right lower limb. An X-ray demonstrated that she also had a femoral metastasis. The pain was only partly controlled by morphine by mouth up to 180 mg a day. Intrathecal block at T12-L1 and L2-L3 interspaces with 2 ml of phenol in 7.5% glycerin led to a considerable reduction of pain. The dose of morphine was subsequently reduced, and remained so for the last six weeks of the patient's life. During this time the limb became hypotonic as a result of the block.

The reduced intake of morphine resulted in both patients becoming more alert, more communicative and experiencing some improvement in appetite. Both, however, remained limited in activity because of the pre-existent functional deficit.

CONCLUSIONS

The treatment of pain in terminal cancer includes the use of neurolytic or anaes-thetic nerve blocks. These techniques bring about a reduction and sometimes complete relief of pain unobtainable by drugs alone in many cases of nerve compres-sion. Though technically simple, nerve blocks are not free from complications. Consequently they should be undertaken only by highly skilled personnel, working at easily accessible institutions distributed throughout the country.

Generally, nerve blocks are not the only treatment indicated, partly because of the presence of multiple pains and partly because of the patients psycho-emotional needs. A multimodality approach should be employed in the patient with terminal cancer. This means that the use of neurolytic blocks should be complemented by systemic analgesics and by life-style and behavioural modifications as indicated.

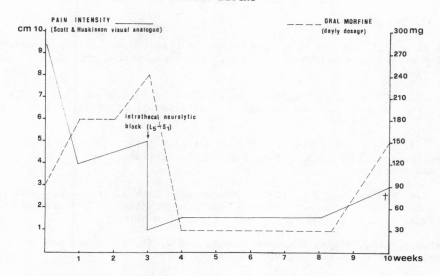

CASE 1 : pt. C.N. , male, age 51 – ca. rectum.

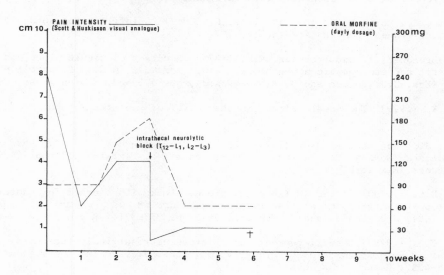

CASE 2 : pt. P.L., female , age 65 – ca. uterus .

Fig. 5

144   V. Ventafridda, C. Fochi and F. De Conno

Bond, M.R. (1971) The relation of pain to the Eysenck Personality Inventory,
Cornell Medical Index and Whitely Index of Hypochondriasis. *Br. J. Psychiatry*,
119, 671-678.

Bonica, J.J. (1979a) Importance of the problem. In: *Advances in Pain Research and
Therapy*, Vol. 2 (Eds. J.J. Bonica and V. Ventafridda), pp. 1-12. Raven Press, New
York.

Bonica, J.J. (1979b) Introduction to nerve blocks. In: *Advances in Pain Research
and Therapy*, Vol. 2 (Eds. J.J. Bonica and V. Ventafridda), pp. 303-310. Raven
Press, New York.

Bonica, J.J. and Madrid, J.L. (1979) Cancer pain in head and neck: role of nerve
blocks. In: *Advances in Pain Research and Therapy* (Eds. J.J. Bonica and V.
Vetafridda), Vol. 2, pp. 537-542. Raven Press, New York.

Brindenbaugh, L.D., Moore, D.C. and Campbell, D.D. (1964) Management of upper
abdominal cancer pain. *J. Am. Med. Ass.* **190**, 877.

Brechner, V.L., Ferrer-Brechner, T. and Allen, G.D. (1977) Anaesthetic measures
in management of pain associated with malignancy. *Seminars in Oncology*, **4**, 99-108.

Ciocatto, E., Moricca, G. and Cavaliere, R. (1967) L'infiltration sous arachnoid-
ienne antalgique. *Cahiers Anesth.* **15**, 747.

Ferrer-Brechner, T. and Brechner, V.L. (1976) Accuracy of needle placement during
diagnostic and therapeutic nerve blocks. In: *Advances in Pain Research and Therapy*,
Vol. 1 (Eds. J.J. Bonica and D. Albe-Fessard), pp. 679-683. Raven Press, New York.

Lewit, K. (1979) The needle effect in the relief of myofascial pain. *Pain*, **6**, 83-
90.

Madrid, J.J. and Bonica, J.J. (1979) Cranial nerve blocks. In: *Advances in Pain
Research and Therapy*, Vol. 2 (Eds. J.J. Bonica and V. Ventafridda), pp. 347-355.
Raven Press, New York.

Moore, D.C. (1979) Celiac (splanchnic) plexus block with alcohol for cancer pain
of the upper intra-abdominal viscera. In: *Advances in Pain Research and Therapy*.
Vol. 2 (Eds. J.J. Bonica and V. Ventafridda), pp. 357-371. Raven Press, New York.

Pagni, C.A. (1979) General comments on ablative neurosurgical procedures. In:
Advances in Pain Research and Therapy, Vol. 2 (Eds. J.J. Bonica and V. Ventafridda),
pp. 405-423. Raven Press, New York.

Papo, I. and Visca, A. (1979) Phenol subarachnoid rhizotomy for the treatment of
cancer pain: a personal account on 290 cases. In: *Advances in Pain Research and
Therapy*, Vol. 2 (Eds. J.J. Bonica and V. Ventafridda), pp. 339-346. Raven Press,
New York.

Scott, J. and Huskisson, E.C. (1979) Graphic representation of pain. *Pain*, **2**,
175-184.

Swerdlow, M. (1979) Subarachnoid and extradural neurolytic blocks. In: *Advances
in Pain Research and Therapy*, Vol. 2 (Eds. J.J. Bonica and V. Ventafridda), pp.
325-337. Raven Press, New York.

Ventafridda, V. and Martino, G. (1976) Clinical evaluation of subarachnoid neuro-lytic blocks in intractable cancer pain. In: *Advances in Pain Research and Therapy*, Vol. 1 (Eds. J.J. Bonica and D. Albe-Fessard), pp. 699-703. Raven Press, New York.

Ventafridda, V., Fochi, C., Sganzerla, E.P. and Tamburini, M. (1979) Neurolytic blocks in perineal pain. In: *Advances in Pain Research and Therapy*, Vol. 2 (Eds. J.J. Bonica and V. Ventafridda), pp. 597-605. Raven Press, New York.

Wood, K.M. (1978) The use of phenol as neurolytic agent: a review. *Pain*, 5, 205-229.

Neurosurgery

J. SIEGFRIED

Neurosurgical Department, University of Zürich, CH - 8091 Zürich, Switzerland

ABSTRACT

One of the cardinal principles for neurosurgical treatment of intractable pain of terminal cancer patients is the use of a procedure
which is devoid of stress, suitable for patients in poor general condition and which can be performed practically on an ambulatory basis.
The percutaneous ablative or augmentative (stimulating) procedures
conform to these criteria and are reviewed. The criteria for indications and choice of the technique are given according to personal
experience and analysis of the literature.

INTRODUCTION

Neurosurgical treatment of terminal cancer pain has definite indications. In the terminal patient, pain has lost its value as a symptom
and in fact has become a disease. However, when the pain is properly
controlled by appropriate drugs without alterations of the consciousness, an operation can be avoided, unless it is the wish of the
patient. Intractable pain is not only total and all encompassing,
but is physiologically detrimental. Although it is necessary to attempt to identify and eliminate the physical source of pain, it is
imperative to acknowledge that pain should be treated on the basis
of a subjective report by the patient. If a satisfactory pain relief
is not obtained with drugs, or at the cost of mental changes or disturbances of the consciousness, neurosurgical treatment can be taken
into consideration.

Neurosurgical treatment of pain is an alternative only when the procedure chosen is devoid of stress, performed with local anesthesia,

is of short duration, with minimal risks and good chances of success. The percutaneous approach to the nervous structures concerned is the only reasonable way to treat neurosurgically intractable pain of terminal cancer patients. In this report open surgery and operations with general anesthesia have been deliberately excluded.

Ablative neurosurgical procedures (destruction of a nerve root, a medullary pathway or a brain target) as well as stimulating neuro-surgical procedures will be reviewed.

ABLATIVE PERCUTANEOUS NEUROSURGICAL PROCEDURES

Rhizotomy

Spinal posterior rhizotomy by way of a laminectomy must be definite-ly banned in cases of terminal cancer patients. To ensure long-lasting relief, a large number of nerve roots must be sectioned and this requires an extensive laminectomy. The percutaneous approach with radiofrequency lesions is a valuable alternative; this proce-dure can be performed under local anesthesia and is not time-consu-ming (Uematsu, 1974). However our own experience in non-cancerous cases has shown that a perfect analgesia is sometimes very difficult to obtain and that the whole procedure for the patient is unpleasant. The indications are limited to localized pain with no tendency for the tumor to spread into surrounding regions (Papo, 1979). The lite-rature does not give any account of the results with percutaneous rhizotomy, but the data for the open rhizotomies can easily be adap-ted to the other technique. For Sindou (1976), certain forms of loca-lized cervical, trunk and pelvic cancer can justify a rhizotomy and an analysis of the literature gives a success rate of about 50 %.

The technical difficulty sometimes experienced in obtaining a good analgesia in the appropriate territory by the percutaneous approach and an expected success rate of only 50 % limits considerably the indications for a rhizotomy.

Percutaneous rhizotomy of 2 cranial nerves can be considered and is certainly an interesting approach to some facial pain due to cancer. Our limited experience with the percutaneous thermocoagulation of the Gasserian ganglion and of the glossopharyngeal nerve is pro-mising with a satisfying pain control in well selected cases (loca-tion of pain in the territory of these nerves, no preexistence of analgesia and/or anesthesia, no deep pain with bone destruction) (Broggi, 1979; Siegfried, 1979a).

Percutaneous cordotomy

High cervical percutaneous cordotomy is certainly one of the most satisfying neurosurgical procedure for intractable cancer pain. In-troduced in 1963 (Mullan) and used in the following years by only very few neurosurgeons, this method became more and more attractive and is today the technique of choice for interruption of the spino-thalamic tract. This operation is absolutely suitable for the treat-

ment of intractable cancer pain of terminally ill patients: the procedure can be carried out with local anesthesia, is of short duration and is devoid of stress. It has a very slight operative risk
and a high percentage of success, since it is possible to control
clinically the best placement of the electrode during the operation.
The technique most frequently used is that of the lateral approach
and radiofrequency lesioning. The early results of percutaneous cordotomy are considered as excellent or good in 75 - 96 % of the cases
in a large review of literature of 3742 operations (Lorenz, 1976).
In a German joint study of 224 cases, the early good results were
evaluated at 85 % (Lorenz, 1975). Failures are caused by difficulties arising from patients'uncooperativeness, impossibility to
achieve correct positioning of the needle, or less frequently, failure to penetrate the spinal cord. Delayed successes are diversely
reported, but it is known already from open cordotomy studies that
pain recurs frequently over the years. In the follow-up study of
350 coagulations, Rosomoff (1971) reported 90 % of good results
6 months after the procedure, but the success rate had fallen to
only 24 % after 36 months. In cases of cancer patients with poor
prognosis or of terminally ill patients, these considerations are
not important.

The main limitation of high cervical percutaneous cordotomy is the
bilaterality of pain. The risk of respiratory inpairment is high
after bilateral high cervical cordotomy, even when the procedure
is performed in two stages. Bilateral cordotomy at the level of
C_1 - C_2 can result in reduction of forced vital capacity, forced
expired volume, maximal breathing capacity, and maximal mid-tidal
thoracic pressure (Kuperman, 1971). Involuntary respiration is suppressed with preservation of voluntary respiratory activity resulting in sleep-induced apnea. Postoperative death after cordotomy is
often caused by this type of apnea (Krieger, 1974). Respiratory
troubles are usually reversible, but sometimes respiratory monitoring
and/or assistance is necessary for up to 3 weeks. In our hands, bilateral high cervical cordotomy will not be considered. The other
complications of cordotomy, like transitory Horner-Syndrome in 50 %
of the cases, ataxia in 30 %, hemiparesis in 10 %, bladder disturbances in 10 % and dys- or paresthesias in 5 % as well as permanent
hemiparesis in 5 % are acceptable.

Stereotactic Lesions

Mesencephalotomy. Spiegel and Wycis (1962) were the first to perform
stereotactic deep brain lesions for intractable pain. They made successful stereotactic lesions in the region of the left spinothalamic
tract and the secondary trigeminal pathway at the level of the superior colliculus for right facial pain. The goal was to attack the
pain pathways in the mesencephalon by interrupting not only the as-
cending spino- and quintothalamic systems but also the spinoreticulo-
thalamic pathways. Properly placed, stereotactic lesions in the dorsal tegmentum of the midbrain will usually relieve bilateral pain on
the head and neck without significant sequelae and is strongly recommended by Nashold (1972) for such intractable pain caused by extensive carcinoma. Also excellent relief of pain for the same indi-

cation is given by Whisler and Voris (1978) in a series of 38 patients with intractable pain secondary to malignant disease. Since
this operation can be performed with local anesthesia, it is devoid
of stress and can be done in patients in very poor general condition.
However, the complication rate is relatively high with possible
changes in ocular motility, transient ocular defects, contralateral
weakness and, particularly, postoperative dysesthesias (Nashold,1977).

Thalamotomies. Three physiological systems of pain projection in the
thalamus can be accepted and chosen as stereotactic therapeutic targets: (1) the specific sensory system with the ventro-postero-latera-
lis group of nuclei; (2) the non-specific polysynaptic systems within
the intralaminar nuclei and their adjacent fibers, and (3) the fron-
to-thalamic system within the dorso-medial group of nuclei. Besides
these classical targets, the pulvinar was included despite a lack
of significant physiological and anatomical evidence of its role in
central nociception. Lesions in the specific sensory nuclei ensure
somatotopic anesthesia in the contralateral part of the body but
anesthesia dolorosa as complication cannot be underestimated (Siegfried, 1972). Intralaminar thalamotomy and pulvinarotomy seem to be
the best targets for alleviating intractable pain. However, the
results vary considerably. Permanent pain relief will be very rarely
achieved; in terminal cancer, thalamotomies can certainly be considered, since the procedure is devoid of stress and performed with
local anesthesia. Our own experience (Siegfried, 1972, 1977) with
different targets shows an immediate beneficial effect, but the tendency to a recurrence of pain after a few weeks or a few months is
important. Similar observations have also been reported by others
(Laitinen, 1977; Sano, 1977). Stereotactic destructive lesions for
the control of pain are becoming increasingly abandonned since a
better effect can be obtained by electrical stimulation of different
brain structures.

STIMULATING NEUROSURGICAL PROCEDURES

Peripheral Nerve and Dorsal Cord Stimulation

Electrical stimulation of peripheral nerves and spinal cord is an attractive treatment of chronic pain. However, this technique has been
so far mainly used in pain of benign origin with normal life expectancy. In cases of terminal cancer patients, this sophisticated
method has not yet demonstrated its real clinical efficacy (Loeser,
1979) and the still high cost of the neurostimulating devices will
limit its use in terminal patients when other methods can be applied
with success.

Deep Brain Stimulation

Deep brain stimulation for pain reduction has become very attractive
in the last few years and rely on convincing animal studies. Mazars
(1973) was the first to advocate in 1962 intermittent stimulation
with implanted electrodes in the sensory thalamic nuclei. Richardson

and Akil (1977) reported subsequently that pain could be reduced by electrical stimulation of the periventricular and periaqueductal gray matter in humans. Since then deep brain stimulation for persistent clinical pain has been applied in a large number of cases. It is generally accepted today that stimulation of sensory thalamic nuclei is particularly effective in cases of deafferentation pain (for instance anesthesia dolorosa) and stimulation of the central gray for other kind of pain. This last procedure could contribute to pain relief by the activation of enkephalinergic and 5-hydroxytryptaminergic neural pathways.

The indication for intermittent deep brain stimulation with implanted electrodes must be strictly defined. Despite the fact that this method is non-destructive with minor surgical risks, cerebral procedures must not be used if another can be proposed as an alternative. Cancer pain with midline and bilateral distribution is suitable for deep brain stimulation considering the lack of other reliable methods. The considerable risk of serious complications with bilateral percutaneous cordotomy has already been mentioned. The introduction of an electrode within the brain can be performed with local anesthesia and is devoid of stress. To avoid the considerable cost of a permanent implantation with a receiver under the skin, one can also introduce percutaneously only one electrode and perform the stimulation with a portable stimulator connected directly to the cables of the electrodes. We have used this technique in 9 cases, none of them suffering from cancer pain. Meyerson (1978) applied independently the same technique in 9 cases of intractable cancer pain and observed in 4 cases a good pain relief and in 3 a moderate one with a significant decrease in their requirements for analgetics. Other good to excellent results were reported by others (Hosobuchi, 1979; Lazorthes, 1979; Richardson, 1977).

Deep brain stimulation for intractable pain of terminal cancer is a good indication (Siegfried, 1979b); this procedure can control widespread and bilateral pain with minimal side effects and minimal surgery. The cost of the whole implant system can limit the use of this technique, but can be solved in patients with a limited expected survival time by introducing percutaneously the electrode only.

CONCLUSIONS

Indications and choice of the procedure in the neurosurgical treatment for intractable pain of terminal cancer cannot be easily standardized since each particular case has to be individually considered. Nevertheless, in view of our own experience and after reviewing the literature, some hints can be given.

The neurosurgical treatment has to be limited to the following indications:
1. Insufficient pain relief by drug therapy.
2. Drug therapy effective, but with excessive side effects and/or alteration of consciousness.
3. Wish of the patient.
When the indication for operation is given, the choice of the neurosurgical procedure is indicated in the following table:

Proposal for neurosurgical procedure:

1. Unilateral pain C_1 - C_2 percutaneous
   below C_4 - C_5 level : cordotomy

2. Unilateral facial pain   . percutaneous rhizotomy
   a) territory of V and IX   : of V and IX

   b) extensive territory   . deep brain stimulation
      and bone pain   : or mesencephalotomy

3. Bilateral or midline   . deep brain stimulation
   pain   : or thalamotomy

With these strict limitations, neurosurgical treatment of terminal
cancer pain can be of great value.

REFERENCES

Broggi, G. and J. Siegfried (1979). Percutaneous differential radio-
    frequency rhizotomy of glossopharyngeal nerve in facial pain due
    to cancer. Advances in Pain Research and Therapy, 2, 469-473.
Hosobuchi, Y., J. Rossier, F.E. Bloom, and R. Guillemin (1979). Sti-
    mulation of human periaqueductal gray for pain relief increases
    immunoreactive β-endorphin in ventricular fluid. Science, 203,
    279-281.
Krieger, A.J., and H.L. Rosomoff (1974). Sleep-induced apnea. I.
    A respiratory and autonomic dysfunction syndrome following bila-
    teral percutaneous cordotomy. J. Neurosurg., 39, 168-180.
Kuperman, A.S., A.J. Krieger, and H.L. Rosomoff (1971). Respiratory
    function after cervical cordotomy. Chest, 59, 128-132.
Lazorthes, Y. (Ed.) (1979). European study on deep brain stimulation.
    Resumé of the 3rd European Workshop on Electrical Neurostimula-
    tion, Mégève, March 30-31.
Laitinen, L. (1977). Anterior pulvinotomy in the treatment of intract-
    able pain. Acta Neurochir., Suppl. 24, 223-225.
Loeser, J.D. (1979). Dorsal column and peripheral nerve stimulation
    for relief of cancer pain. In J.J. Bonica and V. Ventafridda (Ed.)
    Advances in Pain Research and Therapy, Vol. 2, Raven Press, New-
    York. pp. 499-507.
Lorenz, R. (1976). Methods of percutaneous spino-thalamic tract sec-
    tion. In H. Krayenbühl (Ed.), Advances and Technical Standards
    in Neurosurgery, Vol. 3, Springer Verlag, Wien, New-York,
    pp. 123-145.
Lorenz, R., Th. Grumme, H.D. Herrmann, H. Palleske, A. Kühner,
    U. Steude, and J. Zierski (1975). Percutaneous cordotomy. Advan-
    ces in Neurosurgery, 3, 178-185.
Mazars, G., L. Merienne et C. Cioloca (1973). Stimulations thalamiques
    intermittentes antalgiques. Rev. Neurol., 128, 273-279.
Meyerson, B.A., J. Boethius, and A.M. Carlsson (1978). Percutaneous
    central gray stimulation for cancer pain. Appl. Neurophysiol.,
    41, 57-65.

Mullan, S., P.V. Harper, J. Hekmatranah, H. Torres, and G. Dobben
(1963). Percutaneous interruption of spinal-pain tracts by means
of a Strontium-90 needle. J. Neurosurg., 20, 931-939.

Nashold, B.S.jr. (1972). Extensive cephalic and oral pain relieved
by midbrain tractotomy. Confin. neurol., 34, 382-388.

Nashold, B.S.jr., D.G. Slaughter, W.P. Wilson, and D. Zorub (1977).
Stereotactic mesencephalotomy. Progr. neurol. Surg., 8, 35-49.

Papo, J.(1979). Spinal posterior rhizotomy and commissural myelo-
tomy in the treatment of cancer pain. In J.J. Bonica and V. Ventafridda (Ed.), Advances in Pain Research and Therapy, Vol. 2,
Raven Press, New-York, pp. 439-447.

Richardson, D.E., and H. Akil (1977). Pain reduction by electrical
brain stimulation in man. J. Neurosurg., 47, 178-194.

Rosomoff, H.L. (1971). Communication at the 39th Meeting of the
American Association of Neurological Surgeons. Houston/Texas.

Sano, K. (1977). Intralaminar thalamotomy (thalalamolaminotomy) and
postero-medial hypothalamotomy in the treatment of intractable
pain. Progr. neurol. Surg., 8, 50-103.

Siegfried, J. (1972). Thalamic surgery in the treatment of pain.
In I. Fusek and Z. Kunc (Ed.), Present Limits of Neurosurgery,
Vol. 1, Avicenum, Prague, pp. 521-524.

Siegfried, J. (1977). Stereotactic pulvinarotomy in the treatment of
intractable pain. Progr. Neurol. Surg., 8, 104-113.

Siegfried, J. and G. Broggi (1979a). Percutaneous thermocoagulation
of the Gasserian ganglion in the treatment of pain in advanced
cancer. Advances in Pain Research and Therapy, 2, 463-468.

Siegfried, J., Y. Lazorthes and R. Sedan (1979b). Indications and
ethical considerations of deep brain stimulation. Acta Neurochir.,
Suppl., (in press).

Sindou, M., G. Fischer, and L. Mansuy (1976). Posterior spinal
rhizotomy and selective posterior rhizidiotomy. Progr. neurol.
Surg., 7, 201-250.

Spiegel, E.A., and H.T. Wycis (1962). Stereoencephalotomy. Part II,
Grune and Srratton, New-York, pp. 211-216.

Uematsu, S., G.B. Udvarhelyi, D.W. Benson, and A.A. Siebens (1974).
Percutaneous radiofrequency rhizotomy. Surg. Neurol., 2, 319-325.

Whisler, W.W. and H.L. Voris (1978). Mesencephalotomy for intractable
pain due to malignant disease. Appl. Neurophysiol., 41, 52-56.

Neuroadenolysis

G. MORICCA, E. ARCURI and P. MORICCA

Department of Anaesthesiology, Resuscitation and Pain Therapy, Regina Elena
Institute for Cancer Research and Therapy, Rome, Italy

The injection of absolute alcohol into the sella tucica and/or the pituitary gland
through the trans-nasal trans-sphenoidal route was developed in an attempt to
improve on existing methods already in use for combating diffuse intractable pain.
The technique, commonly called neuroadenolysis (NAL), was initially used exclusively
for the treatment of intolerable pain from hormone-dependent tumours (Moricca, 1968).
In only about 30% of cases, however, is the complete relief of pain associated with
an arrest of or improvement in the disease. After several years, the use of NAL
was extended to the treatment of bilateral, very severe pain due to all kinds of
cancer (Moricca, 1973, 1974, 1977). The advantages of NAL are not limited to its
remarkable simplicity, low incidence of side-effects, low cost, uncomplicated
instrumentation and repeatability (Moricca, 1976). They lie, above all, in its
mechanism of action which, though not yet fully understood, suggests that the hypophysectomy itself plays only a secondary role in the relief of pain.

THE ROLE OF NAL IN THE TREATMENT OF TERMINAL PATIENTS

We feel that the main problem in defining therapeutic approaches for terminal
cancer pain lies in establishing the appropriate *moment for acting*. The true
questions to be asked are therefore:

(a) At what point can or should it be decided to abandon the traditional methods
     (antalgic blocks, various combinations of pain-relieving drugs, neuro-
     surgical procedures) and adopt NAL instead?

(b) Does there exist a true borderline between a pre-terminal patient and a
     terminal patient?

It is clear that the significance of these terms, which have no chronological meaning and for which no such meaning is possible, is little more than semantic. Such
terms must, in fact, be taken only and exclusively in a *functional sense*; the
answer to this question is, therefore, not so much *how long*, but simply *how* the
patient will live after treatment.

As a result, there are no rigid criteria for selecting one technique or another;
rather, there is a series of more-or-less related factors which are part of the
dramatic clinical picture of the evolution of the neoplastic disease and which must
be evaluated both separately and together. These factors are the following:

155

(a) *the intensity of pain*, both as expressed by the patient and as it can be
     measured through relatively simple "scores" (semantic, graphical, etc.), or
     more sophisticated methods (e.g. evoked potentials);

(b) *the existing use of drugs*, stressing possible drug dependence and the escal-
     ation in strength of the drugs involved;

(c) *the distribution of pain*: localized, monolateral, bilateral or diffuse;

(d) *the speed of evolution* of existing symptomatology;

(e) *life expectancy*, mainly in terms of *quality*.

The above parameters must therefore guide both the choice of antalgic method and
their association within a rational programme of action. It is noteworthy that a
statistical study by Black (1975) shows that the patients who were treated at the
University of Washington's Pain Clinic underwent an average of 10 operations
without relief of pain, and that a record 43 operations were performed in one case,
with no effect or actually with negative effects.

As a general rule, the use of "light drugs" can be effective where pain is mild or
moderate, especially when it can be controlled by non-narcotic drugs which inhibit
prostaglandin synthesis (high doses of aspirin or non-steroid anti-inflammatory
drugs) or with psychotropic drugs (Twycross, this volume).

Where pain is severe but monolateral and not excessively diffuse, good control can
be obtained with antalgic blocks (Ventafridda, this volume) or percutaneous cordotomy (Siegfried, this volume).

However, when pain is bilateral, diffuse and increasingly severe, the traditional
methods necessarily reach their natural limits. At this stage, it is no longer
acceptable to continue applying blocking techniques in order to "track down" the
pain in different areas as it appears simultaneously or successively. Moreover,
pain due to highly metastisized cancer is often *only apparently* localized because
of the well-known phenomenon of "greater pain" masking and oscuring "lesser pain".
In such cases, as soon as the major pain is under control, minor pain emerges and
the dramatic problem of relieving it is renewed. Only the complete relief of his
pain can renew the confidence and hope of the patient and allow him to develop the
psychological state of mind that is indispensable before he can collaborate with
dignity with his doctors in attempting to deal with his disease while retaining
maximum mental integrity and decisional ability during the remaining days of his
life.

Neuroadenolysis has resolved many doubts concerning the current role of antalgic
blocks and neurosurgery: by reducing the number of cases where such are indicated,
NAL, as an alternative or sequential therapy, has reduced the risks and failures
that were formerly inevitable in borderline cases.

            THE TECHNIQUE

The technique, which has been improved several times, has become both simple and,
in expert hands, entirely safe. That this goal has been achieved is confirmed —
apart from the results — by the fact that NAL is now being applied, without substan-
tial variations, in many countries, by specialists from many backgrounds and
training: anaesthetists, neurosurgeons, otorhinolaryngologists, oncologists, pain
therapists, etc.

The method routinely involves the use of light endotracheal anaesthesia solely for
the brief time necessary to disinfect the nasal cavity and introduce a special
needle through to the final position (Figure 1). Our experience shows that the

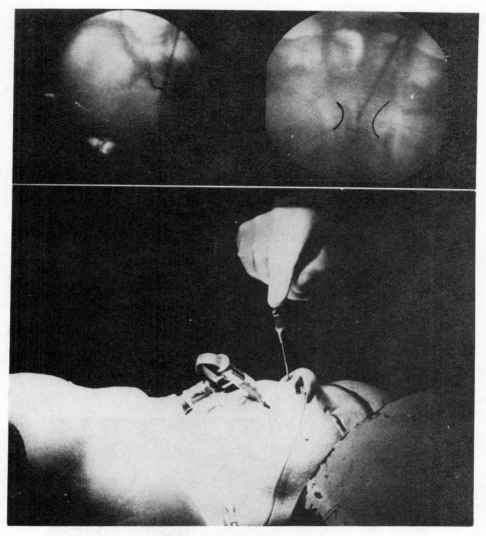

Fig. 1 The lateral projection on the left and the anteroposterior
projection (superimposed) on the right show that the needle is in
the proper position.

time required is about 2–4 minutes for the first insertion and even less for
subsequent insertions if they are carried out homolaterally.

An image intensifier permits easy monitoring of the introduction of the needle as
well as the correction of its path where necessary. Penetration of the needle may
also be monitored by X-ray control.

The needles have small semi-circular notches on the proximal quarter in order to
permit the easier and more precise monitoring of the depth of penetration at each
successive change in position.   Several, even as many as 10 needles
(Fig. 2) may be introduced without difficulty or complications, the aim being to

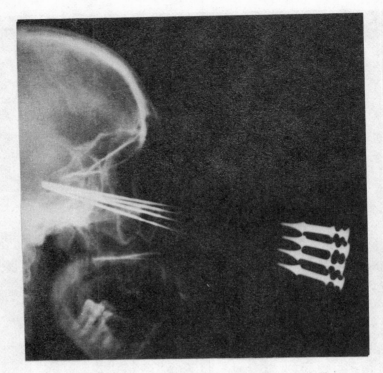

Fig. 2   Neuroadenolysis performed with four needles at
different depths

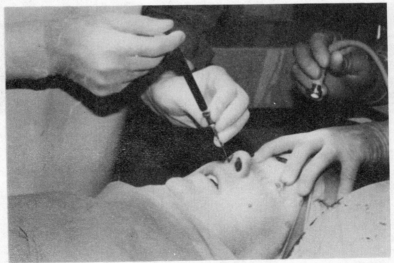

Fig. 3 Pupillary behaviour is monitored during the injection
of alcohol

inject the ethanol into different areas of the gland; in practice, however, the same result can be obtained with a single needle by performing the injections at different depths.

When the needle is in the proper position and the patient is fully awake, the ethanol is injected very slowly. The amount to be injected varies between 0.5 and 5.0 ml, depending on the following:

(a) *intrinsic and extrinsic eye motility*: during the injection, pupillary reaction and eye and palpebral movements are carefully monitored (Fig. 3);

(b) *the size of the sella*;

(c) *resistance to the injection*.

If modifications appear in eye or palpebral movements, the injection is immediately stopped and as much as possible of the ethanol already injected is withdrawn. Alterations will regress rapidly when some spinal fluid is withdrawn — preferably by the cisternal route — and followed by the administration of hydrocortisone by the same route.

A few (3-15) days later a second NAL is generally performed through the other nostril. This is routine procedure for tumours which are classically considered to be hormone-dependent; in the case of other types of tumours, it is done only if the antalgic effect was incomplete.

RESULTS*

Between 1963 and 1978, 2202 patients were treated, involving a total of 8155 alcoholizations and 5953 subsequent applications. Table 1 shows that the vast majority of the cases involve patients with hormone-dependent tumours (91.6%).

TABLE 1   Details of Pituitary Injections

No. of patients treated	2202	
No. of NAL performed	8155	
Hormone-dependent tumours	2015	(91.6%)
Non-hormone-dependent tumours	187	(8.4%)

On the other hand, Table 2 summarizes the breakdown by type of hormone-dependent tumour, with breast cancer clearly in the first place. All these patients had variably associated multiple (bone and visceral) metastases and intractable pain.

Table 3 shows the behaviour of pain relief. In about 70 per cent of patients relief was complete and immediate after the first NAL (59.2%) or the second. If the patients who underwent a third NAL are also considered, the percentage of total pain relief rises to 96.4 per cent. In 80 cases (3.6%) pain relief was incomplete but satisfactory according to subjective judgment: it was possible to stop narcotic drugs and control residual pain with minor analgesics. In many of these patients

*The cases presented here refer exclusively to the patients who had been treated prior to December 1978, in order to obtain a significant perspective. Nor has any account been taken of the patients treated from February 1958 (date of the first NAL's) to December 1963, because these were unequivocal terminal patients and the evaluation of pain relief, which was always observed, would not have any statistical significance in time.

G. Moricca, E. Arcuri and P. Moricca

TABLE 2   Breakdown of Hormone-dependent Tumours

Total patients treated for hormone-dependent cancer from 1963 to 1978	2015
Breast cancer	1650
Prostate cancer	125
Thyroid cancer	75
Endometrium cancer	57
Kidney cancer (clear cells)	55
Chorionephithelioma of testis and ovary	28
Multiple myeloma	25

TABLE 3   Results obtained through Neuroadenolysis   (2202 cases)

Complete and immediate pain relief after the first NAL	1305	(59.2%)
Immediate improvement and complete pain relief after the second NAL	211	(9.5%)
Complete pain relief after the third NAL	616	(27.7%)
Incomplete pain relief after the third NAL	80	(3.6%)

a primary role in the failure to secure complete relief could be attributed to complex psycho-emotional factors and often to a level of drug use that could only be reversed with difficulty.

In about one-third of the patients treated for hormone-dependent tumours, significant clinical improvement or at least a stabilization of the disease was recorded and reported.

Finally, it must be remembered that traditional anti-cancer therapies, whether alone or variously combined, had not been effective or had ceased to be effective for all these patients.

SIDE EFFECTS AND COMPLICATIONS

The side-effects, which are listed in Table 4, are the natural indicators of the effects of the neurolytic on the involved nerve and/or glandular structures. However, they have little to do with the relief or diminishing of pain and they regress spontaneously, generally without need for replacement hormone therapy or special treatments.

TABLE 4   The Side-effects of Neuroadenolysis

Diabetes insipidus	Very frequent
Hypothyroidism	Infrequent
Hypoadrenalism	Infrequent
Hypogonadism	Rare
Hyperphagia	Rare
Hyperthermic crisis	Very rare
Anhydrosis	Exceptional

TABLE 5   The Complications of Neuroadenolysis

Cephalalgia	Very frequent
Rhinorrhea	Very rare
Palpebral ptosis	Exceptional
Diplopia	Exceptional
Hemianopsia	Exceptional

Table 5 lists the complications. *Cephalalgia* is common during the first and some-times the second day, but requires at most the use of minor analgesics. *Rhinorrhoea* is very rarely observed and disappears rapidly and spontaneously. Ocular compli-cations, which were both extremely rare and transient, were generally due to chemical irritation of the nerve structures. Apart from congenital anomalies, they could be attributed to mitakes in applying the technique or placing the needles. Since the improvements described were adopted, ocular complications have not been observed.

ACTION MECHANISMS

In spite of numerous studies, the action mechanisms of NAL are not yet clearly understood. At the present time it appears highly probable that the effectiveness of the technique is due to a complex association of several components which can be outlined as follows:

(1) *Hormonal involvement.* Hormonal subtraction is certainly the cause of the inhibiting effects on the progress of the disease (in tumours that are still hormone-sensitive). The lowering of the levels of many hormones such as frolactin (Vijayane, 1979) artd ADH (De Wied, 1977) could, however, also be linked to the disappearance of pain.   This is undoubtedly true in the case of hypophyseal gonadotropin (LH and FSH) which inteferes with prostaglandin synthesis (Sato, 1975).

(2) *Involvement of the endorphin-enkephalin system.* The difficulty of measuring these peptides in patients who have undergone NAL is the first obstacle to the verification of this hypothesis. One of the main ways in which over-production of endorphins might occur is through the stimulation of antinociceptive structures such as the periaqueductal grey. Some authors (Levin and Katz, 1979), by way of proof, have reported a reversal—albeit temporary—of the antalgic effect of NAL after the intramuscular injection of naloxone, a well-known competitive inhibitor of the link between endorphins and opiate receptors (Terenius and Vahlstrom, 1975). The antalgic effect might also be the result of a hyposecretion of endorphins followed by a modification of the feedback loop between endorphins and enkephalins involving an increase in enkephalins. This hypothesis appears to be supported by the frequent drop (following NAL) of ACTH which is, like beta-MSH, an antagonist of endorphin and enkephalin activity.

(3) *Involvement of nerve pathways.* Hypophyseal-hypothalamic, hypothalamic-cortical and thalamic-cortical pathways may be involved, even partially, by the action of the ethanol (Levin and Katz, 1979). It was very recently demonstrated (in monkeys) that NAL is followed by a significant decrease in the amplitude of cortical potentials evoked by painful stimulus (Yanagida and Corssen, 1979). This decrease was reversed in only 50 per cent of these animals (remaining stable in the others) by injecting naloxone. We feel that this is an expression of two different types of damage which correspond to different ways in which the neuro-lytic can spread.

(4) *Combination of different mechanisms*. This is, to our minds, a reasonably probable hypothesis since all the previously described mechanisms may occur to a certain extent depending on the speed and amount of the injection, the form of the sella or other anatomical or functional cerebral conditions.

CONCLUSIONS

Over 20 years of experience and the many improvements to the technique have made NAL perhaps a delicate but a fully safe technique in expert hands. It provides complete and long-lasting relief of cancer pain, and may also improve the disease itself if the tumour is still hormone-sensitive.

Apart from its effect on pain, the low incidence of complications, repeatability and simplicity of execution are the main reasons for preferring NAL to other antalgic methods. Such advantages are even more significant in the case of the very "poor-risk" patients who are considered, sometimes wrongly, terminal: in such cases, in fact, the relief of pain may permit the return, albeit temporary, ot the patient to his family or to society, and it may coincide with a greater willingness and confidence for collaboration with his doctors in applying proper therapy.

REFERENCES

Black, R.G. (1975) The chronic pain syndrome. *Clin. Med.*, 82(5), 1720).

De Wied, D. (1977) Hormonal influence on motivation learning and memory processes. *Hosp. Pract.*, 12, 123-131.

Levin, A.B. and Katz, J. (1979) Stereotaxic chemical hypophysectomy in the treatment of diffuse metastatic cancer pain. To be published in *Proceedings of the International Symposium on Pain*, Sorrento, June 11-15.

Moricca, G. (1968) Progress in anaesthesiology. In: *Proceedings of IV World Congress of Anaesthesiologists*, p. 268. Excerpta Medica, Amsterdam.

Moricca, G. (1973) Chemolysis of the pituitary in the management of cancer pain. In: *Proceedings of V World Congress of Anaesthesiologists*, pp. 272-275. Excerpta Medica, Amsterdam.

Moricca, G. (1974) Neuroadenolysis for the antalgic treatment of advanced cancer patients. In: *Recent Advances on Pain* (Eds. J. Bonica, P. Procacci and C.A. Pagni), pp. 322-324.

Moricca, G. (1976) Neuroadenolysis for diffuse unbearable cancer pain. In: *Advances in Pain Research and Therapy* (Eds. J.J. Bonica and D. Albe-Fessard), p. 864. Raven Press, New York.

Moricca, G. (1977) Pituitary neuroadenolysis in the treatment of intractable pain from cancer. In: *Persistent Pain*, Vol. 1 (Ed. S. Lipton). Academic Press, London; Grun and Stratton, New York.

Sato, T. (1975) Effect of indomethacin on the inhibitor of prostaglandins synthesis on hypothalamic pituitary system in the rat. *J. Endoc.*, 64(2), 157.

Terenius, L. and Vahlstrom, A. (1975) Morphine-like ligand for opiate receptors in human CSF. *Life Sci.*, 16(12), 1759-1764.

Vijayane, McCann S.M. (1979) In vivo and in vitro effects of substance P and neuro-
tensin on gonadotropin and prolactin release. *Endocrin.*, 105(1), 63-68.

Yanagida, H. and Corssen, G. (1979) Alcohol-induced pituitary adenolysis: how
does it control intractable cancer pain? An experimental study using tooth pulp
evoked potentials in rhesus monkeys. *Anesth. Analg.*, 58, 279-287.

Editor's comment

Because alcohol injection into the pituitary gland is still controversial, we
have appended comments made by Dr Giuseppe Franchi, Director of Pain Therapy
Division, Ospedale Civile Maggiore di Verona, Italy. He raises a number of
practical points relating to the acceptability of the procedure to the patient.
In addition, his results emphasize the fact that other centres have, as yet, not
been able to reproduce completely the excellent results obtained by Dr Moricca
and his associates. In two recently published reports, complete relief was
obtained in half and two-thirds of the patients respectively (Madrid, 1979;
Miles, 1979)

Comment by Giuseppe Franchi, M.D.

For many years I have taken an interest in pain therapy and, in the past, before I
began to use the technique of radiofrequency thermal lesion, I carried out
pituitary ablation with alcohol on many patients with severe cancer pain. I used
the same method as Moricca, who taught me personally. This means I used the same
kind of patients, the same technique, and the same amount of alcohol.

In my experience with more than 120 patients, a reduction, and at times the
complete relief, of pain is observed only in about 20%. Relief lasted for a
period ranging from a few days to several weeks, after which the pain recurred.
A prolonged pain-relieving effect can be obtained by repeating the treatment a
second, third or fourth time. I have noticed, however, that on many occasions
the patient becomes disheartened, depressed and pessimistic, and that neither
relatives nor patient can be persuaded to agree to repeat treatment, despite its
initial pain-relieving effect. Their reluctance relates in particular to memories
of post-treatment headache, the discomfort of the plug in the nasal cavity, and
the after effects of general anaesthesia.

I disagree with Professor Moricca when he states that ablation of the pituitary
with alcohol constitutes a "step forward" in the treatment of diffuse cancer pain,
and that this method has "resolved the many problems and failures of radiofrequency percutaneous cervical cordotomy". In my opinion, this is not so.

Madrid, J.L. (1979) Chemical Hypophysectomy. In *Advances in Pain Research and
Therapy*, Vol.2 (Eds. J.J.Bonica and V.Ventafridda), 381-391. Raven Press, New
York.

Miles, J. (1979) Chemical Hypophysectomy. In *Advances in Pain Research and
Therapy*, Vol. 2 (Eds J.J.Bonica and V.Ventafridda), 373-380. Raven Press, New
York.

IV
SYMPTOM CONTROL

Control of Symptoms Other Than Pain

W. S. NORTON* and S. A. LACK**

*Associate Physician, The Connecticut Hospice, Consulting Physician (Emeritus),
St. Luke's Hospital, New York City, N.Y., USA
**Medical Director, The Connecticut Hospice

The patient with terminal cancer may experience a number of distressing symptoms
(Table 1). These may relate to the cancer or to a co-existent disease. They are
best controlled by a team approach, especially when the patient is at home. The
multidisciplinary team includes physicians, nurses, secretaries, financial adviser,
social worker, chaplain, physical therapist, and volunteers (Lack, 1976).

TABLE 1   Symptoms Recorded in 100 Consecutive Home-Care Patients

Symptom	%
Pain	75
Weakness	71
Constipation	49
Depression	46
Anorexia	38
Nausea	28
Vomiting	24
Dyspnoea	21
Painful decubitus	12
Dysphagia	10
Diarrhoea	6
Dry/sore mouth	5

All symptoms are assessed by taking a detailed history and making a careful docum-
entation of the location of the symptom, its intensity, time of onset, duration,
and its effect on normal body functions. All symptoms should be documented in an
orderly manner on the patient's record. The experienced physician learns quickly
to sort these out and make priorities.. He or she must first deal with those
symptoms which are most distressing and which preoccupy the patient's mind. The
physician must consider symptoms individually and determine how each is related to
the primary disease, if at all. The patient's past history may indicate that he
has had a similar symptom before and, if so, it is important to know its course,
duration, and management.

It requires great patience and judgement on the physician's part to explore all
aspects of each symptom, especially what the symptom means to the patient and the
degree of anxiety it arouses in the family. The physician must be careful not to

emphasize and attach too much unnecessary importance to a symptom for this might
heighten the patient's anxiety. It takes a lot of time to take a careful history,
to do a careful physical examination and to work out a care plan for each symptom.
This cannot always be done on the first assessment visit and it may take a number
of visits. Part of the assessment can be done by the nurse on some of her visits.
Because symptoms may come and go daily, hourly, or in a matter of minutes, care
plans must not be routine. Care plans need to be re-evaluated regularly and so
allow for flexibility on the part of the caregiver whether the caregiver be physician, nurse, family member, or the patient himself. If it is a symptom that cannot be changed, then the physician must take time to explain this to the patient
and family. Having established his credibility, the physician must help the
patient and family face this frustrating situation, accept this conclusion, and
learn to live with it. If the symptoms can be altered favourably or completely
eliminated the plan of care should be energetic and the specific therapy given or
ordered. Symptoms of psychosomatic origin need much time, and reassurance must be
given to achieve understanding and relief.

Understanding the cause and the meaning of symptoms may be very important to some
patients, but of little interest to others. The latter may only want didactic
advice and instant help. Similarly, members of the family vary from this same
attitude to intense involvement in understanding the symptoms, their meaning and
management. Time must be allotted for this dialogue. In terminal disease worry
and fear are the usual concomitant mental and emotional reactions to all symptoms
whether these concerns are verbally expressed or not. Imaginatively try to devise
something that can divert the patient's preoccupation with the symptoms. Here it
is important to understand whether fear, loneliness, or some aspect of guilt is the
problem with which the patient cannot cope. Counselling by nurse, doctor, social
workers or chaplain are essential in the palliative care programme.

WEAKNESS

Weakness as a subjective phenomenon provokes anxiety. When it involves loss of
control and dependency then the family structure is threatened and team care is
needed (Table 2). In approaching the management of weakness, its meaning to the
patient and family must be considered before the care plan can be effective.

TABLE 2   Weakness

Causes	Management
Bedrest	Specific therapy
Secondary to surgery	Hydration
drugs	Nutrition
chemotherapy	Mobilization if possible
radiation	Modification of lifestyle
Fever	Drugs — corticosteroids
Malnutrition	vitamins
Dehydration	Blood transfusion
Anaemia	IV alimentation
Exhaustion	

Efforts to prevent further weakness are important. Changing the patient's position,
getting up in a chair, walking, range of motion exercises, and consultation with a
physical therapist may introduce a positive attitude that is so badly needed. When
assistance is needed, introduce it gradually and by suggestion — since the thought
of helplessness and loss of physical independence is frightening and contributes to
the patient's depression.

Some people today believe that body resistance to cancer depends greatly on a diet of natural foods and vitamin supplements. If this is the case, every effort should be made to see that they are provided. The metabolic effect of corticosteroids can help overcome weakness and anorexia; for example, prednisome 10 mg three times a day initally, tapering to 5 mg two or three times a day after one or two weeks.

ALIMENTARY SYMPTOMS

Symptoms related to the gastrointestinal tract are very common (Table 3).

TABLE 3   Gastro-Intestinal Symptoms

Anorexia	Farting
Dry/sore mouth	Diarrhoea
Bitter taste	Constipation
Dysphagia	Tenesmus
Belching	Distension
Regurgitation	Incontinence
Nausea/vomiting	Cramps

Anorexia

Anorexia may be caused by a variety of factors (Table 4). Management may be as simple as reassurance by an honest caregiver who has time to sit quietly at the bedside. On the other hand the management may require skilled medical intevention and judicious use of specific medication to correct an underlying metabolic abnormality.

TABLE 4   Anorexia — Failure to Eat

Causes	Treatment
Fatigue	Mouth care
Mouth discomfort	Hydration
General discomfort	Small helping of favourite foods
Pain	Getting up
Disease process	Getting dressed
Anxiety	Fresh air
Odours	Change of environment
Unpleasant sights	Family instruction
Dehydration	Drugs — phenothiazines
Malnutrition	caffeine
Constipation	corticosteroids
Uraemia	alcohol
Hyponatraemia	amphetamines
Hypercalcaemia	
Secondary to drugs	
chemotherapy	
radiation	

Nausea and Vomiting

Anorexia may be the prodroma of nausea and vomiting (Table 5). Local irritation to
the lining of the gastrointestinal tract, interference with gastrointestinal motility, mechanical blockage due to tumour or constipation are all possible causes of
reflex nausea and/or vomiting. In the presence of bowel obstruction, vomiting may
be well tolerated in the absence of nausea. Anorexia, nausea or vomiting are managed by first dealing with an identifiable cause. Nausea alone or with infrequent
vomiting often can be controlled with a phenothiazine.

TABLE 5 Nausea and Vomiting

Causes	Management
Alimentary bleeding	Deal with cause
	Vomiting often tolerated in absence of nausea
Vagal stimulation:	Mouth care
gastric irritants	Bowel regulation
blood	Deal with social and emotional factors
drugs	
iron	Drugs:
aspirin	Phenothiazines:
Bowel obstruction	Prochlorperazine (Compazine)
ileus	10-25 mg, tablet or suppository
	Trimethobenzamide (Tigan) 100-250 mg tablet,
Secondary to drugs	suppository 200 mg
chemotherapy	Triethylperazine (Torecan)
opiates	10 mg, tablet or suppository
digitalis	Antihistaminics:
Anxiety	Diphenhydramine (Benadryl)
	50 mg, tablet or injection
Raised intracranial pressure	Dimenhydrinate (Dramamine)
Ketosis	50-100 mg, tablet or suppository
Uraemia	Pyridoxine, 10-50 mg, tablet or injection
Hypercalcaemia	Tetrahydrocannabinol
	Naso-gastric tube?
	Parenteral fluids?

Narcotics cause nausea and vomiting by stimulation of the chemoreceptor trigger
zone of the medulla. This can be controlled by giving prochlorperazine with (or
sometimes one hour before) the morphine. When symptoms are severe medication may
be given per rectum. We use prochlorperazine 25 mg or, when added sedative effect
is needed, promethazine 25-50 mg suppositories repeated six-hourly. Alternatively,
one of the antihistaminics (diphenhydramine 50 mg or dimenhydrimate 50-100 mg)
given intramuscularly every four to six hours will usually control symptoms and
avoid the possible Parkinsonian side effects of some phenothiazines.

Pyridoxine 10-50 mg orally or 50-100 mg by injection (usually given for hyperemesis
gravidarum) is occasionally helpful for post-radiation nausea. There is some
anecdotal evidence that delta-9-tetrahydrocannabinol by mouth or inhaling marihuana
smoke can prevent the anxiety and nausea that follows radiation therapy, and the
nausea that follows treatment with some chemotherapeutic drugs.

Severe dehydration following frequent repeated vomiting may be reversed by a few
days of intravenous fluids. Prolonged hydration and alimentation either by the

intravenous route or via a naso-gastric tube will not reverse the course of terminal
cancer but when given temporarily will provide psychological support. These measures, considered by some to be life-supporting, are usually not employed at the
Connecticut Hospice Home Care Programme.

Dry Mouth

Dry mouth often associated with dehydration or fever is a common finding and often
annoying to the patient with terminal cancer (Table 6). Other distressing symptoms
may be more preoccupying to the patient but simple mouth care can brighten the day.
Even when the patient cannot swallow, rinsing the mouth, gentle removal of sticky
secretions, or sucking a lemon drop will make the patient more comfortable.

TABLE 6   Dry/Painful Mouth

Causes	Management
Monilial infection	Mouth care :
Dehydration	lemon glycerine swabs
	removal of sticky secretions
Mouth breathing	gentle suction
	Ice chips
Malnutrition (hypovitaminosis)	Fluids
	Nutrition
Secondary to drugs:	Ascorbic acid (500 mg twice daily)
anticholinergics	Lemon sugar candy
chemotherapy	Artificial saliva
	Viscous xylocaine rinses
Radiation therapy	Mycostatin in cocoa butter
	Corticosteroids (hydrocortisone pellets)

The burning lesions of a monilial infection usually improve by allowing an insert
of mycostatin in cocoa butter to dissolve in the mouth every four to six hours.
Aphthous ulcers heal more quickly and with less discomfort if cleansed with dilute
zinc chloride mouth washes every three hours.

Constipation

The new patient who has trouble verbalizing his needs, who is weak, eating poorly,
unhappy, moderately dehydrated and restless with abdominal pain, is usually constipated and often impacted. After being bedridden and taking regular analgesic
and narcotic medication for pain, the patient needs daily stool softeners, peristaltic stimulants, and usually assistance from a suppository or enema.

When narcotic analgesics are first prescribed, it is wise to start a bowel regulator as well as ordering adequate fluids, fruit juices, and making efforts to
mobilize the patient. An aggressive preventative regime is less traumatic than
the later use of drastic purges and digital disimpaction.

Table 7 lists those measures employed to prevent constipation and measures for the
management of acute constipation.

We give a stool softener, dioctyl sodium sulfosuccinate (Colace, DSS) 100 mg
three times a day, to most of our patients. Some prefer methyl cellulose with
adequate oral fluids. Most patients also need a peristaltic stimulant —

TABLE 7 Constipation

Causes	Management
Intestinal atony	Hydration and nutrition —
	high residue diet
Reflex inhibition due to	fruit
intestinal disease	Stool softeners — psyllium
Abnormal defaecation reflex:	hydrophilic mucilloid (Metamucil)
	Dioctyl sodium sulfosuccinate
Prolonged physical inactivity —	(DSS Colace)
chronic disease	Lubricants — mineral oil
bedridden	Saline cathartics —
	magnesium sulfate
Malnutrition — low residue diet	sodium phosphate
	milk of magnesia
Dehydration —fever	Peristaltic stimulants —
	cascara, senna
Secondary to drugs —	bisacodyl (Dulcolax) 5 mg
anticholinergics	Suppositories —
analgesics	glycerine
narcotics	bisacodyl
	Enemata —
	tap water
	saline
	soap suds
	oil
	sodium phosphate
	bisacodyl 10 mg

danthron (Dorbane) 25-75 mg; senna (Senokot) or bisacodyl (Dulculax) 5 mg by mouth or 10 mg suppository are effective alternatives.

Diarrhoea

Diarrhoea is not a common symptom (Table 8). Be alert to the patient who has frequent watery or pasty stools in small quantities, accompanied by restlessness and abdominal pain. This is the classic syndrome of faecal impaction.

Drugs with peristaltic action, infiltrating bowel neoplasms and inflammatory intestinal disease are frequent causes of diarrhoea. These must be considered before treatment is given. A rectal examination is part of the assessment.

Proprietary medications such as kaolin and pectin are seldom effective. Initially, we use a narcotic such as codeine 30 mg or morphine 15 mg 4-hourly by mouth. For persistent diarrhoea, when a treatable cause has not been found, we use diphenoxylate with atropine (Lomotil) 2.5 to 10 mg every 4-6 hours, together with a low residue diet.

TABLE 8   Diarrhoea

Causes	Management
Hard fecal mass in rectum	Digital examination of rectum
Increased bowel motility	Low residue diet
High residue or irritating diet	Rehydration

Inflammation —
   bacterial
   post radiation
   parasitic infestation
	<u>Minor drugs</u> (seldom effective)
	Aluminium hydroxide 20-40 ml
	   6-hourly
	Bismuth, Kaolin, Pectin

Secondary to drugs —
   magnesium salts
   peristaltic stimulants
Infiltration of intestine by cancer
	<u>Synthetic opiates</u> (four hourly)
	Diphenoxylate with Atropine
	   (Lomotil) 2.5-10.0 mg
	Loperamide (Imodium) 2 mg

Partial bowel obstruction Tension Fear Anxiety	<u>Opiates</u> (four hourly) Codeine 15-30 mg Paregoric (Camphorated Tincture of Opium) 5 ml Tincture of Opium 3-10 drops Morphine 15-20 mg
	Anticholinergics Tranquilizers Corticosteroid enemas

Dysphagia

Difficulty in swallowing may be caused by cancer of the pharynx or upper mediastinum with infiltration of or pressure on the oesophagus (Table 9). Diet should be semi-liquid or fluid. Medication should also be in liquid or pulverized form.

TABLE 9   Dysphagia

Causes	Management

Obstruction — tumour
            post-operative fibrosis
            inflammation
Mechanical — muscle weakness
            neurogenic
Psychogenic
	Deal with causes — surgery
	                radiation
	                chemotherapy
	                antibiotics
	Education of family and care-givers
	Mouth care
	Pulverize medications
	Liquid medications
	Modified diet
	Celestin tube
	(Gastrostomy)

The patient who is unable to swallow fears starvation. When a person cannot eat, the family is deprived of their role of providing nourishment. Starvation means impending death. Everyone now turns to the physician to make a decision and he must guide the patient and family through a forest of uncertainty, anger and desperation.

If the patient is already in a terminal state, this crisis may be resolved and accepted. If it is a sudden change of status, measures such as radiation or chemotherapy should be considered.

When dysphagia is associated with advanced metastic cancer, gastrostomy or parenteral alimentation may be temporarily life sustaining. These measures are used only where psychological or physical support is an urgent need, such as to gain a few days of life to see a daughter married.

RESPIRATORY SYMPTOMS

Dyspnoea is a very frightening symptoms, particularly if severe (Table 10). Lack of oxygen causes cellular death unless treatment is promply given.

TABLE 10 Dyspnoea

Causes	Management

Hypoxia —
anaemia
heart failure
hypotension
decreased alveolar volume
emphysema
post-pneumonectomy
	Mouth care
	Position of patient
	Deal with cause if possible —
	    thoracentesis
	    tracheo-bronchial suction
	    radiation of tumour
	Oxygen therapy

Hypercapnia — bronchial obstruction obstructive lung disease	Drugs: Bronchodilators Aminophylline 200 mg t.i.d. orally, 500 mg IM or IV
Mechanical — immobility of spine or thorax immobility of diaphragm	Isoproterenol 10-15 mg sublingual Mucolytics SSKI
Lung disease — inflammatory infiltrative	Acetylcysteine (Mucomyst nebulizer) Guaifenesin Syrup N.F. 200 mg t.i.d.
Anxiety	Corticosteroids Prednisone 10-15 mg t.i.d. Tranquillizers Chlordiazepoxide 5-25 mg 4-6 hourly Hyoscine 0.4-0.6 mg Teach patient correct breathing and coughing techniques Emergency care plan

Emergency treatment includes these measures:

1. Clear the airway of any obstruction.
2. Provide oxygen via nasal catheter or mask.
3. Position the patient at about 45 degrees.
4. Deal with reversible causes.
5. Teach breathing and coughing techniques.
6. Provide reassurance for patient and family with frequent follow-up visits. Do not abaondon the patient.
7. Talk over an emergency care plan and alternative methods of care, i.e. hospital.

Cough is common when cancer involves the respiratory tract. Emergency management is to clear the airway of any obstruction or irritation (Table 11). Having evaluated the situation as best he can, the physician must decide whether measures directed towards suppression of the cough or enhancing expectoration are most appropriate. The inspired air should be humid. SSKI by mouth (5-10 drops three times a day) or Mucomyst by nebulizer is used when thick sticky sputum is a problem.

TABLE 11   Cough

Causes	Management

Tracheo-bronchial —
    irritation
    inflammation
    allergy
    infection
    tumour infiltration
	Deal with aetiology —
	    remove irritants
	    radiation of tumour
	    antibiotics for infection
	 Hydration
	 Humidification

Thoracic disease	Decide whether suppression or expectoration is more appropriate
Pleural disease	Mucigogues
Cardiac decompensation	SSKI q.i.d.
Middle ear disease	Guaifenesen Syrup t.i.d.

	Mucolytics
	 Detergent aerosols — Alevaire
	                               Tergemist
	 Proteolytic enzymes — trypsin
	                                   pancreatic
	 Streptokinase, Streptodornase
	 Sulfhydryl — acetylcysteine
	                (Mucomyst nebulizer)

	Depressants Codeine 15-30 mg 4-hourly Morphine 15-30 mg 4-hourly

To allow the patient (and family) to sleep at night, the cough should be suppressed. We use codeine or morphine (15-30 mg 4-hourly by mouth), being careful not to suppress the respiratory centre. Concomitant oxygen therapy will be needed if the respiratory rate falls and the patient becomes cyanosed.

PRURITUS

Itch is a cutaneous sensation that causes restlesness and a desire to scratch (Table 12). In our experience, the most common causes are dry skin, jaundice, allergy, systemic drug toxicity and local irritants including pyogenic, fungal and parasitic infections. Symptom relief depends on eliminating any suspicious systemic and/or local cause, maintaining 60% humidity at the skin surface and lightly rubbing on soothing creams and lotions. These may be non-medicated, such as lanolin, or contain an antihistamine (tripelemamine HCl 2%). A low potency corticosteroid such as hydrocortisone 1.0% or a non-soecific cream such as crotamiton (Eurax) may be tried. It is wise to give each medication several days trial before making a change.

Oral antihistaminics are often helpful, such as chlorpheniramine 4 mg q.i.d., trimeprazine tartrate (Temaril) 2.5 mg q.i.d. or promethazine 25 mg nocte. Corticosteroids by mouth in small doses help to reduce any inflammatory ot allergic component. We use the least expensive, namely prednisone 5-10 mg t.i.d.   Itching

TABLE 12   Itch

Causes	Management

Dry skin —
    low humidity
    hypometabolism
	Discourage scratching
	Allow gentle subbing
	Maintain 60% humidity
	Avoid soap

Malnutrition — hypovitaminosis	Topical care Oil, lanolin

Systemic —
    secondary to drugs
    histamine release by morphine
    uraemia
    malignancy — Hodgkin's
                myeloma
                prostate
	"Alpha Keri"
	Creams, lotions
	Antihistamine cream:
	    Tripelenamine 2% (Pyribenzamine)
	    Crotamiton cream (Eurax)
	Corticosteroids:
	    Hydrocortisone 1%
	    Triamcinolone Acetonide 0.025%
	        (Kenalog 1/4)
	    Fluradrenalone 0.025% (Cordran 1/2)
	    Fluocinolone 0.01% (Synalar 1/2)

Local irritation —
    chemical — soap
              drugs
    thermal
    allergic
    infection — pyogenic
               parasitic
               fungus
	Oral drugs
	Antihistamines:
	    Chlorpheniramine (Chlortrimeton)
	        4 mg q.i.d.
	    Promethazine (Phenergran)
	        25 mg nocte
	    Trimeprazine (Temaril) 2.5 mg q.i.d.
	Prednisolone 5-10 mg q.i.d.
	If associated obstructive jaundice try
	    Cholestyramine (Questran) 4 g q.i.d.

associated with obstructive biliary disease and hyperlipidaemia will often respond
to oral cholestyramine (Questran) 4 gm t.i.d.

When there is associated anxiety and restlessness we use an antihistamine with
sedative properties, for example diphenhydramine (Benadryl) 25-50 mg t.i.d., or
promethazine (Phenergan) 12.5-25 mg t.i.d.   In more marked anxiety one can add
chlordiazopoxide (Librium) 10 mg t.i.d. or diazepam (Valium) 2-10 mg t.i.d.

    DECUBITUS ULCER

Ischaemic necrosis of the skin, deep subcutaneous tissue and muscle due to constant
pressure results in ulceration and infection (Table 13).   For the early lesion,
gentle care of the affected skin avoids cracking and infection. Light, frequent
massage to the areas surrounding the pressure point helps to improve local blood
supply.   Proper positioning and mobilization and placing the patient on an egg
crate mattress, oscillating air mattress or waterbed distributes contact points.

Keep superficial moist lesions dry with unscented talc or by allowing Maalox
(magnesium and aluminium hydroxide) to dry on the affected area. Ulcerated
lesions are cleansed and irrigated thoroughly with sterile saline or non-irritating
disinfectants, especially when the edges are undermined. Applying thin coats of
dextranomer (Debrisan) to the moist ulcer helps decrease local oedema.   Sterile
dressings are applied and, if wet from secretions, changed at least twice and
often four times each 24 hours.

TABLE 13 Bedsores

Causes	Management
Pressure	Relieve pressure:
Tissue ischaemia and necrosis	change patient's position
	mobilize patient
Malnutrition — hypovitaminosis	Massage edges gently to increase
	blood flow
Stages (cp. Burns)	Distribute body contact points:
1. Hyperaemia	egg crate mattress
blanching	sheep skin
non-blanching	oscillating air mattress
	water bed
2. Blister	Clean/dry any secretions:
3. Broken skin	lamp
	hair dryer
4. Penetration	Lotions to dry areas
upper skin layers	Control of infection:
deep ulceration	irrigation
	local disinfectants
	Avoid topical antibiotics
	Vitamin C 1 g q.i.d.
	Vitamin A 25,000 units q.i.d.

Local antibiotics are contraindicated as their use is nearly always followed by reinfection with resistant organisms. Systemic antibiotics are used only when spreading cellulitis is evident. There is good evidence that an adequate, balanced diet improves host resistance and tissue healing. Vitamin C 1.0 g daily and Vitamin A 25,000 units daily may be helpful.

INSOMNIA

Wakeful nights are distressing to the patient and perhaps more so to the family. Control of pain and/or other symptoms does not always result a good night's sleep. Anxiety and/or depression can cause insomnia (Table 14). Important in the management is a careful evaluation of the patient and all the dynamics in the home. It is essential that the care-giver be accepted by the patient and the family. Good nursing care, the bedtime back rub, reassurance, all help to generate confidence and peace of mind and create an atmosphere conducive to sleep. Certainly this is all necessary before a medication is prescribed.

If a combination of anxiety and depression seems to be the cause of the wakefulness, amitriptyline 50 mg at bedtime will often produce a deep sleep. If this does nothing for the insomnia, then the most likely factor is the anxiety. Through dialogue and counselling the cause of anxiety may be identified and dealt with. On the other hand, medication may be the cause, as with one recent patient who was receiving 10 mg cocaine 4-hourly in a Brompton Mixture. When the cocaine was eliminated and the morphine given alone, she slept soundly. Time-tried chloral hydrate 500 mg at bedtime will often be an effective sedative when more modern medications have failed.

TABLE 14 Wakeful Nights and Insomnia

Causes	Management
Uncontrolled distress	Physician reassessment
Anxiety/depression	Quiet environment
	Darkened room
Fear of sleep	Counselling
(loss of control)	Reassurance (fear of dying)
	Relief of pain
Secondary to medications	Back rub
	Hot drink
	Bio-feedback
	Medication
	Phenothiazine:
	Promethazine (Phenegran) 25 mg
	Benzodiazepine:
	Chlordiazepoxide (Librium) 5-25 mg
	Tricyclic antidepressant:
	Amitriptyline (Elavil) 25-50 mg
	Alcohol: Whisky 30-45 ml
	Hypnotics:
	Flurazepam (Dalmane) 15-30 mg
	Chloral hydrate 0.5-1 g
	(tablets or liquids)

SUMMARY

The management of symptoms in terminal cancer depends on:

1. A physician who is comfortable in the presence of the dying patient and who is available day and night.

2. An interdisciplinary team of care-givers, including nursers, social workers, clergy, volunteers, who are always available and who will never abandon the patient.

3. A thorough assessment of each symptom, including the meaning to the patient and family.

4. A therapeutic team with unlimited, imaginative and resourceful measures to deal with each symptom, and with the anxiety it arouses in the patient/family unit.

REFERENCE

Lack, S.A. (1976) Philosophy and organization of a hospice program. In: *First National Training Conference for Physicians on Psychological Care of the Dying Patient* (Ed. C.A. Garfield), University of California School of Medicine, San Francisco.

Confusional States

A. STEDEFORD

Sir Michael Sobell House and Warneford Hospital, Oxford, UK

Mental confusion is common in terminal illness. It is distressing to patients and their relatives, and disturbing to others in the ward. Unless there is an obvious and treatable cause here, patients are too often treated by sedation only, without much investigation, on the assumption that nothing more specific can be done to bring relief. This is partly because doctors commonly feel helpless when confronted with a confused patient as coherent conversation seems impossible and behaviour may be bizarre or disturbing. The majority of these patients can, however, be understood and helped, and it is always worthwhile attempting to do so. When successful we break through the fear and isolation which many confused patients experience, and doing this is an essential part of treatment.

A MODEL OF AWARENESS

Confusional states can be understood in terms of a model in which it is postulated that there is a filter which controls the quantity and quality of stimuli reaching consciousness at any moment. Figure 1 represents the experience of a normal person who is awake. The area within the circle represents the filter determining which stimuli will be allowed into consciousness from the environment via the sense organs, from the body (e.g. pain and excretory needs), and from the unconscious (e.g. memories, hopes and fears). The permeability of the filter varies; in the awake state more stimuli are allowed in from the environment than from the body or the unconscious. Incoming material is further selected according to expectations, memories or fears. A person hears something more readily if he is listening for it. Occasionally, he may misinterpret the sound he actually hears as one which he is expecting. The normal person recognized the course of the various components of his experience; the lines dividing the circle represent barriers which separate these three components.

Figure 2 represents the experience of normal sleep. The filter is now less permeable to stimuli from the environment and the body, so that only those messages that demand a response, such as the ring of the telephone or the sensation of a full bladder, reach awareness. Most of the experience comes from the unconscious as dreams and their content may be partly determined by the patient's current hopes or fears, as well as by memories of the past. The barriers between the three areas are less firm; the sound of the telephone may be woven into a dream before a person wakes up.

A. Stedeford

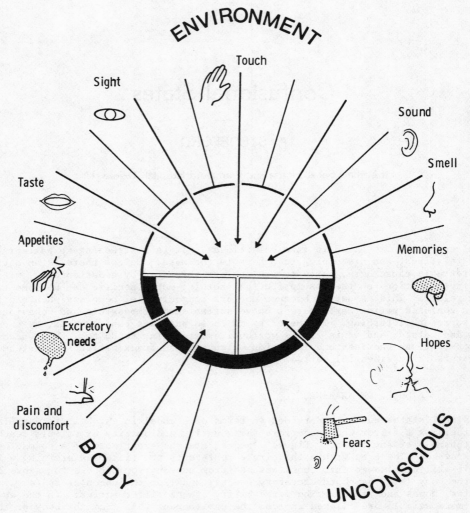

Fig. 1 AWAKE. Within the circle is the experience of the
individual at any one moment. He can choose which stimuli
to attend to and knows from which area they come. He
allows in only as much as he can handle. He selects
according to his purpose (consciously) and according to
his emotional set (unconsciously). Most of this experience
is related to the environment.

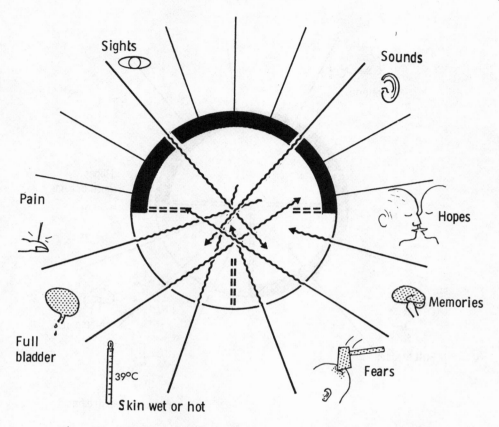

Sights

Sounds

Pain

Hopes

Full
bladder

Memories

39°C

Fears

Skin wet or hot

Fig. 2. ASLEEP. Most experience comes from the unconscious
as dreams. Only urgent stimuli, e.g. 'telephone' from outside or 'full bladder' from the body, are let in. Separation of the sources of stimuli is not so clear — telephones
can get into dreams.

Figure 3 represents confusional states. Drugs, organic and biochemical changes
may all lower the state of consciousness, shown here by the densness of the filter,
allowing less in from the environment. Bodily sensations such as pain enter more
easily, and may be misinterpreted. Unconscious material wells up and may be
experienced as nightmares, hallucinations, and a chaotic mixture of memories. The
barrier separating the components seem to break down so that the patient may not
know whether what he is seeing is happening in the outside world or is part of his
nightmare.

Table 1 shows how this model can be used to explain three abnormal experiences
commonly seen in patients who are terminally ill and confused. The state of consciousness, the physical stimuli, and the emotion set of the memories which the
patient is currently experiencing all combine to produce these experiences. Thus,
patient number 1 may be asleep or heavily sedated, hot and feverish, and frightened,
for instance, of dying. This could produce in him a nightmare of burning to death.
The appropriate management of this patient is to wake him up as fully as possible,
cool him down, and reassure him by explaining that he became frightened because he

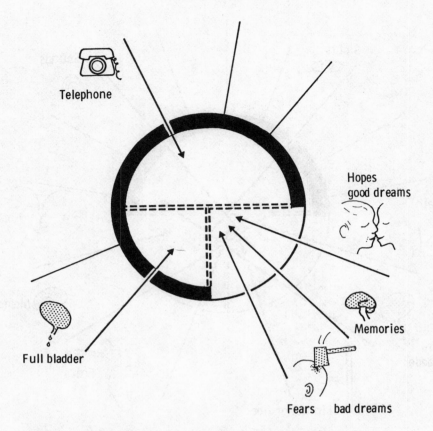

Fig. 3 CONFUSION. As in sleep, less enters from the
environment. Physical sensations and unconscious material
enter awareness more readily, but may be misinterpreted.
The separation between these three sources of experience
is poor.

TABLE 1   Components of Abnormal Experience

Patient	State of consciousness	Physical stimulus	Emotional sets, or memories	Abnormal experience
1	Asleep or sedated	+ Hot and feverish	+ Fear of dying →	Nightmare of burning to death
2	Awake but clouded or drugged	+ Seeing an unfamiliar person	+ Fear or guilt →	Seeing a frightening figure, e.g. a policeman
3	Twilight state or daydream	+ Seeing an unfamiliar person	+ 'Living in the past' or longing to see someone →	Seeing a relative

was very hot and too deeply asleep to realise what was wrong. If he does not accept this explanation and remains frightened, he may need to talk about the underlying fear and he should be given an opportunity to do so.

The second patient may be awake but suffering from clouding of consciousness when an unfamiliar person walks up to his bedside. If he is afraid or feeling guilty he may perceive that person as a frightening figure, for instance, a policeman. This is a misperception; a response to someone who is really there, and who is perceived as frightening because of the patient's mental state. Treating the cause of the clouding, and helping him to cope with his fear or guilt may stop these experiences.

It is common for patients to mistake strangers or hospital staff for near relatives. This comes about when a patient in a twilight state or day dream, living in the past or longing to see someone, misperceives an unfamiliar person as a member of his family. This is not an hallucination and should not be treated as such.

PHYSICAL CAUSES OF CONFUSIONAL STATES

The onset of a confusional state should always be an indication for a careful diagnostic review using as an aide-mémoire a check-list such as that in Table 2. If this is not done, treatable causes may be missed, especially if the development of the confusion is insidious and occurs in a patient who has already been in hospital for some time. The assumption that his confusion is an inevitable part of a general deterioration in his condition can lead to the patient being covered by a "blanket" of chlorpromazine in an attempt to provide symptomatic relief. This can further obscure the diagnosis and may even exacerbate the confusion.

TABLE 2   Common Causes of Confusion

Infection	whether pyrexial or not
Trauma	head injury subdural haematoma
Tumour	cerebral primary cerebral secondary non-metastatic
Cerebrovascular disease	strokes dementia
Cardiac and respiratory failure	anoxia hypercapnia

Biochemical and metabolic	electrolyte imbalance — dehydration
	                                          hyponatraemia
	                                          hypokalaemia
	hypercalcaemia
	uraemia
	hepatic failure
	hypoglycaemia

General discomfort	full bladder or bowel uncomfortable bedding pruritus

When physical examination and appropriate investigations reveal a reversible cause or precipitant this should be treated. Several days may elapse, however, before the treatment is effective and attention should be paid to the symptomatic management, including the psychological aspects, while the confusion persists.

THE USE AND EFFECTS OF DRUGS

Almost all patients are on some medication and an important step in elucidating the cause of any type of confusion is a review of the total intake of drugs. Often this increases as a problem escalates and various doctors prescribe additional drugs in an attempt to bring the situation under control. It is easy to overlook the fact that some analgesics and sedatives summate and night sedation may need to be reduced if narcotic analgesics are prescribed or increased. As a patient's condition deteriorates he may need smaller doses of drugs, especially if he is elderly. Idiosyncratic responses should be considered; for example, a few patients become hallucinated on morphine-like drugs especially pentazocine, and occasionally tricyclic antidepressants produce distressing agitation and nightmares as well as true hallucinations.

Sedatives should not be given routinely at night unless the ward is so noisy that there is no alternative. Instead, drugs should be prescribed to treat whatever symptoms are keeping the patient awake: adequate analgesics for pain; diazepam for anxiety; and tricyclic antidepressants where they are specifically indicated for the sleep disturbance characteristic of depression. Where pain and anxiety occur together chlorpromazine may be the most appropriate drug because it potentiates the analgesics as well as acting as a tranquillizer.

Some anxious agitated patients do well on chlorpromazine and badly on diazepam, or vice versa, so that failure with one is an indication to switch to the other. In extreme anxiety characterized by restlessness, compulsive talking, and a reluctance to be left alone, diazepam seems to be the most effective. Where purely sedative effects are needed, dichloralphenazone or nitrazepam is the drug of choice. Elderly patients sometimes become confused on nitrazepam, however, so it should be used with care. Barbiturates are contraindicated unless the patient has been on them for a long time; to choose a time of crisis and admission to strange surroundings as an opporunity to wean him off them is to invite a worsening of his condition due to withdrawal of the drugs to which he has become habituated.

It is tempting to increase sedation at night if there are recurrent nightmares. However, where fear is the underlying cause sedation does not seem to stop the terrifying dreams but only makes the patient too drowsy or confused to take in the explanations and reassurance that should be given.

In the acute confusional states where consciousness is already clouded but the patient is restless and unmanageable haloperidol is useful because it controls the agitation and any psychotic phenomena with less sedation than chlorpromazine. It may be given orally or by injection. In ill and debilitated patients the dose usually required is between 1.5 and 5 mg given eight-hourly.

THE PSYCHOLOGICAL PHENOMENA OF CONFUSION

The definitions and nomenclature used by different writers to classify confusional states are diverse and confusing. These can be simplified by considering two basic conditions: the acute brain syndrome, which is potentially reversible and often called delirium, and the chronic brain syndrome, which is not fully reversible because there is cell damage or loss and is usually called dementia (Table 3). It is also possible to have a mixture of the two.

TABLE 3   The Two Basic Confusional States

Acute brain syndrome (delirium)	Chronic brain syndrome (dementia)
reversible	irreversible
clouding of consciousness	consciousness usually clear
phenomena result from release	phenomena result from deficit

The acute brain syndrome is always characterized by clouding of consciousness, although this may entail only minor lapses of attention or slight difficulty in concentration. The condition fluctates from time to time, usually being at its worst late in the day and on first waking from sleep. It is a syndrome in which emotions that are usually controlled may be released and unconscious material (both neurotic and psychotic) that is suppressed in health may come into consciousness. Thus the naturally anxious person becomes agitated and the fearful terrified; the depressed person may become suicidal and the suspicious paranoid.

In the clouded state real people and objects are mis-identified and unconscious material that would normally only surface in dreams appears as hallucinations. Occasionally delusions are built up on the basis of these abnormal or distorted sensory experiences. Wolff and Curran (1935) in their classic paper on the nature of delirium and allied states quote a case of a patient who had a psychotic illness in clear consciousness, and then many years later in a toxic state reproduced exactly the same psychosis which cleared soon after the physical condition that precipitated it had resolved. Because the mechanism of symptom production is one of release the picture is a florid one; the emotional response to the experience is poorly controlled resulting in severe agitation and attempts to escape.

In contrast, the patient with the chronic brain syndrome has cell damage and his symptoms are the result of deficit rather than release. He is not usually anxious but shows poverty of affect, his emotions being superficial, inappropriate, and labile (Table 4).

TABLE 4   Clinical Pictures in the Acute and Chronic Brain Syndromes

	Acute brain syndrome	Chronic brain syndrome
Affect	++	—
	Agitation, terror, attempts to escape	Superficial, labile, inappropriate
Misinterpretations	+	+
Hallucinations	++	—
Psychosis	+	—
Reliving the past	Rambling and incoherent, hallucinatory, affect ++	Stereotyped, limited, affect —

Although the clinical pictures of the acute and chronic brain syndromes are so different in the aspects just described, there is a cluster of symptoms related to the cognitive functions of the brain which appears at first sight to be similar in the two conditions. This includes poor concentration, disorientation, impairment of short-term memory, and a tendency to go over the past (Fig. 4).

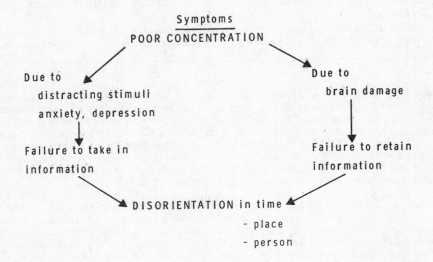

IMPAIRMENT OF

SHORT TERM MEMORY

(RELIVING THE PAST)

Fig. 4   Cognitive disturbances in acute and chronic brain
syndrome.

However, the mechanisms whereby the memory disturbance and so on are produced in
the two conditions are not the same. The patient with the acute brain syndrome has
clouding of consciousness and this together with the distracted emotional state
already described impairs his concentration and attention so that he fails to take
in much of what is going on around him. If he can concentrate well enough to
answer the questions, long-term memory is found to be intact. The patient suffering from the chronic brain syndrome also shows impairment of recent memory, mainly
because cell damage has interfered with his ability to retain information. The
material that has been acquired most recently is most readily lost, so that the
severely demented patient may be incapable of remembering anything that people have
tried to teach him recently but be able to say his tables or recite nursery rhymes
learned in his childhood.

The disorientation that both groups of patients show has two causes. The impairment of recent memory interferes with their learning about their current surroundings so that they may not be able to recognize where they are at present. In
addition, memories of the past may be more vivid for the patient than the stimuli
he is receiving from his environment. This leads him to misidentify places and
people, for instance thinking that he is back in his old home and that staff who
approach him on the ward are relatives he knew long ago.

Both groups of patients tend to relive the past, but the person with the acute
brain syndrome does so in a rambling and incoherent way. Fragments of memory from
different parts of his life seem to come and go with alarming rapidity, although
what he recalls is often closely related to past crises in his life, especially
other illnesses or occasions when he was in danger. The picture may be complicated

by hallucinations and is usually accompanied by emotional distress. In contrast, the demented patient may tell the same story from the past day after day. Sometimes he relives the emotions that accompanied the original event, but more often it is told with little or inappropriate feeling (Table 4).

From the above it is obvious that it is usually possible to make a clear distinction between the acute and chronic brain syndromes. Where this cannot be done the condition is probably a mixed one. The patient with early dementia learns to compensate while he is well and in familiar surroundings. When he is admitted to hospital this compensation breaks down, revealing the full extent of the dementia. He is especially sensitive to the toxic effects of illness and medication, which may then produce a superadded delirium. If such a patient can be cared for at home, some of this deterioration can be avoided. When admission is essential he should be accompanied as much as is practical by a familiar relative or friend and discharged home at the earliest possible opportunity. There he may be able to compensate again and recover almost to his former level.

SYMPTOMATIC MANAGEMENT OF CONFUSED PATIENTS

Delirium and dementia

It is important to distinguish between delirium and dementia because their management is quite different in some respects.

The delirious patient should be nursed in a well lit but quiet room with the minimum of staff changes and a reassuringly constant regimen. He may be helped by a tranquillizer such as diazepam, chlorpromazine, or haloperidol. The demented patient, on the other hand, is often made worse by any kind of sedation since it damps down the function of his already depleted brain cells. Early dementia is common in the elderly and should be tested for as it is easily missed in those patients who present a normal social facade. The quiet demented patient may be wrongly diagnosed as a depressive or may in fact be suffering from both conditions since awareness of mental deterioration can lead to reactive depression. Tricyclic antidepressants can make dementia worse and should be used with caution in these cases. In our limited experience, dexamphetamine 5 mg in the morning may be very effective for some patients. In others it causes irritability or confusion after an initial improvement and has to be discontinued.

Disorientation is a distressing symptom and may lead the delirious patient to suspect that he is becoming senile or even insane. He needs repeated reassurance about this and is more comfortable if his problems can be anticipated. A perplexed expression or a blank smile when he is approached should prompt staff to say who they are and why they have come before he has to ask or attempt to cover up his ignorance. He should be helped to orientate by giving him in the course of conversation the information he needs about where he is and the time of day. His mental state should not be formally reassessed unless it is essential to monitor the progress of his condition to determine changes in treatment. Attention to such details helps him to maintain his self-respect by minimizing the number of occasions when he is confronted by his deficit. He should never be laughed at, although there may be occasions when he is capable of laughing with the staff about mistakes he has made and this type of good humour may make it easier for him to tolerate his disability.

Disorientation in time may include reliving the past; terminally ill patients in particular may be preoccupied with reviewing their lives. If they become confused, their rambling conversation is only understandable to those who know something of their life history and family members should be asked if they can identify the

events and people the patient is talking about. It must be very disconcerting to
be in World War I at one moment and in hospital being offered a meal the next.
Failure to appreciate the perplexity of such a patient can lead to uncooperative
behaviour. He should be helped to reorientate by an explanation that enables him
to separate past and present and realize that the distressing experience happened
long ago.

If it is impossible to understand what is worrying the confused patient, it is
better to be honest with him than to pretend. Even in severe delirium a person may
have a lucid moment, perceive that his doctor is bluffing, and become suspicious.
In susceptible patients paranoid ideas can begin in this way. But the person who
shows concern that he has not understood leaves the patient with the knowledge that
someone sympathizes with his problem and still regards him as a rational being over
whom it is worth taking time and trouble.

Misperception, misinterpretation, and nightmares

Anyone in a general hospital who seems to be hearing voices is usually reported to
be hallucinated. Strictly, a hallucination is a sensory experience that is not
provoked by an outside stimulus, and most of these patients are not suffering from
hallucinations at all. They see or hear something that is really there, but
because of their mental state they experience it as something else. Thus a drowsy
and frightened patient who hears the telephone ringing may think it is a fire alarm
and struggle to get out of bed. Another who overhears snatches of conversation is
too confused to take them in and is worried about himself, so he may say that
people are talking about him. These are not hallucinations or paranoid delusions
but examples of misperception and misinterpretation. Management is often very
simple, as the following case shows:

> A ward sister was called to a women who was terrified and
> very restless. The patient said that she could hear many
> voices and that people were laughing at her. While the
> sister sat with her she too heard the voices and laughter
> which were coming through the thin wall from the adjacent
> kitchen. Moving the patient to a quiet room cured the
> "hallucinations" immediately. When she had partially
> recovered she could return to her previous ward because
> she understood where the voices came from and could dismiss
> them as irrelevant to her.

It is usually thought appropriate to darken a patient's room at night so that he
may go to sleep. However, in conditions where visual misperceptions are common
the room should be kept well lit. Then the patient can easily see the people and
objects around him and is less likely to imagine menacing shapes in the dark
corner or the drape of his dressing-gown on the chair. When distressed he may be
relieved if he can be wakened fully enough to take in the explanation that it is
his illness that is causing his symptoms and that they are likely to subside as he
recovers. When it is impossible to nurse such a patient in a side ward and he has
to be quietened for the sake of others, sedation has to be used and must be given
in sufficiently high doses to be effective. Because one cause of the condition is
impairment of consciousness, a slight increase in sedation may make the patient
worse by disinhibiting him further and causing him to be even less open to
reassurance.

Even heavy sedation may not be effective in relieving the distress of nightmares.
It may make the patient too weak and incoordinated to climb out of bed, but his
muttering and facial expressions signify to the observer that the frightening
experiences are still going on. As in delirium. nightmares are managed best by

waking the patient as fully as possible and reassuring him. If that is ineffective, as it often is, he should be given the opportunity to talk about the fears that may have provoked his dreams. This does not require specialized skill, only time to listen. A remark such as "Your nightmare makes we wonder if there is something real that is worrying you" may be quite sufficient to enable him to begin. In the night, defences that are firm in the day-time may be breached and he may confide, for example, that he has been worrying that he has terminal cancer. Such fears should be accepted and discussed as fully as the person who is there at the time feels he can. Once the subject has been opened up, further discussion with either the same person or a more experienced member of staff can help the patient to accept the reality of his situation. This often results in the cessation of the nightmares.

Hallucinations and delusions

Patients with the acute brain syndrome who present a particularly florid picture are often suffering from what used to be called a toxic psychosis. Common causes of this group of confusional states are the side effects of drugs or their withdrawal as exemplified by delirium tremens. As well as misperception these patients have hallucinations or, more rarely, delusions. Presumably hallucinations come from the unconscious and may be triggered off by the excitation of certain specific areas of the brain as happens when they form part of the seizure pattern in temporal lobe epilepsy. This condition is beyond the scope of this paper except to remind the reader that the diagnosis should be considered in any case where hallucinations are recurrent and stereotyped and there is reason to suspect a focal brain lesion. The distinction is important because these hallucinations are more likely to be controlled by antiepileptic drugs than by phenothiazines.

Patients experience auditory and visual hallucinations exactly as if they are real and it is frightening to the person who has insight to know that no one else can hear or see those things of which he is so compellingly aware. He often suspects that he is going mad and is usually relieved when others acknowledge the reality of the experience for him, explaining that it is his tumour, drugs, or illness that is causing it. In our experience patients find it more acceptable to know the cause of their symptoms even when it is a brain tumour, than to live with the fear of insanity. Some seem able to separate the concepts of 'myself' and 'my illness' and respond to regular reassurance that, however bizarre their experiences or behaviour may be, the staff still regard them as sane.

Patients who are hallucinated are sometimes relieved, at least temporarily, by surprisingly simple measures. A man who was convinced that there was a deep pit beside his bed into which he was about to fall lost this sensation when moved to another room.

Where medication is required chlorpromazine should be used if sedation would also be desirable. Trifluoperazine or haloperidol is preferable if the patient is already drowsy.

It is sometimes thought that all hallucinations are a sign of either drug effects or organic or psychiatric illness. Some normal people experience visual hallucinations in the twilight state before they fall asleep and many patients who have clouding of consciousness do the same. These are usually called hypnagogic hallucinations. It is also normal in the early stages of bereavement for people to experience hallucinations of the presence of the person who has recently died. As Wolff and Curran (1935) pointed out, the content of abnormal experiences is "primarily determined by ... the individual equipment and experience of the subject". This is well illustrated by the following case:

> A woman of 59 who has been suffering from disseminated
> breast cancer for a number of years began to have recurrent
> nightmares in which she was lying flat trapped in a box and
> struggling to push up the lid and get out. The experience
> also occurred in the day-time when it would come on suddenly
> while she was sitting alone but not asleep. The episodes
> made her pale and trembling. She was a very tense, anxious
> woman, but steadfastly denied that she had any unusual
> worries. In an attempt to break through this denial she was
> asked what she thought about telling people the truth about
> their illnesses. She replied: "It would be bad to know that
> you might be going to die soon because it would make you
> worry and have bad dreams." She was accurately describing
> herself, but she was not at that stage able to acknowledge
> the connection between her illness and her experiences.
> Within a few weeks she did come to accept her prognosis.
> Her anxiety became less and the hallucinations and night-
> mares ceased and did not recur in the remaining 7 months
> of her life.

On rare occasions it is right to accept a patient's beliefs or experiences as if
they were real:

> An elderly woman with bowel carcinoma had a well organized
> delusional system in which she believed there was a communist
> plot against the doctors. Attempts to reason with her made
> her distressed and antagonized her so that she refused all
> medication and wanted to discharge herself. Acceptance of
> her delusional system and reassurance that the matter was
> being taken care of brought peace.

Trial and error reveal which is the best course in each case, but management based
on reality should be tried first especially if the patient is likely to recover.

After a delirium or a psychotic episode some patients, as part of their total
recovery, go over their experiences trying to understand what has happened to them.
Explanations and reassurance that seemed ineffective when given may be recalled and
used at this stage, showing that they did in fact make an impression although there
was no response at the time. Tactless remarks made on the assumption that the
patient was too ill to understand may be remembered too. Therefore it is best to
assume that a person is aware of what is being said, however disturbed or deeply
unconcious he appears to be.

NEGATIVISM

Uncooperative behaviour often occurs in confused patients. The commonest cause is
simple failure to understand what they are required to do; in this case careful
and repeated explanations may solve the problem. Negativism in general may be the
way a patient expresses his anger and frustration at his plight and his desire to
maintain more control over events. Not since infancy have other people decided
when he will have his bath or go to the toilet and it is very irksome indeed to
have his freedom so drastically curtailed. Staff should constantly question how
much conformity is essential and allow each patient the maximum independence compatible with the smooth running of the ward. Irritability and impossible demands
are more easily tolerated by staff and relatives if they are able to recognize
that the patient's hostility is not necessarily directed at them personally. It
is easier for him to find fault with those around him and be angry with them than

to accept the reality that he is seriously ill or dying and be angry with fate or God or whoever he regards as responsible. Psychotherapy aimed at undoing this displacement and redirecting the anger onto its appropriate target enables the patient to face his situation and through catharsis and mourning reach acceptance. This often results in considerable improvement in his mood and relationships.

REFUSAL OF MEDICATION

Negativism often includes refusal of medication and the reason for this should always be sought. Occasionally patients find the side effects of drugs more unpleasant than the symptoms they are supposed to relieve and it may be appropriate to respect their refusal. In terminal illness in particular they should have the freedom and opportunity to say so if they think unpleasant treatment should come to an end. Many patients are reluctant to appear critical of the staff and hide fears such as that their medication is making them worse. On some occasions they are correct in their suspicions and on others they are confusing the effects of the drugs with the symptoms of their illness. Terminally ill patients may believe that certain medicines hasten death simply because they have seen a neighbouring patient die within a few days of starting a given mixture.

When refusal persists without good reason and the medication in question is essential, ways of persuading the patient should be varied according to his mental state. Coaxing as one would a child may be appropriate to the demented or regressed but is insulting to others. Disguising unwanted pills in something the patient likes is often satisfactory but is contraindicated if there is any tendency to paranoia. If such a patient discovered the trick, it would confirm his worst suspicions about the staff and he might then refuse food and drink also. Sometimes the paranoid or deluded patient can still trust a relative or one particular member of the staff and his help should be enlisted. There is almost always some way round the problem and force should never be used except on those rare occasions when patients are so disturbed that they have to be on an order for the safety of themselves or others.

When a patient makes a scene by threatening to be violent or walk out it is natural for extra staff members to come to the bedside to help. If possible, one person should handle the situation since confused and distraught patients feel very threatened by numbers. They feel much safer with one person, preferably sitting rather than standing beside them. The staff member in his turn may feel less comfortable and the understanding between colleagues should be such that he or she can count on someone else staying near at hand, able to intervene if necessary but out of sight of the patient until peace is restored.

FAMILY INVOLVEMENT

Mention has been made of relatives several times in this paper and their importance in the management of confusion should be clear. They may be reluctant to visit if they are afraid the patient will not recognize them or will behave strangely, since this naturally causes them distress. Sympathy from the staff together with an explanation of the cause of the confusion and what is being done to help may enable them to cope. They need to feel useful and their assistance should be sought in trying to understand what is worrying the patient and in reassuring him. They should be told that confused and stuporous patients hear and understand more than those around them suspect and that it is worth continuing to visit expecially if they can come at the time of day when the patient is at his best.

Families of patients who have been slowly deteriorating have often become adept in handling them and know the best ways of managing them without confrontation. Staff should be prepared to learn from relatives and to make use of them to gain the patient's confidence and cooperation.

Occasionally, confused patients seem to deteriorate markedly when visited, especially if a particular member of the family appears. This is not usually coincidental and a discreet enquiry may reveal that, for example, the marriage has been an unhappy one. If this is so and the partner concerned is coming mainly from motives of duty or guilt, a tactful suggestion that visiting need not be so long or frequent can bring relief to both.

THE AIM OF CARE

There are many confused patients for whom we can do nothing to treat the underlying condition and efforts must be concentrated on relieving their distress and that of their relatives. Some surprisingly good results can be obtained, as the following case history illustrates.

Mrs RG was a 58-year-old woman with a slowly growing parietal lobe tumour who was admitted when her hemiplegia became too severe for her to be cared for at home. The family found her very irritable and difficult; in hospital this behaviour alternated with periods of apathy and complete withdrawal. She knew her diagnosis and was preoccupied with thoughts of the tumour growing in her head. One day she seemed quite mad, sitting in her chair and angrily shaking a large watch that she had on a ribbon around her neck. Conversation was limited because of dysphasia; however, it eventually became evident that she was disorientated in time and was aware of it, but she displaced her anger onto the watch which she said was always wrong. Having been assured that it was not the fault of the watch she said something about "100 minutes".

Remembering how difficult brain-damaged people found transition to decimal currency, she was asked if she wondered whether time had been similarly changed. She did! She was looking for something on which to blame her disorientation and if "they" had decimalized time that would account for it. Having been told that they had not, she was quiet for a long interval and then said: "It's only a matter of time." This was taken up and this strange conversation switched to her realization that her time would soon come and that she could not know how long she had left to live. Through a tortuous route she came to express and accept this painful truth.

Following this conversation her whole attitude gradually changed; she became more friendly and cooperative and a rewarding patient to nurse. The episodes of confusion persisted but they no longer distressed her. In a lucid moment she said "I think it is perfectly logical that I should be confused", thereby indicating very astutely that she had reached that level of acceptance and peace that should be the aim of all care in confused but incurable patients.

ACKNOWLEDGEMENT

I am grateful to the Editor of the *British Journal of Hospital Medicine* for permission to print those parts of this paper which first appeared in Stedeford, A., "Understanding Confusional States", 20/6 December, 1978.

REFERENCE

Wolff, H.G. and Curran, D. (1935) *Archives of Neurology and Psychiatry*, <u>33</u>, 1175.

Physical Therapy and Rehabilitation

R. ZANOLLA and G. MARTINO

Istituto Nazionale per lo Studio e la Curie dei Tumori, Milan, Italy

INTRODUCTION

Lack of knowledge and scarcity of aids to make continued home care practical
cause patients and their families to seek admission, in the belief that being in
hospital guarantees the best support and care. Rehabilitation is not, however, an
automatic service offered by hospitals and, moreover, there is a reluctance to
engage in "patient re-education" in far-advanced cancer. This is a pity because
feelings of exclusion and isolation tend to increase during time in hospital as any
form of privacy with the family is discouraged and, when a person gets worse, he is
often segregated from the other inpatients.

Doctors, too, fail to recognise the place of rehabilitation in the care of patients
with cancer, and even centres equipped for physiotherapy are reluctant to admit
such patients. This disinclination is even more marked when the patient is terminal.
Yet, even when terminal, cancer patients benefit from rehabilitative skills, because
rehabilitation offers an extremely positive form of psychological support. With
these patients, the primary goals are:

1. occupational therapy;
2. prevention and management of the side effects of immobility;
3. continuation of such treatments in the patient's home, if feasible.

If the second goal can be achieved with a minimum of education there is a real
possibility of the patient being cared for again at home or in some form of
sheltered accommodation.

In this chapter, we describe the assistance given at the Division of Pain Therapy
and Rehabilitation of the Istituto Nazionale dei Tumori, Milano, to both outpatients
and inpatients who were admitted to the Division, despite failure to respond to
anti-tumour treatment.

METHODS

Physiotherapeutic procedures used in terminal cancer do not differ essentially from
those utilized for patients who need rehabilitation at earlier stages. Mobilization
and massage is used methodically for paraplegic and bedridden patients as the main
measures for the prevention and treatment of immobilization syndrome (Farneti, 1972).

193

This consists of venous stasis, stiffness of the joints, tendon contractions, respiratory insufficiency and bedsores. Without continued physiotherapy, the development of this syndrome may cause considerable discomfort, resulting in greater feelings of dejection and social isolation. Re-education of the bladder is instituted in paraplegic patients to reduce the risk of urinary infections (Archimbaud, 1974; Pearman and England, 1975; Zanollo and Redaelli, 1972). This consists of inducing the patient to urinate every two hours with Crede's and Valsalva's manoeuvres and giving him parasympathomimetic drugs that stimulate contraction of the detrusor muscle. These simple procedures produce a fairly good recovery of bladder function and may allow the catheter to be removed. Measurement of residual bladder volume and urine culture are, however, both necessary at regular intervals.

In terminal post-mastectomy patients, increasing lymphoedema of the ipsilateral arm may develop. This is sometimes accompanied by intense pain due partly to circulation stasis and partly to the weight of the limb. In addition, the weight can exacerbate the pain of an osteolytic lesion at the shoulder or of brachial plexus nerve compression. Our records include 20 patients with lymphoedema of whom 16 showed other complications such as pain, limited function of the scapulohumeral joint, brachial plexus palsy and carcinomatous lymphatic obstruction. Lymphoedema was treated with manual and mechanical massage. The device we use is a sleeve connected to a pump that exerts pressure rhythmically on the whole limb and removes excess fluid from the tissues. After each treatment the patient should in daytime wear an elastic support that exerts pressure on the limb continuously (Beninson, 1962; MacCaughey, 1968; Patrick Leis et al., 1966; Sanderson et al., 1965; Zanolla, 1977).

Motor deficit was treated by segmental mobilization, by electrostimulation with rectangular or triangular pulse currents of deficient muscles and by applications of splints intended to preserve adequate muscle function and to reduce scapulo-humeral joint block (Basso Ricci et al., 1976; Castaigne et al., 1969; Stevens, 1965; Wynn Parry, 1966, 1978). Supraclavicular or limb iontophoresis was used to reduce local inflammation.

Where pain was very intense treatment consisted of a series of local anaesthetic infiltrations of the stellate ganglion to produce a chemical sympathectomy and a consequential increase in the blood supply to the limb. This method was used in all cases in which the pain was thought to depend primarily on ischaemia. If the patient experienced paraesthesia or neuritic pain, transcutaneous electrostimulation was performed with direct current and rectangular pulses whose intensity, rate and duration varied with patients. The electrostimulator was positioned on the trigger point or along the cutaneous irradiation region of the involved trunks (Long, 1974; Ventafridda et al., 1979a). This treatment was always supplemented with a drug therapy including antidepressants (amitriptyline) and tranquillizers (fluphenazine) (Ventafridda, 1979b). Antibiotics and corticosteroids were administered to patients with lymphangitis.

Out of 20 patients with complications from progressive lymphoedema, only two patients failed to receive any benefit. Complete remission of oedema occured in four patients and a partial reduction of the limb's circumference with considerable subjective improvement was obtained in fourteen. In the group of ten patients reporting pain, complete remission was obtained in three and, in the other seven, pain was reduced to such an extent as to permit its control simply by means of anti-inflammatory agents. Only two out of thirteen patients with scapulohumeral joint block did not benefit at all from treatment. In the six patients with brachial plexus palsy almost no recovery in motor function was obtained. All patients with lymphatic obstruction achieved execellent resolution of associated inflammation, and thus of pain.

The best results were obtained with ostomy patients who, when first seen, were commonly in a state of absolute mental and physical isolation because of faecal incontinence, skin complications as a result of ill-fitting bags, and general lack of care through ignorance. If possible, re-education of the colostomy was achieved initially by means of irrigations. In all cases we tried to preserve skin and to treat its complications by means of individually chosen colostomy bags, protective patches and the topical application of mucosa and skin-protecting preparations (American Cancer Society, 1964; Gustosky, 1972; Muldoon, 1965; Postel et al., 1965; Rowbotham, 1970; Ventafridda and Zanolla, 1976).

Our records include 39 patients with an ileostomy or a colostomy: 31 were re-educated by means of daily stoma irrigations and eight treated simply with suitable topical applications to the surrounding skin. Twenty-four of the 31 cases treated with irrigations responded very well as far as the control of bowel function was concerned but seven patients did not benefit by the treatment or had to discontinue it on account of marked general deterioration. The skin problems of the eight patients were all solved by means of protective patches and appropriate bags.

The most difficult cases we have had to treat are patients with a fistula caused by neoplastic necrosis or as a severe after-effect of radiotherapy. In addition to a calorie-rich diet administered parenterally to improve the patient's general state, the discharge from a fistula must be kept from contact with the skin by using a suitable drain. This will help prevent further complications such as local pain, ulceration and infection. A good skin barrier can be obtained by combinations of a modern stoma appliance, karaya gum or paste and "Stomahesive" (a compressed wafer of gelatin, pectin and methylcellulose which can be cut to shape around the fistulous opening) (Knighton and co-workers, 1976; Gross and Irving, 1977). These were used with good effect in every case.

Finally, we should like to stress that, until death, we adopt a combined psychological and physical approach to the terminally ill patient and his family, trying to create both a technical and a personal relationship with the patient and so satisfy his actual needs (Martino, 1979). Moreover, where possible the patient was encouraged to engage in occupational therapy for diversional purposes. Psychological benefit was undoubtedly derived from this type of activity and consisted of a definite reduction of both pain and feelings of isolation and fear.

CONCLUSIONS

The terminal cancer patient can and should receive rehabilitative care in order to minimize physical and mental isolation. Our results demonstrate that rehabilitative goals can be achieved with such patients. It much be emphasized, however, that physical therapy and rehabilitation should not be used on their own but only within the context of total patient care, including adequate psychosocial support.

REFERENCES

American Cancer Society (1964) *Care of Your Colostomy: a Source Book of Information.* New York: American Cancer Society.

Archimbaud, J.P. (1974) Les dysfunctionements vesico-sphincteriens neurologiques. 68 Session Association Francaise d'urologie. Masson (Paris).

Basso Ricci, S., Ventafridda, V., Zanolla, R. Cassani, A., Spreafico, R. (1976) Presentazioni di 25 casi di lesione post-irradiatoria del plesso brachiale e loro trattamento. *Tumori*, 62.

Beninson, J. (1961) Six years of pressure, gradient therapy. *Angiology*, 12.

Castaigne, P., Laplane, D., Degos, J.D., Ammoumi, J.A. (1969) A proposes des paralysies du plexus brachial après cancer du sein. *Presse Med.*, 77, 1801-1804.

Farneti, P. (1972) Terapia Fisica e Riabilitazione. Pubblicazione A. Wasserman, 11.

Gross, E. and Irving, M. (1977) Protection of the skin around intestinal fistulas. *Br. J. Surg.*, 64, 258-263.

Gustosky, F. (1972) Ostomy procedure nursing care before and after. *Am. J. Nurs.* 72(2).

Knighton, D.R., Burus, K. and Nyhus, L.M. (1976) The use of stomahesive in the care of the skin of enterocutaneous fistulas. *Surg. Synec. Obstet.*, 143, 449.

Irving, M. (1977) Local and surgical management of enterocutaneous fistulas. *Br. J. Surg.*, 64, 690-694.

Long, D.M. (1974) External electrical stimulation as a treatment of chronic pain. *Min Med.*, 57, 195-198.

MacCaughey, A.M. (1968) A comprehensive physical therapy program for the post-mastectomy lymphedema patient. *45th Annual American Physical Therapy Association Conference*, Chicago, June 30.

Martino, G. (1979) Aspetti sociali, familiari ed internieristici nel trattamento del cancro in fase molto avanzata. In: *La Chemioterapia del Tumori Solidi* (Ed. Pannuti), Vol. 11, 786-790.

Muldoon, J.P. (1965) A new concept in patient care: abdominal stomal therapy. *Mich. Med.*, 64, 664.

Patrick Leis, M., Bowers, J.M.J., Dursi, J. (1966) Postmastectomy edema of arm. *N.Y. State J. Med.*, 66.

Pearman, J.W., England, E.J. (1975) *The Urological Management of the Patient Following Spinal Cord Injury*. Charles C. Thomas (USA).

Postel, A.H., Grier, W.R.N., Localio, S.A. (1965) The rehabilitation of the colostomy patient. In: *A Conference on Research Needs in the Rehabilitation of Persons with Disabilities Resulting from Cancer*. U.S. Dept. H.E.W. Vocational Rehabilitation Adm. and Institute of Physical Medicine and Rehabilitation, New York Univ. Medical Center.

Rowbotham, J.L. (1970) The stoma rehabilitation clinic. *Dis. Colon Rectum*, 13, 59.

Sanderson, R.G., William, S., Fletcher (1965) Conservative management of primary lymphedema. *Northwest Med.*, 64, 584-588.

Stevens, J.H. (1965) Brachial plexus paralysis. In: *The Shoulder* (Ed. E.A. Codman), pp. 332-399. Boston, Mass.   (2nd Edition)

Ventafridda, V., Zanoola, R. (1976) La riabilitazione dei colostomizzati. *Minerva Chirurgica*, 3(8), 368-374.

Ventafridda, V., Sganzerla, E.P., Fochi, C., Pozzi, G., Cordini, G. (1979a) Transcutaneous nerve stimulation in cancer pain. *Adv. Pain Res. Ther.*, 2, 509-514.

Ventafridda, V., Sganzerla, E.P. and Fochi, C. (1979b) Considerazioni sull'uso di sostanze psicotrope ad azione antidepressiva in terapia antalgica. *Minerva Med.*, 70.

Wynn Parry, C.B. (1966) *Rehabilitation of the Hand*. London: Butterworth.

Wynn Parry, C.B. (1978) Management of peripheral nerve injuries and traction lesions of the brachial plexus. *Internat. Rehab. Med.*, 1(1), 9-20.

Zanollo, A. and Redaelli, E. (1972) Profilassi et terapia delle complicazioni settiche del cistoplegico da lesione midollare. *La Riabilitazione*, 5(2).

Zanolla, R. (1977) La riabilitazione fisica delle pazienti mastectomizzate. In: *I Tumori della Mammella* (Eds. U. Veronesi, A. Perussia, H. Emanuelli and M. De Lena), pp. 401-407. C.E.A.

V
NUTRITION

Enteral (Tube) Feeding

M. E. SHILS

Departments of Medicine, Memorial Sloan-Kettering Cancer Center and Cornell
University Medical College, New York City, New York, USA

ABSTRACT

When voluntary and adequate ingestion of food by mouth is not possible,
alternative routes of feeding the cancer patient must be utilized in order to
prevent or treat malnutrition. The alternatives are enteral (tube) or intravenous
feeding. If the intestinal tract is patent, tube feeding is an attractive
alternative to the parenteral route. The factors of feasibility, safety and
potential complications, expertise, patient receptivity, duration of treatment and
costs to patient and hospital must be considered in deciding which alternative
to use. Enteral feeding is useful in conditions when there is 1) severe and
persistant anorexia, 2) presence of a fistula or obstruction of the upper
alimentary tract when the tube can be placed to bypass them and 3) severe
malabsorption requiring slow and continuous administration of a liquid formula to
permit absorption. Tubes may be placed via the nasopharnygeal, esophagostomy,
gastrostomy or jejunostomy routes. The composition of the formula to be fed will
depend upon the absorptive capacity of the patient and coexisting physiologic
and metabolic status. Many useful commercial formulas (defined formula diets for
medical use) are now available. Their proper use requires knowledge of composition,
cost and an awareness of nutritional and metabolic needs of the individual.

INTRODUCTION

While it is desirable to have patients voluntarily ingesting an adequate diet
orally, a significant number of cancer patients are not able to do so. Alternative
routes must be considered and appropriate action taken when depletion is already
present, when a potentially debilitating situation is likely to be extended
without expectation of immediate significant improvement, or when plans for cancer
treatment are likely to prelude adequate oral intake or absorption for a
significant time.

The development of malnutrition often presents a major problem in terms of patient
well-being and management. A large number of undesirable metabolic and physiologic
problems occur which express themselves in progressive weakness, weight loss,

M.E. Shils

increased susceptibility to infection and interference with the treatment program (Shils, 1979).

When either tube or intravenous route is necessary, the preferable alternative will depend on an assessment of a number of variables. The factors of feasibility, safety and potential complications, expertise at hand, patient receptivity, duration of treatment, and cost to the hospital and patient must be considered in determining these alternatives.

If the small intestine is patent, and if the patient is unable to ingest food orally, tube feeding into the alimentary tract is an attractive alternative if aspiration is not a significant potential danger. Situations in which tube feeding should be considered as the alternative include (1) severe and persistent anorexia; (2) a fistula or obstruction in the upper alimentary tract where feeding may be given through a tube so placed as to bypass the fistula or obstruction; and (3) severe malabsorption requiring the administration of a formula that must be fed slowly over many hours to permit absorption.

TUBE FEEDING SITES

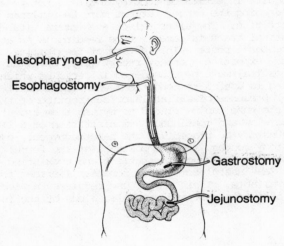

Fig. 1

ENTRY SITES FOR TUBES (Figure 1)

A nasopharyngeal tube should have its tip in the lower esophagus rather than in the stomach to avoid interference with the lower esophageal sphincter thus reducing the chance of reflux especially when the patient is supine. In the majority of patients such a tube is easily and safely placed and replaced. When required for long periods, patients can be taught to remove and reinsert the tubes themselves after each feeding.

Many cancer patients have had prior experience with nasal tubes for aspiration following surgery and are opposed to further encounters with them. We have found that small caliber silicone elastomer (silastic) or other pliable plastic tubes are much better tolerated than are the usual larger and more rigid polyethylene or rubber feeding tubes. Very small catheters of the type used for central venous cannulation are also well tolerated. Once induced to allow insertion of a small tube, the patient is often willing to keep it in place, even in the presence of esophagitis. If they tend to be expelled on regurgitation or coughing, this may be overcome by using mercury weighted tubes. Small-bore tubes require a finely dispersed formula to prevent plugging of the tube.

The potential for aspiration of formula must always be considered. This hazard is increased in debilitated patients having depressed cough reflexes and a preexisting pulmonary problem and may require intravenous feeding. To minimize aspiration in all tube-fed patients, it is essential that strict procedures be adhered to by the staff. These include preliminary testing with water and then dilution of the formula at slow infusion rates and progressive increases while monitoring the ability of the patient to tolerate the formula. The patient should be in a semi-sitting or sitting position during the feeding and for a period afterwards. The potential for aspiration is decreased by slow drip feeding from a bag or bottle and by passage of a mercury-weighted tube into the jejunum.

An esophagostomy tube may be inserted into the esophagus through the lower neck as an alternative to nasopharyngeal or gastrostomy tubes for long-term feeding. This procedure is simpler to perform than a gastrostomy and eliminates the psychological and social problems faced by a patient who has to walk around with a tube protruding from his nose. It is an alternative to a jejunostomy tube for unobstructed patients who have had a subtotal gastrectomy or esophagogastrectomy with the stomach drawn up into the chest.

The gastrostomy tube is valuable for patients who are likely to need tube feedings for prolonged periods of time. The Stamm gastrostomy closes quickly when the tube has been removed. Directions to nursing staff, patient and family are necessary to prevent leakage around the tube and to insure proper skin care at the entry site.

A jejunostomy tube is indicated when there is obstruction at a higher level. The availability of finely dispersed formulas that flow easily through fine bore tubes has made feasible the use of a very small catheter inserted at surgery through the intestinal wall by means of a needle (Page, Ryan and Hoff, 1976).

Rapid entry of hyperosmolar solutions into the jejunum may lead to the "dumping syndrome." This potential problem can be prevented by initially infusing the formula at reduced concentration and rate with increases as tolerance is demonstrated. Use is recommended of complete liquid formulas of relatively low osmolality. Intrajejunal feeding presents the possibility of inadequate mixing of the formula with bile and pancreatic juice with resultant depressed digestion. While usually not a significant problem, it can be overcome by employing certain ingredients such as pancreatic extract, medium-chain triglycerides, oligosaccharides, protein hydrolysate or free amino acids which can be absorbed without further digestion by pancreatic enzymes.

FORMULA COMPOSITION

A wide variety of foods in blended or finely dispersed form may be used in the tube feeding of those patients in whom digestion and absorption are normal.

Knowledge of the widespread occurrence of lactose intolerance in various population groups and in those with bowel disease has resulted in marked modification of
the usual hospital tube formula which was,in the past, based primarily on milk and
milk products. Hospital tube formulas with lower milk concentrations have been
developed with the added advantage that various nutrients, such as fat, sodium,
and potassium can be easily modified (Shils, Bloch and Chernoff, 1976). Commercial formulas with little or no lactose are available. Some patients accustomed
to regular bowel elimination may be unhappy with low residue formulas that cause
them to be "constipated."

Physicians and dietitians should give consideration to the costs as well as the
composition of tube feeding formulas for in-patients and out-patients. Those
patients requiring tube feeding who do not have absorptive disorders do not need
expensive "chemically defined" type diets with crystalline amino acids and their
special constituents.

DEFINED-FORMULA DIETS FOR MEDICAL PURPOSES

In recent years there has been an outpouring from the pharmaceutical industry of
special liquid formulations. Some have been termed "elemental" or "chemically
defined" diets but I prefer the more general term "defined-formula" diets. Their
numbers and diversity in composition have created a field requiring special expertise on the part of the physician and dietitian who are faced with decisions on
their use. Many are claimed by the manufacturers to be complete in all essential
nutrients, but little data have been published on nutrient stability with storage
under various conditions. Some are composed of purified amino acids (both essential and non-essential) with only small amounts of fat as polyunsaturated fats and
with carbohydrates as glucose oligosaccharides. Others have their amino acids
predominantly in the form of hydrolysed protein with amino acid supplementation.
Others incorporate intact proteins. Fat is present usually as long chain triglycerides high in polyunsaturates; in some preparations there is a proportion of
medium-chain triglycerides. Carbohydrates vary in type and quantity. All have
added minerals, trace elements and vitamins. A compendium of available commercial
defined-formula diets has been published (Shils, Bloch and Chernoff, 1976).

Such commercial diets are both a boon and a problem to the physician and dietitian.
They are nutritionally complete and are easy to store, order, and administer.
Serious problem, however, may arise because such formulas are of "fixed" compo-
sitions. Patients with certain metabolic conditions may be unable to tolerate
the amounts of one or more nutrients when a formula is given in the volume necessary to meet overall nutritional requirements. Such a formulation may, in fact,
be hazardous for such patients because of the development of adverse effects.
This is true, for example, of patients with renal disease who cannot tolerate the
levels of protein, sodium, potassium, phosphate or magnesium present in the diet.
The physician must be aware of specific composition and possible contraindications.
In these situations, the dietitian must modify the formula by either adding desired ingredients, which dilute the undesirable ingredients, or preparing a completely different preparation from specific nutrients.

The hospital dietitian should be able to prepare nutritionally adequate formulations designed to meet special metabolic needs according to the physician's prescription. Purified individual nutrients (e.g. amino acids, protein, protein
hydrolysates, oligosaccharides and other carbohydrates, fats and vitamins and
minerals) are commercially available and can be combined as required (Shils,
Bloch and Chernoff, 1976).

OTHER PRECAUTIONS IN FEEDING

The volume, calories and nutritional composition of the formula supplied should meet the needs of the individual. There is a serious tendency on the part of many physicians, nurses and family to underfeed patients via tube even though precise recommendations have been made by the nutrition team. Continuing education and oversight are essential to ensure achievement of nutritional goals. When serious absorption problems exist, slow continuous feeding utilizing a pump is often essential. Because large amounts of water, protein, carbohydrate and other nutrients may be involved in the use of some defined-formula diets, the patient should be followed initially as closely as those started on intravenous feeding. The formula should be stayed in decreased concentration and at reduced volume per time period. Serial physical examination, laboratory studies, urine fractionals, and weighing should be standard practice with frequency dictated by the patient's response. Hyperosmolar nonketotic coma may occur in diabetic patients on high carbonhdrate tube-fed formulas when adequate precautions are not taken. There may be exacerbation of metabolic problems related to protein intake in patients with renal and hepatic disorders. Serious losses of water and electrolytes may result from diarrhea with tube feedings in patients with serious malabsorption secondary to bowel fistulas or the short bowel syndrome.

SPECIAL USES OF DEFINED-FORMULA DIETS

Effects on enteric organism. The possibility of markedly reducing the concentration and types of microorganisms in the large bowel through the use of defined-formula diets was one of the initial claims (Winitz, Adams, Seedman etal, 1970). Subsequent reports have been unable to duplicate these results (Shils, 1977). It has been uniformly found that the concentration of bacteria in the feces was unaffected by the test diet; however, since the fecal volume was markedly decreased, the total number of organisms delivered from the large bowel also declined during the feedings. Nevertheless, the numbers of organisms in the large bowel were still enormous.

Preventing intestinal epithelial damage. There are conflicting claims concerning a possible protective effect of certain defined-formula diets against the deleterious effects of chemotherapeutic agents on intestinal epithelium of small experimental animals. More data on this subject is necessary.

Gastric and pancreatic secretion. It may be desirable to minimize pancreatic secretions in cancer patients with pancreatic fistulas or with large intestinal fluid losses following bowel damage by radiation and resection. Data obtained in dogs using various formulas with casein hydrolysate or purified amino acids indicate that gastric secretion is reduced, compared with regular diets. Intrajejunal administration of such formula diets reduces pancreatic secretion; however, intravenous feeding is more effective than intrajejunal feeding in reducing secretion (Shils, 1977).

Treatment of fistulas of the alimentary tract. These formulations are useful as a source of nutrition fed through a tube with its tip placed beyond high bowel fistulas, such as those in the esophagus, duodenum, or upper jejunum. During maintenance of good nutrition such fistulas may and often do close spontaneously. When an upper fistula cannot be by-passed or when tube feedings lead to serious fluid losses and skin excoriation, parenteral nutrition is preferable. When the fistula is present in distal small bowel or colon, slow tube feedings are often useful in maintaining nutrition and providing opportunity for fistula closure. It should be remembered that a patient with a resected, by-passed of damaged terminal ileum is unable to reabsorb efficiently his conjugated bile salts. The entry of bile salts into the colon may result in diarrhea. This "choleretic diarrhea" may respond dramatically to cholestyramine.

Malabsorption syndromes. The requirement for and successful use of defined-form-ula diets will depend on the degree of malabsorption. Those patients who have such severe malabsorption that they cannot be successfully maintained even on an optimum tube formulation will require supplementary intravenous feeding or total intravenous feeding. For patients with somewhat lesser degrees of malabsorption "pre-digested" types of formulations may be useful particularly when fed slowly. Crystalline amino acids, short chain peptides or hydrolyzed protein may be used in conjunction with mixtures of mono, di and oligosaccharides and sufficient water, vitamins, minerals and trace elements to make up for expected losses in stool or fistula drainage. Initially, fats should be restricted and then gradually added as tolerance is demonstrated. MCT may be useful in such patients. Lactose-con-taining foods should be added cautiously until tolerance is proven. At the other end of the spectrum are those with mild to moderate malabsorption who do not re-quire the highly purified formulations and who do well with more normal types of diets taken by mouth or tube and with supplements of defined-formula diets of proper composition and rate of feeding. Tube feedings can be administered suc-cessfully in very young infants with malabsorption as well as in children and adults.

Treatment of organ failure. Because of depressed appetite, frequent nausea, and lethargy seen in patients with serious renal dysfunction, oral intake of diets with restricted protein and electrolytes is often poor. Administration of form-ulas by tube may therefore be highly desirable. Special diets with essential amino acids including histidine are now available for those with advanced renal failure; however, diets containing restricted amounts of intake protein may do just as well provided caloric intake is adequate. Recent research indicates that patients with hepatic failure and porto-caval shunting (Fischer etal,1976) and those with serious sepsis (Freund, Ryand and Fischer,1978) may benefit by feeding amino acid mixtures with increased amounts of branched-chain amino acids and lesser amounts of aromatic amino acids. Formulation with such composition are becoming available for oral or tube feedings.

ROUTE OF FEEDING AND INTESTINAL EPITHELIUM

Short-term fasting leads to decreases in weight, DNA, protein, glycolytic enzyme and disaccharidase concentrations of the small bowel. Entry of food into the alimentary tract increases hyperplasia of the epithelium of intact and postresec-tion residual bowel when compared to the situation when nutrition is supplied solely by the intravenous route. An important factor in maintaining organ mass and composition is the passage of food through the alimentary tract with its stim-ulus to endocrine and paracrine secretions and consequent trophic effects. There is also evidence that intraluminal nutrition augments small intestinal mass by direct contact with eipthelial cells and indirect effects of hormonal or neuor-vascular stimuli (Williamson, 1978).

REFERENCES

Fischer, J.E., H.M. Rosen, A.M. Eibeid, J.H. James, J.M. Keane, and T.P. Soeters (1976). The effect of normalization of plasma amino acids on hepatic enceph-alopathy in man. Surgery, 80, 77-90.
Freund, H.R., J.A. Ryan Jr, and J.E. Fischer: Amino acid derangements in patients with sepsis: treatment with branched chain amino acid rich infusions. Ann. Surg., 188, 423-429 (1978).

Page, C.P., J.A. Ryan, Jr., R.C. Haff (1976). Continual catheter administration
    of an elemental diet. Surg. Gynecol. Obstet. 142, 184-188.
Shils, M.E. (1977). Enteral nutrition by tube. Cancer Res. 37, 2432-2439.
Shils, M.E. (1979). Principles of nutritional therapy. Cancer, 43, 2093-2102.
Williamson, R.C.N. (1978). Intestinal adaptation. New Engl. J. Med.298, Pt.1,
    1293-1402; Pt. 2, 1444-1450.

Parenteral Nutrition at Home

M. E. SHILS

Departments of Medicine, Memorial Sloan-Kettering Cancer Center and Cornell
University Medical College, New York City, New York, USA

ABSTRACT

Advances in human nutrition enable long-term maintenance of patients in good
nutritional status entirely by the intravenous route. The technique of home
total parenteral nutrition (HTPN) is applicable to patients with persistant
severe malabsorption, obstruction and vomiting. The technique of HTPN requires
an indwelling central venous catheter, meticulous attention to prevent infection
and provision of adequate nutrients, fluid, electrolytes, trace elements and
vitamins. Patients are taught to make their own solutions and to administer them
at home. The criteria for eligibility for HTPN, special needs and procedures for
catheter change and infection management are described.

The great majority of patients on total parenteral nutrition (TPN) in the usual
hospital setting do not require this type of feeding for more than one month. In
our experience this is 85 percent of the patients. However, a small but
significant percentage of the patients require TPN for more than two or three
months. These patients usually have one or more of the conditions listed in
Table 1.

TABLE 1 Clinical States Requiring Prolonged TPN

1. Severe malabsorption and fluid and electrolyte
   losses not responding to oral and/or tube feeding in:

   a. Inflammatory bowel disease with bowel resection
   b. Severe radiation enteritis with bowel resection
   c. Massive bowel resection
   d. Small bowel fistula

2. Persistent bowel obstruction or ileus

3. Persistent nausea and vomiting - usually with long term
   high dose chemotherapy

There are common objectives in providing parenteral nutrition for both short term and long term patients. These are listed in Table 2. However, these goals become particularly important for long term patients. For example, one might be willing to perform a percutaneous insertion of a venous catheter into a subclavian vein once a week for two or three weeks but one would not wish to do this over many months because of the increasing danger to the patient of pneumothorax and of damage to the endothelium of the blood vessel. Since one can never be absolutely certain that a potential short term patient will not develop into a long term patient, one must try to meet the objectives in Table 2 from the initiation of TPN.

TABLE 2 Objectives of Long Term TPN
- In Hospital and at Home -

1. Long term patent CVC with minimal endothelial damage

2. Protection against infection, toxicity, and particulate matter

3. Provision of all nutritional needs

To avoid frequent percutaneous insertion of new central venous catheters, I have for many years exchanged catheters over a sterile flexible steel guidewire whenever the catheter is functioning poorly or when septicemia is suspected. This procedure has virtually eliminated pneumothoraces, subclavian thrombosis, and improperly placed catheters. The technique is simple and rapid. Catheters can be replaced frequently if one is concerned about continuing sepsis. Changes over a guidewire are preformed on in-patients and out-patients.

To help protect against extraneous infection and particulate matter in solutions, in-line filters are used. We know that the particulate matter is present in solutions in the form of cellulose fibers and tiny particles of rubber and glass. It seems to be important to remove these so that they do not end up in the lungs of the patients on long-term feeding.

To further minimize risk of infection, the filter and the tubing from the filter to the central venous catheter and the dressings over the catheter are changed twice weekly by trained nurses using sterile technique.

Blood sampling may not be performed or blood given through the central venous catheter; however, we allow other solutions, particularly electrolyte solutions to be given through the filter. For the long term patients we are careful to avoid overdosage of Vitamins A and D. We monitor frequently the blood levels of all of the electrolytes as well as trace elements. Copper and manganese are given to patients with biliary obstruction with caution and with serial blood determinations since the bile is the major source of excretion of these two potentially toxic trace elements.

To insure that all nutritional needs are met, nutrients are provided from the initiation of TPN since many of the patients are already malnourished when we see them in consultation. Patients with large gastrointestinal fluid losses are particularly likely to be deficient in potassium, magnesium, and zinc. Our vitamin regimen includes biotin and all other water soluble and fat soluble vitamins believed to be essential for man. In order to provide essential fatty acids, these are given once or twice weekly as 500 ml of 10 percent intravenous fat emulsion. A sample of a formulation for a long term TPN patient is given in Table 3.

TABLE 3 Example of a TPN Formulation for Long-Term Use*

	Volume (ml)	kcal	Na (mEq)	K (mEq)	Mg (mEq)	Ca (mEq)	P (mg)
Amino Acids (10%)	750	400					
Dextrose (50%)-water	750	1700					
Sodium chloride (0.9%). . . .	750		117				
Potassium chloride(2mEq/ml)	20			40			
Potassium phosphate	5			22			420
Sodium acetate (2mEq/ml). . .	20		40				
Magnesium sulfate (50%) . . .	6				26		
Calcium gluconate (10%) . . .	30					14	
TOTAL	2331	2100	157	62	26	14	420

Additives per week: MVI, 5ml x2; Berocca C; 2ml x1; Folate, 1.5mg x2; B$_{12}$, 100mcg x1, Vitamin K, 2mg x1; Zn^{++}, 18mg; Cu^{++}, 5mg; Mn^{++}, 0.25mg; I$^-$, 0.05mg; Cr^{+++}, 0.06mg; 10% Intralipid, 500ml.

*Short bowel syndrome; diarrhea 0.75L/day; normal weight

For the patients on TPN who are diabetic for whatever reason, regular insulin is given intravenously in the TPN solutions. Such patients also have urine glucose measured every six hours with coverage of regular insulin as required in the event that a patient develops increased insulin needs with the sudden onset of infection.

Additional problems and needs arise for the patient who is considered a candidate for home TPN (HTPN). My criteria for suitability for discharge on HTPN are in-dicated in Table 4. Patients vary greatly in their clinical status and prognosis, their will to live, the need and degree of support of their family members, and, sometimes, the outcome of an illness is much in doubt. Consequently, I prefer not to be too rigid in some of these criteria and place words like "reasonable" and "many" in quotation marks to indicate that this is a flexible matter depend-ing on the individual situation. Another reason for not being too rigid is the fact that we know relatively little concerning how patients with advanced cancer will live with or without antitumor treatment so long as adequate nutrition is provided. This is a type of patient that has never existed before and I believe that we can learn from such patients.

TABLE 4 Patient Suitability Criteria for Home Total Parenteral Nutrition

1. Relatively stable clinical state
2. Expectancy of "reasonably" comfortable home life for "many" months
3. Supportive home environment
4. Presence of another individual competent in HTPN techniques
5. Initial availability of a trained visiting nurse
6. Availability of a physician and other clinical support services

Assuming that a patient has met these criteria, one must consider additional needs which are listed in Table 5. One does not make the decision for HTPN lightly since it imposes serious problems and obligations for the patient, the physician and the hospital. My policy has been to have the patient or member of the family prepare the nutrient solutions at home from commercial parenteral solutions and pharmaceuticals supplied by the hospital. Such solutions are added to sterile plastic bags. Even with this procedure the cost to the patient without any profit to the hospital is at least $50. per day. If the patient is required to obtain the mixed solution from the hospital pharmacy, the price will be double or triple this amount. There are additional costs of an infusion pump, laboratory analyses and visits to the physician. On the other hand, this is a life saving procedure which, if the underlying disease permits, will allow long survival in good physical condition.

TABLE 5 Special Needs for Home Total Parenteral Nutrition (HTPN)

1. Patient-family education in HTPN
2. Assurance of safe preparation and administration of solutions
3. Adequate provision of nutrients, supplies and equipment
4. Assurance of adequate medical follow-up and emergency care
5. Allowance of as normal a life-style as possible
6. Meeting economic and social needs

My service has a team of trained physicians, dietitians, nurses and pharmacists who educate the patient and families of all aspects of HTPN including preparation and administration of the solution and closing the catheter with a heparin lock. The majority of patients infuse the solutions over eight to twelve hours at night and are then free of solutions and tubing for the rest of the twenty-four hours.

Patients are seen initially once weekly following discharge and then at increasingly longer intervals up to every four to five months.

It has been my policy since we initiated HTPN to utilize a central venous catheter inserted by percutaneous venopuncture into the subclavian or jugular veins. I believe that it is essential to change a catheter rapidly and without the need for a surgical procedure for patients who develop fever or have a catheter problem. As indicated above the change is over a guidewire.

Our TPN nurse acts as the first contact in case a patient has a problem at home.

We recognize only one emergency and that is the sudden onset of chills and fever. This requires an immediate visit to our emergency room, evaluation of the patient (including urinalysis, chemistries, white count and chest X-ray), change of the central venous catheter over a guidewire and the taking of blood for culture. If sepsis is believed to be present, antibiotics are initiated. In the early years of our HTPN program all such patients were admitted to the hospital. However, we have gained such assurance by our experience that now only elderly patients or those with unstable cardiovascular-pulmonary systems are admitted. All others are started on broad spectrum antibiotic coverage and sent home. They prepare and infuse their own antibiotic solutions on a prescribed schedule through their central catheters. The patient telephones daily with a progress report. The status of the cultures in the laboratory are followed daily and antibiotics are stopped, continued or modified on the basis of the reports. If the patient has not improved within 24 to 36 hours he/she is admitted. For those patients who are admitted, the duration of stay is only long enough to obtain a definitive culture report and insure clinical stability. The patient is then discharged either with no antibiotics or on the antibiotics indicated by the culture reports.

With the exception of myself, all other physicians in the U.S.A. or Canada who have patients on HTPN use a subcutaneously tunnelled catheter which is then inserted into the entry vessel. This may originate in the lower chest and enter the subclavian vein as is done using the Broviac-Scribner catheter or enter the upper chest with insertion into a facial vein as is done by a group in Toronto. Insertion and removal of these catheters almost always require a surgical procedure in the operating room.

Is any increased safety attributable to the subcutaneously channelled catheter? If one looks through the literature there is very little information to give guidance on this subject. However, as a result of information obtained in a questionnaire sent out by the Registry of Patients on Home Total Parenteral Nutrition, it appears that there are significant problems with these tunnelled catheters. The Broviac-Scribner catheter is difficult to clear of a blood clot, will perforate in the subcutaneous tissues if undue pressure is exerted on it and is associated with its share of infection.

In my series of fifty patients who have been discharged, there has been only two deaths attributable to sepsis, both of these occured in elderly women who delayed for several days following onset of fever in coming to the hospital; when they were admitted they were in septic shock and did not respond to treatment. A number of our patients are known to have chronic infection secondary to partially obstructed ureters, damaged bladders secondary to pelvic radiation and draining abdominal fistulas; hence, a certain amount of infection is to be expected. Using the procedures I have outlined above, infection is relatively infrequent and is readily managed. It tends to be individualized since some patients with chronic infection will go for periods of a year or more without an episode of infection while some will come in with recurrent infection in a cyclical fashion.

It is essential to permit the patient to have as normal a life-style as possible. This is made possible by infusing TPN solutions at night and utilizing a heparin lock during the day. Almost all of the adult male patients that I have had on TPN have been able to work full time and the women have been able to work or to carry on homemaking responsibilities and care for their children.

Others have reported that a significant number of their patients on HTPN who have symptomatic debilitating inflammatory bowel disease have improved to the point where they have restored their oral intake. A certain percentage of others with serious malabsorption have had improved absorption to the point where they are able to be maintained by tube or oral feeding. Some but not all of the patients with extensive tumor prior to antitumor therapy who have been on HTPN had recurrence of tumor and died.

Intravenous Feeding

F. BOZZETTI

Division of Clinical Oncology, Istituto Nazionale per lo Studio e la Cura dei Tumori,
Milan, Italy

ABSTRACT

Cancer patients who have reached the terminal stage of their disease and are
dying from widespread metastases usually do not need any special nutritional
support. There are, however, patients who might be considered "terminal" either
because serious malnutrition prevents them from receiving specific anti-cancer
treatment or because their condition of nutritional failure represents the primary
cause of death, even though their life expectancy in relation to metastatic spread
could be fairly good. Nutritional support is strongly recommended in the first
group of patients whereas, in the second group, treatment should be planned
individually after a careful evaluation of all the aspects of the problem. In the
first group, the nutritional requirements of the patients should be met by delivering, via a central vein, a caloric regimen of about 1.6 times the measured
resting metabolic expenditure (about 50 kcal/kg/day plus 1.5 g amino acid/kg/day).
In the second group, some patients exhibit marked hypermetabolism and require high
doses of dextrose and amino acids. On the contrary, other patients have a normal
resting metabolic rate, a low nitrogen requirement and are well adapted to their
condition of chronic starvation. These patients can be maintained in a steady
state with almost iso-osmolar infusions via a peripheral vein.

INTRODUCTION

Clinicians who take care of the nutritional status of terminal cancer patients are
faced with a difficult task. The word "terminal" may be somewhat misleading since
it includes a heterogeneous number of patients who can be divided into three groups
with respect to the prognosis and treatment:

1. Patients who are dying of widespread metastases.

2. Patients with advanced cancer who have such a marked depletion of caloric and
    protein stores that they would not tolerate, with an acceptable risk, any form
    of palliative treatment.

3. Patients with advanced cancer in which protein-calorie malnutrition is so
    serious as to represent the first immediate cause of death.

F. Bozzetti

GROUP I

In this group, when the disease has progressed far beyond every change of cure and palliation and there is only a short life expectancy, the best policy is to discontinue intensive central venous nutrition and to plan a more straightforward peripheral nutrition. This means the use of isotonic solutions of dextrose, amino acids, electrolytes and vitamins in a volume of about 2 to 2.5 litres of water per day via a peripheral vein. The advantages of this kind of nutritional support include:

1. The patient will not die of thirst.
2. Treatment is not expensive or difficult.
3. It can be performed easily at home.
4. It partly satisfies the clinician's sense of duty and relieves the relatives' anxiety because adequate nutritional support is given for as long as possible.

GROUP II

If malnutrition is so serious as to prevent any change of palliation, effective nutritional support is strongly recommended. These patients often have cancer of the gastrointestinal tract or huge abdominal masses that could be palliated surgically, if surgical exploration did not imply an extremely high risk. This group includes also patients with extrinsic compression of the gastrointestinal tract by radiosensitive tumours, such as lymphoma or sarcoma, who would be candidates for radiation therapy if the patient's general status did not contraindicate it. Similarly, patients with hepatic or diffuse metastases could benefit from hepatic intra-arterial infusion or systemic chemotherapy but because of their nutritional depletion are unlikely to complete the course of treatment. The aim of nutritional support in these patients is not only to maintain the status quo but to replenish the lean body mass and to increase the energy reserves.

Previous work (Bozzetti, 1979) has shown that many of these patients are hypermetabolic, and that excessive energy expenditure and loss of adaptation to fasting are important factors in the pathogenesis of cancer malnutrition (Table 1). In fact, assuming that loss of body weight is a parameter of malnutrition, a statistically significant correlation exists between resting metabolic expenditure (RME) and weight loss (Figure 1). It is therefore necessary to deliver large amounts of calories to replenish these patients.

TABLE 1 Resting Metabolic Expenditure in 65 Patients with Advanced Cancer

RME	No. of patients	%
≤20	27	42
≥21 – ≤40	19	29
≥41 – ≤60	12	18
≥61 – ≤80	7	11

From a second study on 16 adult cancer patients treated by total parenteral nutrition for a mean period of 12 days (Bozzetti, 1980), we have determined the optimum number of calories to achieve the best weight gain without overloading the patients. We found that the weight gain achieved by patients in Group B (Table 2) was statistically different from those in Group A ($p < 0.05$) but not from Group C. Group B patients received 1.6 times more calories than their RME, which corresponds to about 50 non-protein kcal and 1.5 g amino acid/kg/day. This can be accomplished in most cases by delivering 1 to 1.5 g of 50% and 1 to 1.5 g of 8.5-10% amino acids.

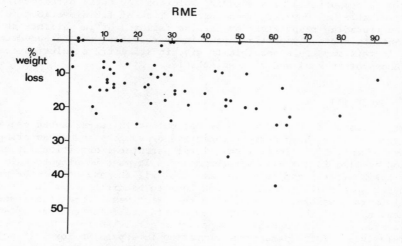

Fig. 1   Correlation between weight loss and resting metabolic
expenditure (RME) in 65 cancer patients (r = 0·41; p < 0.01)

TABLE 2   Determination of the Optimal Caloric Support in Cancer Patients

Group	n	Infusion Regimen				Weight change	
		kcal/RME	kcal/kg	Aa/kg	Fluid load ml/kg	kg	(%)
A	5	1.33	39	1.5	35.4	−0.04	(−0.07)
B	6	1.67	50	1.5	37.6	+0.32	(+0.56)
C	5	1.87	54	1.8	40.2	+0.07	(+0.13)

TABLE 3   Daily Total Parenteral Nutrition Infusion Regimen

Glucose	15 g/kg	Vitamin A	3300 IU
Amino acods	1-2 g/kg	Vitamin D	200 IU
Water	40-50 ml/kg	Vitamin E	10 IU
		Vitamin K	5-10 mg
Sodium	60-125 mEq	Thiamine	3 mg
Chloride	70-200 mEq	Riboflavin	3.6 mg
Potassium	80-120 mEq	Pyridoxine	4 mg
Magnesium	10-32 mEq	Niacin	40 mg
Calcium	5-30 mEq	Pantothenic acid	15 mg
Phosphate	20-80 mEq	Ascorbic acid	>100 mg
Sulphate	10-20 mEq	Vitamin B_{12}	30 μg
Acetate	25-156 mEq	Folic acid	40 mg
Gluconate	11-20 mEq	Choline	500-900 mg
Iron	1 mg	Biotin	1.5-3 mg
Trace elements	1-2 plasma per week	Aminobenzoic acid	2 mg
		Linoleic acid	0.5-1 g

The approximate composition of a standard solution for total parenteral nutrition
is set out in Table 3. However, when there is risk of fluid overload (elderly
patients and impending respiratory or cardiac failure) or in patients able to take
some nutrients by mouth, lyophilized protein hydrolysates can be added to the
dextrose. In this way it is possible to give in 1.5 litre a solution containing
some 2500 non-protein kcal and 75 g amino acids.

GROUP III

A different approach is adopted in those patients with far-advanced cancer who are
no longer suitable for chemotherapy, radiation or surgery and whose primary and
direct cause of death is malnutrition. Total parenteral nutrition for an undeter-
mined period of time is not always recommended. It must be planned only on an
individual basis after a complete evaluation of all the aspects of the problem.
Many of these aspects are not medical and have to be discussed with the patient
himself, if it is possible, and also with the relatives. First the wishes and
psychological needs of the patient must be considered. The patient often, however,
ignores his true condition and this compels the clinician to discuss matters only
with the relatives. Total parenteral nutrition is expensive for both patient and
hospital and can only be done at home for the privileged.

Some of these patients are, in fact, hypermetabolic and they need a high-calorie
high-protein infusion regimen, as with Group II patients. Others, however, are
well adapted to fasting and in these short-term nutritional support is easier and
more practical. These patients may be treated with amino acids (50-100 g), low
amounts of dextrose (150-300 g) without insulin and, if possible, 10% lipids (500
ml). This treatment, which does not attempt to replenish the lean body mass, can
easily be performed at home and, for a limited period of time, will achieve
nutritional balance.

REFERENCES

Bozzetti, F. (1979) Correlation between resting metabolic expenditure and weight
loss in cancer patients. *IRCS* 7, 89.

Bozzetti, F. (1980) Determination of the caloric requirements of patients with
cancer. *Surg. Gyn. Obst.* (in press).

VI
MANAGEMENT AND ORGANIZATION

Introduction

C. VETERE

Ministry of Health, Office for the establishment of the N.H.S., Rome, Italy

In health organization jargon "continuing care" means a comprehensive health system assuring patients of a continuous and rational approach, an ongoing flow of information with data bank linkage and feed-back. It represents the opposite of a haphazard series of contacts and therapeutic approaches, and a lack of interest in the social and emotional problems of the patient, a feature which characterizes much present medical care.

Recently, in the AngloSaxon medical world, a similar trend has developed in relation to terminal care, with the establishment of "Hospices" and "Continuing Care Units", mainly for patients with a limited prognosis suffering from painful diseases. There is sometimes an associated day-hospital and in some places like Sheffield, England, the presence in the day hospital of both cancer and stroke patients serves to emphasize that occupational therapy is an important tool for self-realization even with terminal cancer patients.

The basic philosophy of these units is:

1. The establishment of an atmosphere of "empathy" and the encouragement of free expression of feelings, fears and pain. Sometimes patients draw "murals" while the staff, who accept the Simontons' idea on the relationship between cancer and psycho-emotive patterns, help the patients to localize the painful part of the body and visualize the growth of the cancer. Denial of disease and silence are often symptoms of depression which enhances the development of the cancer and reduces the natural defences of the body. Biofeedback and other behavioural techniques appear promising at least in relation to the self-control of pain.

2. The full involvement of the family not only for obtaining close cooperation in home care but for preventing the so-called "excessive mourning reaction", often a cause of premature death after the loss of a loved one. Here, a holistic approach to medical care allows the enrolment of volunteers from among the relatives of dying patients.

3. The utilization of volunteers whose role may be limited to the very important task of listening to the patients' feelings. It is important to teach the volunteers the basic physiology of pain and about psychological reactions to pain and to the loss of a relative. In such a way they can become a monitoring source and possibly give important information to the medical team in the difficult task of "tailoring" the dose of narcotic analgesics and other drugs to the needs of

different patients. Doctors and nurses too require special training because the
main difference between the old "incurable patients ward" and the new hospital and
outpatient clinics is the attitude of the staff. Some minor structural modifications can reduce the usual alienating atmosphere of hospitals and are much more
important for the terminally ill than for those with acute disorders. In other
words, the more recent experience of Anglo-Saxon Continuing Care wards shows that
it is possible to improve the quality of life for terminal patients and to die
"well" even away from the family home.

In Italy, we are beginning to build up a new health system which is intended to be
based mainly on the users' participation. Limiting factors are not only financial
but relate also to the lack of tained nurses and experienced doctors. There is a
trend towards total decentralization of medical care. This is the best solution.
provided specialized teams can then act in a consultative capacity and research
centres where training can be undertaken are also developed, and are able to survive
in the face of a trend to curtail any kind of "special interest" service. Reduction
in the use of analgesics and the development of alternative means of pain control
present other obstacles. However, the influence of patients' organizations can
counteract such a trend, and my wish is that our medical records could be stamped
"died satisfied". Until the last war there was such a stamp in the Army Quarter-
master's office for identifying soldiers who died in action and who had received
their wages, though maybe not fully satisfied at the premature loss of their lives!

A Terminal Care Service in a General Hospital

B. M. MOUNT

Director, Palliative Care Service, Royal Victoria Hospital, Montreal,
Quebec, Canada

ABSTRACT

The experience, since its opening in January 1975, of the Palliative
Care Service (PCS) at the Royal Victoria Hospital (RVH), a 1,000 bed
McGill University teaching hospital, is presented. A trained multidisciplinary team is oriented toward meeting the physical, psychosocial and spiritual needs of patients with advanced disease and their
families through a home care service in the community, a consultation
team throughout the hospital, an outpatient clinic, a palliative care
ward and a bereavement follow-up program. The PCS has been effective
in improving the control of pain and other symptoms, providing psychosocial support to patients and families, and, with the increased
ability of the patient to remain at home, shortening the length of
terminal hospital admission without excessive additional health care
costs. The advantages of such a service being located within a
general hospital rather than as a free-standing "hospice" are
examined.

INTRODUCTION

The last decade has clarified both endemic deficiencies in the health
care of the terminally ill and the great potential of special services
created to more effectively assist these patients. That this health
care problem is both serious (Duff 1968, Hinton 1972, Kubler-Ross 1969,
Mount 1973) and sizeable (70 percent die in institutions) (Statistics
Canada 1973) can no longer be questioned. That answers have already
been carefully worked out to many of the issues facing these patients
and their families is well established (Melzack 1976, Melzack 1979,
Parkes 1972, Saunders 1978).

The bereaved constitute a further sector of health care neglect.
They are now known to be a high risk population with an increased
incidence of suicide, cardiovascular deaths, GI complaints, anxiety,
depression, functional disorders and visits to the family physician,
and yet their needs are usually ignored. (Parkes 1972)

The central factor responsible for this unnecessary and unacceptable suffering has been shown to be, not the quantity or quality of the motivation of health care professionals, but the orientation of their motivation. Under great pressure to maintain excellence in the midst of ever-increasing medical knowledge we are sharply focused towards investigating, diagnosing, prolonging life and curing, skills that are largely irrelevant to these patients for whom further therapy aimed at modifying the natural history of the disease is inappropriate. Surrounded as they are by a health care team whose hard won expertise is irrelevant to their needs, the dying find themselves isolated and neglected (Mount 1976).

The challenges of the day then, must be: (a) to further evaluate the impact of specialized palliative care or "hospice" programs and (b) to define optimal models of care which will make improved care of this type available to the large proportion of the population who stand to benefit.

The last decade has witnessed new interest in the development of specialized facilities aimed toward the resolution of these problems. Several features distinguish these programs as significant departures from the traditional medical model.

1. While the physical care of the patient and excellence of symptom control are of prime concern, once these ends are accomplished psychological, social and spiritual issues are accepted as being of central importance. Whole person health care is seen as mandatory.
2. The patient and family, not simply the patient alone, constitute the unit of care.
3. Terminal care is viewed as a prelude to bereavement follow-up.
4. Institutional depersonalization is ever present. It is watched for and minimized while recognizing that "efficiency is very comforting."
5. A relaxation of institutional regulations concerning visitors, food, pets and other details of daily life promotes a relaxed atmosphere.
6. The length of life, being beyond control, is seen as a peripheral concern. The focus is not on dying but on the quality of remaining life. The arena of terminal illness is recognized as being a setting of great potential for personal growth, integration, reconciliation of relationships and a heightened sense of purpose and fulfillment.
7. All involved in the therapeutic triad -- the patient, family and care giver are recognized as being at risk for significant stress. Each requires clearly defined support mechanisms.

8.   The traditional hierarchical, physician dominated, health
     care team is inadequate for this task. Such multidimen-
     sional care requires significant multidisciplinary input
     by a team with new operational patterns.
9.   A blurring of traditional professional roles is accepted --
     necessitating patience, skilled listening and a minimum of
     professional insecurity.

While a variety of models may be appropriate in the many different
settings in which these patients live, serious questions must be
asked if there is to be a widespread and optimal application of
"hospice care" throughout our society. Is the free-standing hospice
really an appropriate model in a country with an over-extended health
care dollar and a 65 percent bed utilization rate in many communities?
Should existing strictures defining permissable bed utilization in
acute care institutions, and present reimbursement patterns be determinants which outweigh other considerations in defining the models
for improving care? What of quality control? The "hospice movement"
must avoid a recreation of the nursing home scandal. Will this be
most effectively fostered by erecting free-standing hospices that are
developed totally separate from traditional health care services,
easily accessible to entrepreneurs and less accountable to existing
quality controls and peer review? How can the humanizing impact of
hospice care be most readily transferred to the acute care system;
from a free-standing unit or by an integrated service within the
institution?

This communication examines the experience gained since January 1975
at the Royal Victoria Hospital (RVH), a 1,000 bed McGill University
teaching hospital, in integrating a Palliative Care Service (PCS) designed to deliver "hospice care" within the general hospital setting
(PCS 1976). Research and teaching activities complement the five
clinical arms of the service, the palliative care unit, the symptom
control (consultation) team, the palliative care clinic, the home
care service and the bereavement follow-up program.

Figure 1 outlines the staffing patterns of these services and their
administrative relationships within the institution. The differences
between the orientation of traditional general hospital goals and
those of a palliative care service make it mandatory that the hospital administrators, director of nursing and others responsible for
policy within the institution, have a clear understanding of the principles underlying good palliative care if such a service is to have
sufficient freedom to function effectively. The maintenance of a
satisfactory staff-patient ratio on the PCS will only be possible if
the nursing department accepts the principle that goals related to
the psychosocial and spiritual well-being of the patient and family
must have equal priority weighting on a palliative care ward to the
more traditional nursing tasks oriented towards problems of pathophysiology. As part of the nursing department in a general hospital,
the palliative care nursing team will occasionally be asked to

respond to an unexpected nursing shortage on an active treatment ward,
by supplying a nurse to help out for that shift. By the same token
the PCS may go to the department of nursing for help in staffing the
Palliative Care Unit (PCU) when illness or other unexpected absentee-
ism occurs. If unacceptable demands for PCS nurses to work on other
wards are to be avoided, however, there must be acceptance of the
notion that PCU nurses, like nurses on psychiatric wards, have specialized skills that have been developed in order to respond to a different sort of patient and family need.

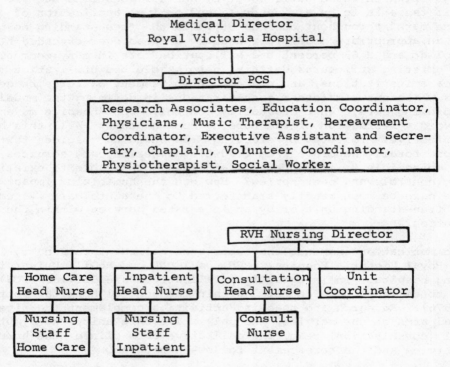

NOTE: Chaplain, Volunteer Coordinator, Physiotherapist and Social
        Worker are responsible to their respective hospital direc-
        tors in terms of professional quality of their work -- but
        responsible to PCS Director in terms of content of work.

Fig. 1 Organization Chart

A further implication of the institutional location of a PCS is the
inherent accountability and peer review that such a setting provides.
In addition there are readily available consultants as well as diagnostic and therapeutic resources not found in a free-standing hospice.
A decompression laminectomy becomes an immediately available option
for the acutely paretic patient; focal irradiation involves a stret-
cher ride down the hall rather than a trip by ambulance across town.
The dermatologist may be asked to drop in during his regular hospital
rounds to see the patient with a troublesome rash.

It is not just the PCS that benefits from the service being within
the institution. Experience suggests that the benefits go both ways.
The presence of the PCS has led to an increased emphasis on whole person medical care throughout the institution in the opinion of independent evaluators within the RVH. Furthermore, since the transition
from active anticancer treatment to palliative care is often unclear,
difficult, or delayed, the presence of the PCS team within the institution is particularly useful since it facilitates their early involvement and lessens the trauma attached to this shift in therapeutic
goals. When the decision is made that further treatment aimed at
cure or prolonging life is inappropriate it is frequently reassuring
to the patient to know that the hospital has specialized facilities
providing skill in symptom control and other aspects of his present
needs and that he is not going to be discharged and "written off" by
those previously involved in care, but transferred to a ward within
the hospital where his own doctor can still visit regularly.

A further beneficial impact of the PCS, presumably related to the
improved symptom control and home care it provides, is seen in the
significant shortening of terminal care admissions at the RVH since
the service started. During the same interval there was also a marked
increase in the number of cancer patients dying in hospital, reflect-
ing the larger flow of patients through the oncology clinics. It has
been highly significant for our hospital with its pressured acute
care beds, that in spite of the large increase in oncology, and the
attendant increase in the number of cancer patients dying in the RVH,
the number of terminal cancer days has not increased in parallel but
has instead decreased dramatically. This change would appear to reflect the impact of the improved symptom control and home care provided by the PCS, since there are no other adequate explanations for
this important shift in the dynamics of patient care (Table 5).

        PATIENT POPULATION

Palliative Care Service patients are those for whom further treatment
aimed at modifying the natural history of the disease is no longer
appropriate. While patients with advanced malignant disease constitute the majority of the patients cared for, those with progressive
neurologic deficit and other forms of end stage medical disease, e.g.:
renal, respiratory and cardiac are included, space and resources permitting.

In the course of malignant disease three primary treatment aims are
recognized -- to cure, to prolong life, and when these are no longer
relevant, treatment exclusively aimed at improving the quality of remaining life. Patients still receiving chemotherapy or other forms of
therapy aimed at modifying the disease trajectory may be followed by
the consultation team, on the home care program, and in the palliative
care clinic, but they are not, in general, accepted for transfer to
the palliative care unit. PCS team involvement in this phase of the
disease is beneficial as it allows the formation of supportive relationships with the palliative care team that facilitate a smooth con-
tinuum of care when the patient's condition deteriorates.

THE PALLIATIVE CARE UNIT (PCU)

Patients are selected for admission to the PCU from the previously described pool of RVH patients. Priority is given to: 1) Patients requiring admission from the home care program and 2) Hospitalized patients difficult to manage in other departments because of poorly controlled physical symptoms or difficult psychosocial problems. Concern
for the well-being of the family is considered an acceptable indication for admission of a patient to the PCU. It has been observed that
a brief "respite admission" of several days "to give the family a rest",
frequently pays rich dividends in renewed physical and emotional resources for those giving home care, thus enabling a greater portion
of families to care for their loved ones at home until the end.

Table 1 documents the admissions to the PCU by sex and referring department. 362 admissions (53%) were by transfer from elsewhere in
the hospital while 318 (42%) were direct admissions from home care or
from the Montreal Neurologic Institute. Table 2 gives the distribution for pathologic diagnoses for PCU cancer patients.

TABLE 1 Admissions No./%, Jan. '75 to June 30/79

	TOTAL	SEX		REFERRING DEPARTMENT						READM'N.
		M	F	MED.	SURG.	GYN.	NEURO.	ONCOL.	OTHER	
PCU	680 (100)	328 (48)	352 (52)	132 (20)	240 (35)	28 (4)	23 (3)	161 (24)	34 (5)	62 (9)
HOME CARE	528 (100)	236 (45)	292 (55)	77 (14)	94 (18)	14 (3)	11 (2)	183 (35)	32 21 (6) (4) PCU	96 (18)

TABLE 2   Diagnosis PCS Oncology Patients

Diagnosis: (By Primary Site)	Home Care Male	Female	Total	PCU Male	Female	Total
Lung	68	25	93	86	23	109
Breast	-	90	90	-	92	92
Large Bowel	38	27	65	50	39	89
Female Reproductive System	-	35	35	-	63	63
Stomach	9	9	18	13	23	36
Head & Neck	12	5	17	21	11	32
Pancreas	11	11	22	14	17	31
Kidney, Bladder	14	2	16	23	6	29
Other	22	25	47	30	18	48
Prostate	11	-	11	20	-	20
Malignant Melanoma	1	2	3	13	6	19
Lymphatic System	3	4	7	8	9	17
Esophagus	5	-	5	8	3	11
Liver	4	2	6	4	5	9
Sarcoma	2	1	3	4	4	8
Hematopoietic System	3	4	7	1	4	5
TOTAL	203	242	445	295	323	618

Twelve percent of PCU patients have been discharged home for follow-up by the home care nurses. This is possible (Table 3) when symptoms have been brought under control and patient and family feel able to cope. The fact that PCS home care patients have a priority listing should readmission be required, facilitates the decision to discharge the patient and lessens the anxiety for both patient and family.

TABLE 3   Discharges, No./(%), Jan. '75 to June 30/79

	TOTAL	SEX M	F	DIED IN PCU	DIED AT HOME	TRANSFER TO NURSING HOME OR OTHER HOSP.	TRANSFER OFF SERVICE
PCU	668 (100)	323 (48)	345 (52)	577 (86)	78 (12)	2 (-)	11 (2)
HOME CARE	506 (100)	233 (46)	273 (54)	202 (40)	62 (12)	33 (7)	22 (4)

Two percent of PCU patients have been transferred off service, usually
to take advantage of specialized expertise in some form of palliative
medical care elsewhere in the hospital.

Table 4 gives the distribution of length of stays for PCU patients.
The mean length of stay has been approximately 23 days while the median
has been 10 days.

TABLE 4   Total Length of Stay on Unit, In Weeks Per Patient
          to June 30/79 (Including 1 or more admissions per
          patient)

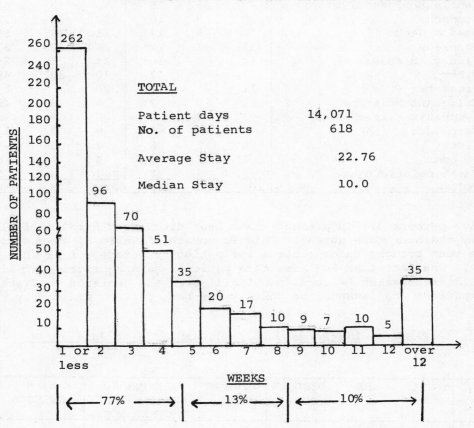

The number of palliative care beds needed in a general hospital will
depend on variables such as the volume of oncology practiced in the
institution, the mix of other types of medical care beds, e.g.: presence or absence of paediatrics, obstetrics, etc., and the availability
of specialized services such as a consultation team and a home care
service. Extrapolating from the RVH experience, one may conclude that
a general hospital with an active oncology program and with both consult and home care services available may have an ongoing need for

2-3 palliative care beds per 100 acute care beds in the institution.

While the patient may be admitted to the PCU under the name of the referring doctor for reimbursement purposes, day-to-day management is directed, and all orders written, by the PCS physician. The referring physician is encouraged to continue his involvement as a consultant.

Prior to admission the patient or a family member is invited to visit the unit. Such a visit may serve to dispel any fears about the nature of the ward. At the time of transfer, a staff member goes to the floor to accompany the patient to the unit.

When the patient is admitted from home, he is transported directly to the unit on arrival at the hospital. Only after the patient is settled and comfortable does the family go to the admitting office to complete necessary forms. The goal of the admission procedure is to give the patient a sense of welcome to a place where people care for the patient as an individual. Use of personal name cards, greetings by name, and bedside flowers symbolize this individual concern. Both patient and family are familiarized with ward routines and the family is reassured that they may continue to be involved in the patient's care to the degree they feel comfortable with. There are no "visiting hour" restrictions and no age minimum for visitors. A family member may stay overnight if the need arises. A pet may visit if it is important to the patient. The family is encouraged to bring in the patient's favourite foods -- there is a microwave oven, refrigerator, etc. for preparing meals and snacks.

Good palliative care means attention to detail and excellence in symptom control. These goals are achieved by a health care team knowledgable in clinical pharmacology. Many patients with advanced malignant diseases have heard their medical team say, verbally or non-verbally, "there is nothing more that can be done." Those working in palliative care declare by their actions and orientation that there is much that can and must be done. The physical, social, psychological, and spiritual components of "total pain" are attacked in the context of a supportive milieu. Patient and family together are considered the focus of care. The multidisciplinary team is made up of physicians, nursing staff, social worker, ward clerk, dietician, physiotherapist, chaplains, recreational therapist, music therapist, and volunteers.

As death approaches, the attention of the team is focused on giving maximum reassurance and comfort to both patient and family. When death has occurred, the family is encouraged to grieve at the bedside in a viewing room located on the unit.

HOME CARE PROGRAM

As noted above the home care team accepts patients who are still receiving active treatment aimed at tumour response (such as chemotherapy)
as well as those for whom such therapy is no longer appropriate. In
such a situation the referring physician continues to supervise the
active treatment while the palliative care physician is in charge of
pain and symptom control. In this situation, should hospital admission be required, it is to the referring doctor's service, not to the
palliative care unit.

Patients requiring admission who are not receiving active therapy are
admitted to the PCU if a bed is available. Otherwise they are readmitted to the service of the referring physician, to be transferred
to the PCU when a bed becomes available. The home care team also follows patients who are discharged home from the Palliative Care Unit.

The home care staff at present consists of four nurses and a physician.
They cover nights and weekends on rotation to supply continuous coverage. In addition, volunteers, the physiotherapist, and the social
worker make home visits and are involved in home care patient and
family problems when the need arises. Coordination of community resources is the joint responsibility of home care nurses and the social
worker.

As in the PCU, palliative care in the home includes the control of
pain and symptoms as well as seeking resolution of emotional, interpersonal, spiritual, and financial difficulties.

Tables 1,2, and 3 document demographic data relating to this arm of
the PCS. The average length of stay on the home care service was 54.9
days. (Mean approximately 33.0 days).

Since 1975, the home care nurses have made 8,061 home visits, an average of 14.9 visits per nurse per week. This average could be expected
to be considerably higher for a home care service relating to a community hospital serving a more compact geographic area.[1] In spite of
the relatively low number of visits per nurse per day, this arm of the
service has made a valuable contribution in reducing the pressure on
acute treatment beds as discussed above. (Table 5). This effect was
predicted in a 1976 review of the PCS home care service that suggested
that at least 50 percent of home care patient days would have been
spent in hospital, had it not been for the home care service (Report,
RVH, 1976).

---

[1]The PCS home care area is approximately 600 square miles. The region
is completely urban. A further factor influencing the work capacity of
the nurses is the Quebec nursing 36.25 hour work week with 4 weeks paid
vacation and 13 statutory holidays annually.

TABLE 5   RVH Oncology Statistics, Pre-PCS (1971, 1972,1973), Post-PCS (1977, 1978)

CANCER PATIENTS	PRE-PCS			POST-PCS	
	1971	1972	1973	1977	1978
Admissions	2,277	2,518	2,765	2,682	2,662
Radiation Therapy	25,307	27,655	28,294	15,553	16,278
Clinic Visits*	7,487	7,957	7,624	20,979	18,388
Deaths In Hospital	225	274	220	391	479
Terminal Days	7,986	8,234	5,163	4,262	5,260
Mean Duration, Terminal Adm'n.	30	32	24	10.9	10.9

*(Neuro Clinic Visits Omitted)

The majority of nursing visits, 6,439 (80%) were for primary nursing care in the home while other visits were for assessment 449 (6%), crisis intervention related to medical or psychosocial emergencies 166 (2%), bereavement counselling 169 (2%), consultation 59 (1%), and follow up of hospitalized home care patients 779 (9%).

THE CONSULTATION TEAM

Patients are seen in consultation at the request of their attending physician or the ward staff concerned. The PCS physician and two consultation nurses are assisted by an experienced team of volunteers as well as the PCS chaplain, social worker and music therapist. They assist the referring doctors and nurses in symptom control and in the development of a comprehensive care plan which may include transfer to the unit or to home care. (Table 6).

TABLE 6   Consultation by Palliative Care Service Team to June 30, 1979

MONTH	TTL NO. CONSUL-TATIONS	TRANS-FERRED TO PCU	TRANS-FERRED HOME CARE	TRANS-FERRED OTHER HOME CARE*	FOLL-OWED OFF SER-VICE	TR.HOME/ NURSING HOME	SIN-GLE VISIT	DIED OFF SER-VICE
Ttl. To June 30/79	1,334	353	216	136	380	69	54	279
%	(100)	(26)	(16)	(10)	(28)	(5)	(4)	(21)

* Outside Palliative Care Service Home Care Area.

In addition to their clinical function, the consultation nurses are
heavily involved in teaching the principles and philosophies of palliative care throughout the hospital and the community. In addition, they
participate in frequent group discussions with nursing staff on the
acute care wards and thus are able to provide staff support as well as
advice regarding patient care. The most significant teaching frequently takes place on a one-to-one basis as the referring staff witness an
improvement in patient/family care as a result of a new care plan or
lessened staff stress.

The consultation service or symptom control team has proven to be an
effective catalyst in furthering quality palliative care throughout
the hospital. In many cases the combined efforts of the consult team
and the staff on the referring ward lead to excellence of care without transfer to the PCU. The aim is to complement and support existing resources and relationships on the referring ward, not to take
their place.

While the impact of such a consultation team is considerable, a significant number of patients -- those with particularly complex psychosocial needs or difficult and uncontrolled symptoms -- can be more
successfully managed in the PCU with the consistent approach and the
controlled therapeutic milieu it provides. The enhanced capability
of a unit as compared to a consultation team alone is suggested by
the improved pain control found in the PCU as compared to that achieved on the private ward accommodations of our hospital (Melzack 1976).

A frequently voiced concern regarding the development of "hospices" or
"PCUs" is that they may serve to isolate and ghettoize the terminally
ill. Perhaps such risk is lessened if these patients are cared for
in specialized facilities within the referring hospital rather than in
a free-standing hospice. Wherever the setting, the risk does exist,
however, if the unit is merely an inadequately staffed dumping ground
for unwanted terminally ill patients. It is ironic that it is precisely in the lessening of the isolation these patients and their
families experience that a PCU has advantage over the consult team
alone as a palliative care tool in many problem cases.

The consultation team acts as a lynch pin, coordinating the responsi-
veness of a complex service (the consult service itself, the home care
service, the PCU clinic and bereavement program) to the needs of the
terminally ill in the institution and in the community. The flexibility and the impact on the remainder of the health care system that
such a model provides cannot be approached by other models of hospice
care including the solitary symptom control team, the isolated home
care service or the free-standing hospice.

BEREAVEMENT FOLLOW-UP

Bereavement leads to a period of crisis.   In the Palliative Care Service, families are encouraged to acknowledge the realities of impending loss. Members of the team are supportive, and open to discussion as they assist anticipatory grief.

Key family members particularly close to the patient (key persons) are assessed prospectively for risk of impairment of health and psychosocial adjustment. Those considered at particular risk are followed while others may or may not be followed by the Palliative Care Service staff after the death of the patient.

As part of a federally funded research program trained nurses and volunteers are currently participating in a supervised, standardized bereavement follow-up program calling for contacts with the key person within the first three weeks of bereavement and subsequently as appropriate up to approximately six months. A memorial card is sent to the key person on the anniversary of the death.

PALLIATIVE CARE CLINIC

The PCS has recently added a fifth clinical arm in the form of a palliative care clinic for the follow-up of outpatients and their families. Patients include those from the PCS home care program and other RVH patients with advanced disease. The initial visits to the PCS clinic may be held while patients are still being followed in the active treatment oncology clinics. This facilitates the transition from life prolonging to palliative intervention by building a supporting network of relations with those whose expertise will be increasingly relevant to the patient and family as health deteriorates.

A team of trained volunteers, the social worker, physiotherapist, chaplain, music therapist as well as consult and home care nurses complement the efforts of the PCS clinic physician and nurses as required. Once again the focus is on whole person health care considering the patient in the context of his family.

FINANCIAL CONSIDERATIONS

The overriding variables influencing the practicality of the PCS in the RVH are that:

- there is a comprehensive program of health care in Quebec, in which hospital costs, including staffing and laboratory investigations, are paid for by a single hospital global budget.
- physicians may be salaried by the Quebec Department of Social Affairs.
- general hospitals in Quebec are required to have 20 percent of beds occupied by chronic patients.

- bed utilization rates in Quebec general hospitals approach 100 percent. There is a particularly heavy pressure on beds within a teaching hospital such as the RVH, thus any increase in efficiency of bed utilization enabling more effective use of acute care beds is welcome.
- in the RVH experience PCU patients have a higher "nursing dependancy rating" (Report, RVH, 1976) than those on all other hospital wards save for those in medical and surgical intensive care facilities (Table 7).[2] Thus a higher staff-to-patient ratio would be justifiable on the PCU on the basis of physical nursing care requirements alone.

TABLE 7   Nursing Dependancy Rating (NDR) and Staffing
          Patterns by Ward (Medical Wing)

	PCU	GEN. MED 5	CARDIAC UNIT	GEN. MED 7	ONCOL. & GEN.	GEN. MED 9	DERM.	GEN. MED 10	TRANS- PLANT
NDR (Per Patient Day)	12.2	7.3	N/A	8.2	9.6	8.6	6.8	9.0	10.8
(Ttl. Hrs. Care Per Patient Day	6.1	3.1	14.8	4.5	5.1	4.7	2.7	4.7	7.2

When one adds psychosocial and spiritual concerns as priority issues in the setting of terminal illness an even higher ratio is clearly called for. In spite of this the PCU staffing pattern (Table 7) has been similar to that seen on some other hospital wards and considerably lower than the 9 nursing hours per patient per day initially projected.

Personnel salaries account for 75-80 percent of hospital expenses. The "cost" of palliative care thus depends largely on this important variable. Laboratory service and investigations represent a second significant area of expenditure, 11-17 percent of global budget.[3] These two parameters were selected for analysis in assessing the cost on in-patient care for a selected group of patients from the Palliative Care Unit and a matched group of patients dying elsewhere in the

---

[2] The nursing dependancy rating (NDR) is a measure of nursing requirements in patient care. The NDR is calculated for all hospitalized patients on a daily basis by the Department of Nursing.

[3] These figures are not mutually exclusive since the figure for laboratory services includes personnel salaries.

RVH. Since randomization of patient admissions to the PCU was not
feasible, an attempt was made to minimize patient selection criteria
as factors prejudicing the results of this study by developing matched
pairs of patients drawn from the PCU and general hospital patient pools.
Strict matching criteria were observed including tumour type, age, sex,
marital status and length of terminal admission.

The data generated demonstrate that the small increase in cost related
to the slightly higher nurse-to-patient ratio on the PCU was more than
offset by the savings accrued through the curtailment of irrelevant investigations if the patient died on the PCU.

COMMENT

In the four and one half years since its inception the RVH PCS has
demonstrated that a multidisciplinary team trained to meet the complex needs of those facing terminal illness can provide better control of pain and other symptoms, enabling these patients to stay at
home for longer periods, often to die at home. This improvement in
care can be achieved with little additional cost.

The RVH PCS has shown that "hospice" type services may be integrated
into the general hospital setting with significant gains accrued for
all concerned.

While home care, consultation service and outpatient clinic programs
may each contribute significantly to patient care and may, in selected
cases, each be sufficient to provide optimal support for the patient
and family, experience suggests that many patients benefit from more
than one arm of the service, while a significant percent have sufficiently complex needs so as to be controlled only with the aid of a
therapeutic milieu provided by a specialized unit such as the PCU.

Such a ward is not appropriate or necessary for all patients, nor are
those involved the only professionals skilled in meeting the needs of
these patients, yet experience clearly suggests that important advances have been made possible by the development of such a service.
Commonly encountered, yet often unperceived suffering at death is now
recognized more frequently in our hospitals and is seen to be largely
unnecessary. New fields of research have been opened. A foundation
has been laid on which can be refined a new health care model. A
model that recognizes medical technology as a means to an end rather
than an end in itself; that recognizes the personhood of the patient
and the special potential for growth encountered by all involved in
the therapeutic triad (patient, family and care giver) when confronting death.

238   B.M. Mount

REFERENCES

Duff, R.S., Hollingshead, A.B. (1968), Dying and Death in <u>Sickness and Society</u>, Harper Row, New York, Chapt. 15

Hinton, J. (1972),<u>Dying</u>, 2nd Edition, Penguin, Harmondsworth, England

Kubler-Ross, E., (1969), <u>On Death and Dying</u>,MacMillan, New York

Melzack, R., Mount, B.M., Gordon, J.M. (1979), The Brompton Mixture Versus Morphine Solution Given Orally: Effects on Pain, <u>CMAJ</u>, 120, pp. 435-438

Melzack, R., Ofiesh, J.G., Mount, B.M., (1976) The Brompton Mixture: Effects on Pain in Cancer Patients, <u>CMAJ</u>, 115, pp. 125-128

Mount, B.M., (1973), Part III, Case Studies in unpublished report, Medical Advisory Board of Royal Victoria Hospital by ad hoc committee on thanatology

Mount, B.M. (1976) The Problem of Caring for the Dying in a General Hospital; The Palliative Care Unit as a Possible Solution, <u>CMAJ</u>, 115, pp. 119-121

Palliative Care Service, October 1976 Report, Royal Victoria Hospital, Unpublished Data, Appendix 20, Table 7, p. 315

Ibid., Appendix 20, Addendum 1, p. 316

Parkes, C.M. (1972) <u>Bereavement</u>, Studies of Grief in Adult Life, Tavistock Publications, London

Saunders, C. (1978) <u>The Management of Terminal Disease,</u> Edward Arnold, London

Statistics Canada: Vital Statistics Bull., 3:61, 1973

Home Care

W. S. NORTON* and S. A. LACK**

*Associate Physician, The Connecticut Hospice, Consulting Physician (Emeritus),
St. Luke's Hospital, New York City, N.Y., USA
**Medical Director, The Connecticut Hospice

As municipal and voluntary hospitals have become more crowded, and orientated towards acute care, the patient with terminal disease has received less than adequate care and less attention from the staff. The patient with a terminal disease needs a quiet environment and care from concerned and unhurried attendants. "The dying person should be allowed to choose to finish his life at home, surrounded by a compassionate family, amid his own possessions and in a setting that can maximize psychological comfort" (Krant, 1978). Home is a refuge, and the urge to remain in one's lair during periods of crisis is innate.

Although Home Care is not for all, it is an alternative that has historic tradition and has proved to be a well received option in contemporary communities. In the Connecticut Hospice, the Home Care program was started in March, 1974. Care is being provided for patients and their families in 19 towns in the greater New Haven area, comprising a population of more than half a million.

The high quality of hospice home care has prompted tremendous verbal and financial support from the community. Since March 1974, 825 patient/family units have been served. In the past year 74% of the patients died at home, as they wished. Families receive bereavement follow-up for at least a year after a patient's death. The 35% of our patients who are of Italian origin are proportionate to the 39% in our catchment area. One-third of the patients are referred to the program by neighborhood physicians; one-third by one of three major general hospitals in the area or by the visiting nurse programs, and one-third have been referred by their physicians at the urging of the patients themselves, neighbors, or members of families of former patients who have been on the program.

The referral is received by the Admissions Registrar and reviewed by our Home Care Team Co-ordinator. A telephone call is made to the referring physician and a medical abstract requested. The local visiting nurse service is contacted to ascertain if this patient is known to them and, if so, the extent of their involvement in the patient's care. If there are major nursing needs, requiring daily home visits, or if counselling is needed for patient and family, then the services of the visiting nurse and the Hospice Home Care Team can be co-ordinated. Hospice aims to supplement existing Home Care services and not duplicate them. A family member is contacted and an appointment is made for a nurse to see the patient as soon as possible whether still in hospital or already at home. This initial nursing assessment should include a history, a physical evaluation of the patient, interview with the family, and the identification of a primary care person. This is usually a member

239

of the family who is living in the home, and who will assume the major responsibility for the patient's 24-hour care. However, the most essential task attempted at
the assessment visit is the establishment of human contact and laying the ground
work for a therapeutic relationship between nurse and patient/family. This task
outweighs the mere gathering of information.

The referring physician provides the initial orders and care plan. Needed equipment
is ordered from a pharmacy or from the suppliers in the area. Medications are given
as per the physician's order. A financial planner visits the home to make a family
financial assessment, to determine if the patient has health insurance coverage and
to establish a rate schedule for Hospice reimbursement. Patients are accepted on
the program on the basis of need, and not the ability to pay. Early in Hospice
involvement the nurse determines if there are members of the family or friends who
live nearby who can assume some responsibility for care of the patient or who might
be available in an emergency.

A telephone call is made to the referring physician to inform him of the patient's
condition and the proposed care plan. The Hospice nurse also asks whether the
patient is to make further visits to the doctor's office or if the doctor will make
home visits, emergency visits and a pronouncement visit when the patient dies. If
the referring physician is unable to fulfill any or all of these needs, then permission is obtained for one of the Hospice physicians to fulfill these duties.

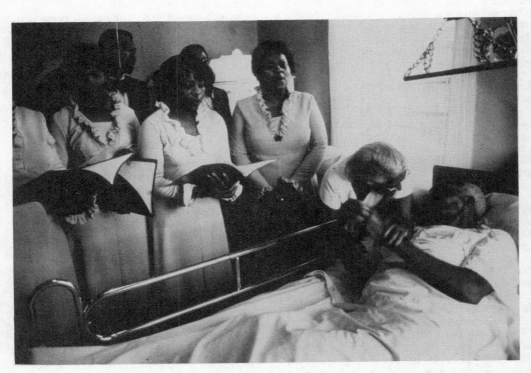

Fig. 1 Not all symptoms need medication. The pain of this man's bone
metastases was quickly relieved by morphine, but the pain of his isolation, his inability to attend church and sing with the choir, was
helped immensely when this group of friends came to him. The Hospice
nurse who was present described his radiant face, the motion of his lips
as the choir sang and his tears of happiness in gratitude.

TABLE 1   Characteristics of a Hospice Home Care Program

1.	Patient and family = the unit of care
2.	Physician directed services
3.	Patient selection on the basis of need, not ability to pay
4.	Skilled control of symptoms (Fig. 1)
5.	Care by an interdisciplinary team (Fig. 2)
6.	Volunteers at all levels of care (Fig. 3)
7.	Service 24 hours a day, 7 days a week
8.	Supplement, not duplicate, patient services
9.	Keep patient at home as long as possible (Figs. 4 & 5)
10.	Bereavement follow-up
11.	Staff support and communication system

THE INTERDISCIPLINARY TEAM

It is impossible for an individual physician or nurse to give adequate time to fulfill all the needs of those who need these services. To be effective for a large number of patients in a widely scattered community, a physician-directed multidisciplinary team must function under an organized Hospice administration in order to meet the physical and emotional needs of the patient and family. At the present time, the Connecticut Hospice has the personnel to provide comprehensive care for approximately 40 patient/family units. Without the supplementary services of a coordinator, a registrar, a financial consultant and other office workers, we could not function.

Physicians

The Home Care Team is under the leadership of physicians. The physicians at the Connecticut Hospice are certified or qualified in internal medicine or family practice and between them have had many years of experience with terminal cancer patients living at home. There are at present three physicians, one 80% time, one 50% time and the third, a volunteer physician, 25% time. One of these is on call all the time.

A physician whose clinical experience has been in the protective security of the well-staffed medical centre may feel insecure and helpless when he finds himself alone with a housebound patient who is experiencing many of the uncomfortable symptoms commonly seen in terminal cancer. Physician acceptance of the responsibility for the care of the patient with terminal disease implies willingness to "change gear" and make a commitment of time. Time to get to know the patient and the family, while they, in turn, are getting to know him, and time to develop mutual trust.

Hospice care requires mature judgment by the physician, for he must first deal with himself to be sure he is comfortable with the patient dying. Only then will he be able to give effective physical care, support and counsel that will sustain the hope and spirit of the patient and family throughout the terminal illness and bereavement.

Nurses

The ultimate comprehensive qualities and skills that characterize the ideal hospice nurses are acquired partly from prior education and training, but mainly from on-the-job experience working with the multidisciplinary team. Most of our new

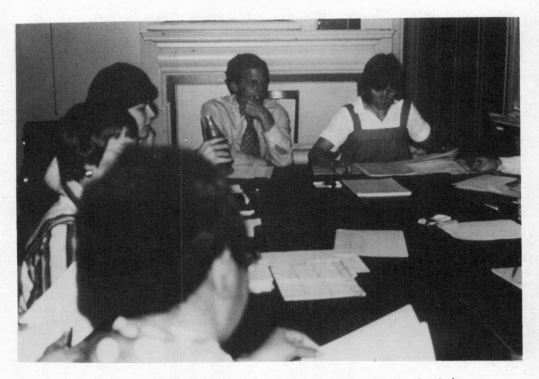

Fig. 2 Every Tuesday, physicians, nurses, social workers, chaplain,
secretary and volunteers meet to re-evaluate all patient/family problems
and care plans.

nurses come with some experience with the dying cancer patient in the home setting.
It is important that they are good listeners and are aware of their limitations in
therapeutics and counselling. Expertise and confidence in these areas may take up
to two years to acquire.

At present, Connecticut Hospice has six full-time and four part-time registered
nurses on the team. They work two shifts: the day shift from 8.00 a.m. – 4.00 p.m.
and the evening shift from 4.00 p.m. – 11.00 p.m. At night a nurse is on call.
Our nurses know how to use a stethoscope, a reflex hammer and an otoscope. They
are able to interpret physical signs and give treatment traditionally assigned to
physicians such as inserting urethral catheters in persons of either sex. On the
other hand, on a number of occasions, the social worker and chaplain have willingly
and effectively performed simple nursing services, and physicians have run errands,
rubbed backs, shaved beards and given enemas.

Social Work

Identifying and formulating a care plan is initially the role of the primary nurse
and the referring physician. The social worker's role is primarily to help the
Team interpret the meaning of the illness and its symptoms to the patient, the
family and the care-givers. The qualified social worker needs to be a good listener,
to be accepting and non-judgmental, and to be able to allow the individual to make
up his own mind.

In addition to the traditional knowledge of community resources for the patient and family, the social workers supervises the delivery of financial counselling, supervises volunteer social workers, provides social work education, and relative consultations. About four families are seen each week in the office. These are families where the patient lives outside the service area, or where the patient declines hospice and the family wants help. The social worker can be particularly effective when he/she is comfortable and helpful with children. Children need a confidant in whom they can express distressing feelings and when fear and bewilderment causes inappropriate behavior. Helping the Team to understand these dynamics improves the Team's effectiveness.

Pastoral Care

In the presence of terminal illness there are basic pastoral issues facing the patient, family and care-givers. An alert, open care-giver, whether secretary, nurse or physical therapist, can help bring these issues into focus. Dealing with feelings of loneliness, insecurity, uncertainty and loss of control are major challenges to all Team members. The Chaplain is especially able to help address these issues with patient, family, Hospice staff and community clergy. A particular joy is experienced when a patient or family member finds his fragmented inner faith and allows it to become a supporting personal religion. Although Hospice has strong Christian roots, the Chaplain can assume a secular role in fostering a calm, creative, environment in which patient and family can deal with their concerns.

Volunteers

Under a Director of Volunteers, we have 40 who have been trained to work with our families. Today, Hospice Home Care breaks with the established health care system and dares to provide innovative skilled medical, nursing and social services by trained volunteers and family members functioning as part of the health care team. Volunteers help the family with daily household chores, and can stay with the patient while the spouse goes shopping. The volunteer forms a close friendly relationship with the family and often becomes the first close confidant of the patient. Volunteer physicians and nurses from the community give part-time services in the home. Lay volunteers have become skilled observers of changing physical signs and have alerted a Team nurse at a critical moment. A volunteer has solved the logistical maze of a hospital admission system and swiftly expedited moving an acutely ill patient from ambulance to nursing unit. The Home Care Team is unique and in its individual roles often expands to meet the immediate needs of the patient (Lack and Buckingham, 1978).

SUPPORTING PERSONNEL

For the care-giver, difficulty coping or searching for answers inevitably produces stressful feelings. These can be resolved by belief in one's own standards, a strong sense of personal and professional identity and a willingness to interact with the patient and family as persons worthy of love. The patient, as a source of strength, must not be overlooked and the care-givers must allow themselves to be cared for by those they seek to serve.

Physicians and nurses dealing with terminally ill patients must become interested in symptom control and skilled in the home management of these distressing complaints. There is never a time when "nothing more can be done". The physician must have an imaginative and extensive supply of remedies. Effective counselling

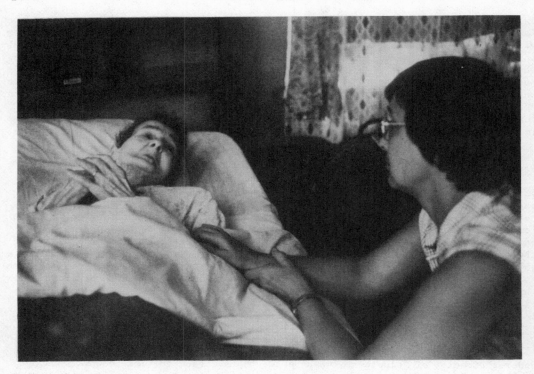

Fig. 3   A volunteer visiting a patient in her home

TABLE 2   Connecticut Hospice Home Care — Statistics for Recent 12-Month Period

Total number of patient/family units	195
Average "case load" at any one time	42
Median length of time on program (range 6 hours – 36 months)	29 days
Number of patients over 60 years of age	70%
Male	44%
Female	56%
Married	64%
Widowed	24%
Bedridden initially	23%
Average total amount of time spent in homes	22.75 hours
Average duration of physician visit	47 minutes
Average duration of nursing visit	67 minutes
Average duration of social work visit	98 minutes
Average number of visits to each patient/family by:	
Physician	1.5
Nurse	11.5
Visiting nurse	2.2
Home health aide	6.2
Social worker	0.5
Pastoral	0.2

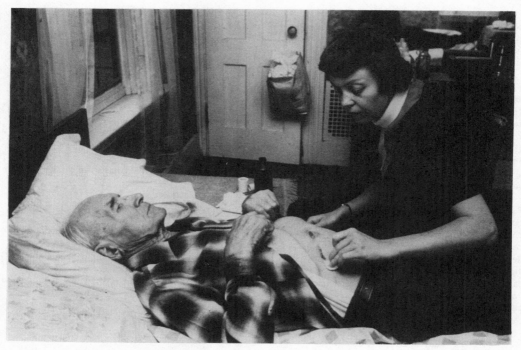

Figs. 4 & 5 A dressing is changed at home. Although weak, the patient is able to be up and about in the garden with his wife.

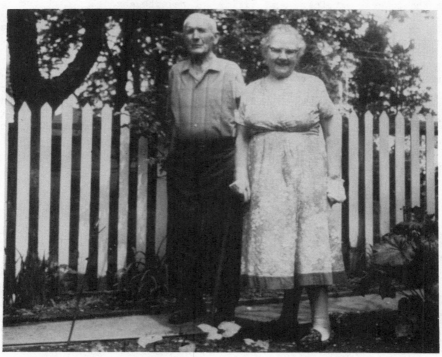

cannot be given to a patient who is uncomfortable. Severe cancer pain can be
controlled. A great deal can be done for other symptoms, but to be effective the
physician and nurses must be positive in attitude and honest in their expectations.
Team goals are to relieve symptoms and allow the patient to live up to his full
physical ability until he dies. These goals are realistic.

A team member may form a close relationship with the patient or a family member.
When this happens it is potentially an added source of stress. New team members
are selected who have handled past personal stress well, have strong support from
family and friends, and have diverting outside interests and hobbies. Time off,
one-to-one and group conferences, time to express feelings, time to play, celebra-
tions, birthday parties, humour and teasing at appropriate times all serve as support for this closely knit community: the Home Care Team Hospice is not, however,
a sheltered workshop; it exists for the care of patients and families and must not
become focused primarily on looking after the staff.

Part of the Home Care Team organization and function is to have a daily report
conference at 3.30 p.m. when the nursing shifts change. Once a week, on Tuesdays,
the entire Home Care Team meets in a conference room to discuss new patients,
reassess specific patient problems and review the care plan of all the patients.
Representatives of other vital community agencies involves in a patient's care,
such as the Visiting Nurses Association, attend regularly. Recent deaths are
discussed, with time allowed for staff members to express their feelings about the
care given and the personal relationships that have been made, and what role a
team member will have in the bereavement follow-up.

                    BEREAVEMENT FOLLOW-UP

Home Care does not stop when the patient dies. The primary nurse may attend the
wake and the funeral service. Home visits and telephone contact with the family
continues for a year or until there is an acceptable adjustment to the psychological
suffering caused by the separation. Opportunity for the spouse, parents, and
children to express their grief and talk about the illness and death does much to
relieve guilt and depression.

Bereavement follow-up is carried on by a team of volunteers who have been carefully
selected and trained. This team meets regularly as a group with close supervision
from a psychologist and back-up consultation from a psychiatrist. The volunteer
who is going to do the bereavement follow-up is often introduced to the family a
few days before the patient's death. In this way, there is a smoother transfer
when the nurse hands over the bereavement care to the bereavement team member.

                    REFERENCES

Krant. M.J. (1978) Sounding board, the Hospice Movement. *New Engl. J. Med.* 299,
546-549.

Lack, S.A. and Buckingham, R.W. (1978) *First American Hospice — Three Years of
Home Care*. Connecticut Hospice, New Haven, Conn.

Total Community Approach to Psychosocial Support

A. H. SCHMALE

University of Rochester Cancer Center, Rochester, N.Y., USA

ABSTRACT

The awareness, tolerance and acceptance of the reality of dying is difficult for
the cancer patient, family and health professional. In order to provide emotional
support and somatic comfort for this final phase of life, there must be an understanding of these difficulties and how to approach them. A community-wide effort
involving several unique resources is available in Rochester, New York, U.S.A.,
which will make it possible to provide meaningful choices and flexibility in
achieving the maximum of care for the patient's comfort and psychosocial support.

GENERAL CONSIDERATIONS

Emotional support for the dying cancer patient requires special consideration.
Ordinarily, emotional support is thought of in terms of what a person needs or
expects to have provided by another in order to achieve or maintain a sense of
well being. Is it easy to see how, in the case of a child, the "something" a
mother provides is emotional support, especially when the child is sick or hurt.
Such support takes the form of the mother holding the child close to her, speaking
soothing words, examining the damaged area and, if possible, removing the child
from the dangerous hurting environment. Emotional support for the dying child
requires this same kind of care. What about the terminally ill adult cancer
patient? What kind of support does he or she need for a sense of well being? Is
there not the same need for physical closeness to specific others, the words of
those who matter who say, "I will share your hurt", and who in action will try to
provide as much comfort as is possible?

How do we recognize the specific "hurt" and determine what will provide the most
comfort? In reality these are the same critical questions we must answer as
health professionals in all our diagnostic and therapeutic work. Once it is
recognized that the "hurt" that is being faced is a progressive, irreversible
disease process and death is inevitable, then the question of what will provide the
most comfort takes on a new meaning. At such times patients and health professionals are no longer willing to tolerate the discomfort associated with specific
procedures and treatments directed towards trying to reverse or slow down the

Supported by grants CA 19681, CA 11198 and CA 17988 awarded by the National Cancer
Institute, Department of Health, Education and Welfare

disease process. The concern become one of what can be done to make the patient comfortable.

Problems arise when either the patient or the health professional is unwilling to recognize and then to accept that the disease is no longer treatable and death is inevitable in the near future. What does the patient do when he accepts the inevitability of dying and the physician is not yet able to? Most patients have difficulty being direct and raising such a question with their physician. They assume that the physician has a better view of their condition than they do. More often than not they will say nothing and the treatment program will continue as before unless the physician provides them with an opportunity that permits them to indicate their awareness even if it is stated as a question. Not infrequently, the patient will discuss this with the family or with another member of the treatment group such as a nurse, social worker or the receptionist. It is important for whoever hears the concern expressed to get the message back to the patient's physician. He can then consider the logic and reality of the patient's perception and concern. If the physician is the first to recognize and tries to communicate the uselessness of further treatment to the patient but the patient is unable to recognize this reality, it is important for the physician to suggest a consultation with another physician in order to get an independent view of what is happening. Such a consultation is most important or at least the offer to have the patient seen by someone else is of importance whenever the physician and patient perceive things differently.

The greatest personal anguish for both the physician and patient occurs in a situation where the disease is recognized to be untreatable but both are unwilling to accept the reality that death in the near future is inevitable. If the patient and physician are struggling with the problem of accepting the reality of dying at the same time, they can decide that some treatment for the disease is in order and thus can temporarily ignore the reality of the dying. When physician and patient are on different wave lengths or have a different reality, the physician must be careful that he does not try to impose his reality onto the patient without finding out the nature and reasons for the patient thinking and perceiving the way he or she does.

It is difficult for the physician to put himself in the patient role, particularly in today's world and particularly when the disease is cancer. We are living in a time of great scientific and technological achievement while at the same time cancer is a disease(s) for which the cause(s) and the cure(s) for the most part elude us. Thus when treating cancer the physician is pushed, even forced, into being an experimental scientist. This is particularly true for the oncologist. For him one day's experimental trial therapy may be the next day's established treatment of choice (or so he and the patient hope).

What can or should be done to protect the reality of the dying cancer patient? Should the patient be faced with his dying if he has shown no interest in or awareness of knowing. The physician must make sure the patient has been given the opportunity to discuss his reality. The importance of a consultation at such a time has already been discussed. Such a consultation lets the patient know that his physician is interested in another opinion, he has a chance to voice and discuss his concerns with another expert, and finally he and his physician have the opportunity to discuss any new options that may have entered the picture. All these opportunities for the patient to think and talk out his understanding of his reality and to learn from others more experienced than he about their perception of his reality is important. Thus, the consultation may help both the patient and the physician some to the realization that the therapies directed to the cancer are not working. Once the physician is convinced that the patient has acknowledged that he has heard the information that the disease is no longer treatable, the physician must be prepared to help the patient tolerate the reality of dying. Many physicians have not been prepared to do this, prepared in the sense of their own self awareness

and sensitivity as to what it is the patient experiences at such a time. The
knowledge about the dying process can only be meaningfully acquired and applied by
those who have been sensitized by their own experience and can tolerate the inevitability of the idea of dying.

Since dying is a process, the awareness, meaning and reactions to the process are
constantly changing. Such change is based on the individual's self image, its
relationship to what is happening to his body, and what is happening in his
relationships with the external world. All this will in turn influence how his
body functions and how he feels about himself. Initially and periodically thereafter the individual who knows that he is dying will show a disinterest in knowing
this or may even avoid and sometimes appear as if he does not know of such a
reality. This may confuse the consultant or the physician or nurse who only has a
brief contact with the patient. It is well established that some patients are very
selective and will discuss the reality of their dying only with a few individuals.
Some patients will reveal that they cannot discuss dying with their own physician
or specific family members because they are afraid this will be too difficult for
them. "The physician will think he has failed me", "My mom could not take it".
Sometimes the patient is correct in his assumption, other times only partly correct.
Frequently, such discussions initiated by the patient will produce an immediate
discomfort and distress which is then followed by a greater closeness with a more
open expression of thoughts and feelings by all concerned.

Part of the reality of the dying process for both the patient and physician is an
acceptance that the disease oriented therapy is not effective and that there needs
to be a shift to another form of medical care which focuses very specifically on
the comfort and emotional support of the patient. Such an approach includes
physical, mental, social and spiritual support. We have come to call this level of
medical care "comfort care only", and it is designed to give the patient a sense of
control over his existence however limited it may be (Schmale and Patterson, 1978).
The patient decides how much intervention is desired for his comfort and the level
of consciousness that he wishes to maintain. The physician and other health
professionals must appreciate that the symptoms of the dying patient take on
special meaning. The pain, nausea, constipation, confusion and incontinence not
only have their biological significance but usually express the patient's frustration, fear and even despair about life itself. To understand these symbolic or
metaphorical elements requires an awareness and a special listening to what the
patient says. For the physician to appreciate when the patient says "I'm just one
big pain" that the patient may be talking about his thoughts of being a burden or
that life itself is unpleasant makes it possible for the physician to understand
why his somatic therapies are only partially effective. Sometimes the relationship
of the patient with the physician not only starts but remains at the symbolic body
language level. There are some physicians who are either unaware of such aspects
of language and its meaning or are uninterested or unable to provide this level of
medical care and will insist that this care is not consistent with the medical model.
These physicians feel that their knowledge and skill should be directed towards
curing or at least slowing down or delaying the progress of cancer and when they
can no longer do this they want to step aside and have others involved with the
dying. It is important to have people involved, whether social workers, trained
volunteers, clergy, etc., who can provide relationships and other supportive help
to family and health professionals. These people. however, should not be seen as a
substitute for the physician and nurse who must be involved to establish and maintain the effectiveness of the patient's "comfort care only" medical therapy. Many
patients, contrary to popular opinion, once they are aware and acknowledge the
untreatable state of their disease, have less pain and discomfort in general and
require a minimum of medical supervision. Again, this emphasizes how much the
previously experienced bodily symptoms were magnified and distorted by the anguish
of uncertainty and not knowing what to think or do.

C.C.T.C.—K

It should be evident that the physician and all health professionals struggle with
emotional issues in their work with dying patients. Their own self image which
includes professional and personal identities, their family and other experiences
of sickness, will determine how they react and how effective they can be in working
with dying patients.

The patient's beliefs and expectations about his disease and its treatability as
well as age, marital status, religion and cultural background will influence the
perception of dying. It may seem ironic, but it is not uncommon for a dying
patient to give support to the physician when he senses the physician is upset over
an inability to provide a disease-oriented treatment. The physician's concern may
be evident in his attitude and actions even though he tries to be reassuring by
what he says. Thus, the physician should be prepared to learn about the meaning of
health, sickness and the process of dying from his patients and to expect that each
will bring something personal and unique to the process. This is one of the rewards
that the physician receives for what he is able to give and share. A more detailed
account of the reactions the physician, patient and family may experience as they
share in the patient's dying have been written about elsewhere (Schmale, in press).
How does an awareness of dying get translated into effective communication and care
in a community setting?

IMPLEMENTATION OF A COMMUNITY APPROACH

This community of Rochester, New York, has a long history of creative and innovative
planning for health services which have served as a model for other communities and
governmental policy. It is in this context that the interest in the hospice concept and what could and should be done to educate the community and to provide
meaningful services evolved.

The actual planning took place on several fronts, one within the University of
Rochester and its Cancer Center, another involved one of the community hospitals
affiliated with the University, Highland Hospital, and other efforts in the community which were in great part organized through the Genesee Region Home Care Association (a home health agency with a long history of serving the sick including the
terminally ill at home).

The University's Cancer Center along with the Strong Memorial Hospital medical
director's interest in understanding the specific needs of the dying patient led to
the formation of a Palliative Care Consultation Committee made up of representatives
from all the hospital's clinical services. This group reviewed the then current
practices and identified the needs of the dying patient and family (Patterson and
Ravizza, 1977). This committee has made itself available to physicians who have
sought support or help in understanding the reality of their patients' perceptions
and how to establish a "comfort care only" medical treatment program. As a part of
this group's deliberations it has recognized the need to make available specific
recommendations for symptom control, skin and mouth care, etc. It has become
evident that the patient, the family and the health professionals all need a set of
guidelines and principles to follow in order to make this form of therapy legitimate medical care.

The Highland Hospital decided they had space available for an in-patient hospice
unit and did a survey of need within their setting. Data from this as well as
other information from the community led to a proposal for a ten-bed facility with
an open admission policy (Cooper and Weider, 1979). It was initially decided such
a facility would be appropriate for this community of approximately one million
people of whom 6,028 died in 1977 and 22.5 per cent of those who died had cancer.
It was estimated that 803 hospitalized cancer patients a year could benefit from
the various levels of hospice care that might be available in the community.

Whether the communities' physicians and the various governmental bodies will
support such a facility is yet to be decided. In the meantime the university
hospital as well as the community hospitals are trying to implement guidelines
which will make it possible for dying patients to get hospice-type care when they
need hospitalization.

The hospice-type care for those dying at home has been organized in great part by
the Genesee Region Home Care Association, Inc., which has contractual arrangements
with institutional and non-institutional providers of health care in the community.
The agency provides central administration, intake, assessor/evaluator/coordinator
services and discharge planning for health care provided in the home (Amado, 1979).
Most of these services are paid for through third party payers. Private health
insurance plans such as Blue Cross and more recently limited support by federally-
funded programs are available (Medicare for those age 65 and over and Medicaid for
those considered poor and unable to pay for their health care). This agency under-
took a study of the appropriateness of existing home health services and the
reimbursement that was provided for the needs of the patient dying at home. The
first study was a three-month study done in 1977 which included 33 terminal cancer
patients. The patients received an average of 39 days of home care at a cost of
$26.19 per day. Roughly half of these patients died at home, a third returned to
the hospital and the others did not die and remained at home during the period of
observation. It was discovered on review of the records that all of those who
returned to the hospital probably did so because they had used up all of their
health insurance benefits. The family could not afford to pay for the type of
professional services that they continued to need.

As a result of these findings, a three-month demonstration home hospice service was
established which included a private insurance reimbursement to provide 24-hour
seven-days-a-week skilled nursing and ancillary home health support. This study
involved 17 patients whose physicians indicated they had a life expectancy of less
than serveral weeks. The patients were provided with 162 days of care at an
average cost of $85.75. All of these 17 patients died at home. This study indic-
ated that cancer patients could and would stay home to die if given the appropriate
support and services. This was accomplished at a cost much less than if such care
had been provided in a hospital. With these findings, then, a home hospice program
was undertaken in April 1978 and has been offered as an alternative to patients and
families who formerly had only the hospital as the place where they could afford to
die. In the first nine months this home care hospice service was offered, 150
dying patients received such service. Ninety-five were classified as imminently
terminal (Stage 2 — within two weeks of death) and they received all the nursing,
physical, occupational therapy, equipment, medication, transportation and home-
health aids needed. Thirty-four of this group received maximum private insurance
support which averaged $132.51 per day. Of the total 150, there were 55 patients
considered not as close to death (Stage 1 — within two months of death) and they
received less intensive services. Nineteen of this latter group were maximally
supported by private insurance coverage for an average cost of $48.36 per day.
This home hospice service has been approved at local, state and federal levels as
a demonstration project and thus now qualifies for support under the governmental
programs mentioned above as well as the private ones. Post death bereavement
counseling is also offered to all families whether the patient was receiving Stage
1 or 2 hospice care at the time of death. The patients receiving home hospice care
in the initial demonstration did so at an average cost of $87.73 per day. Eleven
per cent of the cost went for public health nurse or social work planning and supervision of the care in the home. Thirty-three per cent was spent for the home health
aid services actually rendered in the home and 42 per cent was spent for professional
nursing services provided. Ten per cent was spent on equipment, supplies and transportation and the final four per cent was for drugs, oxygen and laboratory studies.

Another resource which has become available in the community is the Home-Health

Care Team supported by a federal government grant. This is an experimental program for chronically or seriously ill patients (not just cancer patients) who are home bound and have difficulty in getting to a physician's office or a hospital (Groth-Juncker, 1979). The team consists of a physician, nurse-clinician and social worker. Members of the team are on call 24 hours a day, seven days a week, for home visits. Ninety patients have been cared for at home in this program in the past year. There were 23 of these patients who were cancer patients and 14 of them died at home (Groth-Juncker, 1979).

In all of these programs the physicians provide services to the patient at home and charge directly the participating private and public health plans for these services. How are these services coordinated to provide the maximum of psychosocial support? Several examples will be given to illustrate how these programs and individuals inter-relate in order to provide the desired terminal care.

CASE EXAMPLES

1. *Mrs. I.A.M.*, age 71, was of Russian-Jewish background, with a son recently married and a husband age 80 who was a retired salesman. She had undergone surgical debulking and one course of chemotherapy for her lymphoma which was Stage 4 and existed both above and below the diaphragm. The tumor had continued to grow in spite of nine months of chemotherapy.

She was referred by her medical oncologist for radiation therapy, and a decision was made that a course of radiation therapy was appropriate as a possible means to control the tumor. The patient and her husband were advised of this recommendation, but the patient's immediate response was that she was against such therapy. This decision she attributed to having heard of someone who had suffered from radiation burns. Her personal physician as well as the oncologists met with her on several occasions. They introduced her to several patients had had similar cancers and similar treatment without difficulty in order to reassure her of the benefits which they thought outweighed any possible discomfort that might occur. She was suffi-ciently reassured finally to consent to the treatment. However, while getting off the treatment table at the time of her first treatment she had a black-out. This led her to again change her mind and to decide to have no further treatment. She was hospitalized to evaluate her reaction and to consider possible alternatives. It was in this setting that the hospital's Palliative Care Consultation Committee was called to see her. Her personal physician had hoped that the group would be able to talk her into resuming treatment. The patient and her husband were seen on several occasions by various members of the team including a social worker, nurse and psychiatrist. The patient also talked by phone to her son in another city on several occasions, and her rabbi visited her during this period. In putting together all the information that the patient had told various individuals, it was learned that the patient retrospectively felt her oncologist had been wrong in his initial estimation of the possible effectiveness of chemotherapy. She felt that he had falsely guaranteed that her disease would be controlled by the chemotherapy. During this period she had lost some ten pounds and had had great difficulty in eating, particularly for the week after each chemotherapy session. She had become increasingly weaker to the point where she had become totally useless as a home-maker. In addition, there was the story of her marriage which also played a role in her decision not to seek further therapy. She had had full responsibility for raising her son because her husband's work took him away from home for weeks at a time. Because of this she shared all her time and interests with her son and when the husband was home he spent much of his time with his mother and unmarried sister whom he helped to support. Now that her son was grown and on his own, her husband's mother and sister were dead and he was retired, there was little left in life but to take care of him.

Her decision to have no further treatment was based not only on the cancer and the price she had paid for the treatment which had not worked, but also on her age, the limited rewards she had received in her marriage and her physical inability to be in control of her own life and home. At the time of the consultation she had pain and nausea controlled by medication. She was considered oriented and rational. Her husband, however, felt she was crazy for not wanting to be treated and refused to consider having her at home.

The hospital staff and consultation team, by contrast, however, saw her as a warm, thoughtful, sensitive person who had given a lot to her son, her husband and others in her life. The consultation team was able to convince her personal physician that she should be allowed to live her life in as dignified a way as possible. To give her as much sense of control as her disease would allow with no further treatment directed to the disease itself as she had requested. Her husband had difficulty in accepting this. His first response was to say that he could not manage her at home and that, indeed, she would have to go directly from the hospital to a nursing home.

Her personal physician asked for a Home Care evaluation. With the help of a public health nurse, it was decided that a health aide four hours a day, five days a week, would be all the help that would be needed to maintain her at home. She received medication for her constipation and small doses of methadone orally several times a day for a period of approximately six weeks. Her physician was in telephone contact with her and also received weekly reports from the visiting health nurse. At the end of six weeks it was evident that she was weaker, was not interested in eating or getting up and was in need of supportive care around the clock. She was changed to a Home-Care Hospice program, Stage 2. She died within the week following the institution of this more intensive medical help which included a registered nurse two shifts a day. She died on a day after a visit from her son and his wife. Her husband never really accepted her choice and, indeed, was angry with her even to the point of directly telling her he thought that she was depriving him of the care he deserved. The patient, however, would make light of this. She recognized this was in part a way of getting back at him for some of the hurt and loneliness she had felt for years. Her response to his complaints and, indeed, increase in angina was one of reminding him that he had always managed to work out things to his advantage and that she was sure that within six months of her death that he would find another woman to take care of him. A social worker established a relationship with the patient and her husband during her final weeks and will be available to help support the husband if needed.

2. *Mrs. M.R.*, age 55, of Italian extraction, was a mother of four with a three-year history of a large cell anaplastic lung cancer and a 40-year history of two-pack-a-day cigarette smoking. She had had chronic lung disease for some nine years, and this had limited her physicial activity but had not changed her life appreciably up until the time the lung cancer was diagnosed. She received radiation therapy and did well for approximately a year. Mediastinal spread of the disease was then treated with a combination of chemotherapy agents. Within the next several months pain, cough and shortness of breath plus leukopenia led to a decision to discontinue chemotherapy.

Her first contact with the University of Rochester Cancer Center came with her admission to Strong Memorial for evaluation of increasing dyspnea and cough which had been productive of bloody sputum for several weeks. On examination she was found to have bilateral pleural effusion and an organized blood clot which was causing a partial obstruction of her superior vena cava. She was put on an anti-coagulant and oxygen but refused a regular pain control regimen. She would only take Percodan when the pain became disruptive of sleep. Bronchoscopy, pleural fluid, brain and liver scan showed no evidence of tumor. Review of her situation revealed that she had received the maximum in specific tumor therapy and could only be given whatever would be necessary for symptom control. This plan was discussed with the patient, her husband and her personal physician. The physician had the greatest difficulty in accepting this reality. He repeatedly found himself emphasizing that there was little evidence of new disease and minimized the extent of the untreatable disease that was present.

The patient acknowledged the untreatable nature of her disease but hoped for a miracle. She did not want a Home Care evaluation and did not want a health aide in the home. She preferred to manage at home with the help of her extended family. Her husband rented a hospital bed and equipment to provide oxygen because of her breathing difficulties. At the patient's request her mother and sister took turns in helping her during the day while her husband was at work. Other members of the family would visit regularly in the evenings and week-ends. The patient was proud of the fact that she could manage on her own several hours a day. With her sister's help she was also able to wash and set her hair once a week. Over the next three months, there were several brief hospitalizations or emergency room visits for re-evaluation of her pain and dyspnea and, indeed, there was evidence that the disease was progressing. The patient continued to insist that she did not want to die but acknowledged she was in God's hands. She had difficulty in breathing even with the continuous use of oxygen. In this same period she lost more weight because of difficulty breathing, swallowing and no appetite. She attributed this to her increased consumption of Percodan. Following her youngest child's return to school in the fall, she began having difficulty sleeping and because of increased breathing difficulty only slept for minutes at a time. Nevertheless, she had established a routine for herself which included TV viewing, visits with family members or friends on schedule each day. This was her way of maintaining control.

The Palliative Care Consultation Team at the University hospital was called a month before she died to see if there was anything further that could be done to help her maintain her independence in the face of her decreasing physical strength. Again, she and her husband declined the possibility of having anyone in the home from the Home-Care program. Of all the things that were considered, it appeared that an extension phone placed by her bed seemed to be the one thing that she was willing to add to continue her sense of control. During this period it was possible for her to call the physician or for him to call her. However, in every instance the only calls made were those by the physician and were prearranged in terms of time. The last week of her life she was too weak and dyspneic to talk on the phone but listened as her physician talked to her. She also had difficulty in asking her mother or sisters to help with some of the more personal forms of care that she needed now that she was occasionally incontinent. The last day of her life she was having difficulty remaining awake and seemed confused. The family considered having a nurse brought in to help, but she died in a "twilight sleep", as her husband called it, before this could be arranged. She died at home with her family in attendance and as she and they had wanted. Follow-up telephone call one month after the patient's death revealed her husband and other members of the surviving family were busy at work but keeping in close contact with each other. Even though they missed the patient they considered this had been a "good" experience for all of them.

        CONCLUSION

A description of comfort care and the problems in recognizing the participating in such care has been described. A community-wide program of hospice services have been organized for the patient who is recognized as dying. This program which includes both education and service components has the support of a Cancer Center in a medical school setting, a university hospital with its palliative care committee and associated community hospitals, an organized home care agency as well as individual physicians practising in the community. This hospice approach gives a range of options for the health care and emotional support of the dying cancer patient. From the initial experience, it appears that most patients when given these options prefer to maintain the maximum of independence and control which usually means staying at home if at all possible. The availability of such choices not only maximizes the emotional support when needed but prevents the unnecessary use of health resources and reduces the cost of dying.

REFERENCES

Amado, A.T. (1979) Genesee Regional Home Care Association Home Hospice Service Application. Anthony T. Amado, Administrator; Roger J. Boulay, Medical Director.

Cooper, R. and Weider, M., *et al.* (1979) Hospice Care in the Finger Lakes Region: A Cooperative Effort to Advance Terminal Care. Proposal submitted by University of Rochester Cancer Center, Genesee Regional Home Care Association and Highland Hospital.

Groth-Juncker, A. (1979) Home Health Care Team: A Choice. A research proposal suggested by HEW grant HSO3030 to the National Center for Health Service Research, OACH.

Patterson, W.B. and Ravizza, C. (1977) Proposal for the establishment of a hospice unit at Strong Memorial Hospital — Study supported by the Monroe County Cancer and Leukemia Association 1975-76 and final report of Palliative Care Consultation Group's recommendation made on March 8, 1977.

Schmale, A.H. (in press). Psychodynamic Processes and Psychotherapeutic Interventions in Life Threatened Illness. Chapter on "The Dying Patient" to appear in *Advances in Psychosomatic Medicine*, Vol. 10.

Schmale, A.H. and Patterson, W.B. (1978) Comfort care only — treatment guidelines for the terminal patient. Chapter 2 in *Psychosocial Care of the Dying Patient* (Ed. C.A. Garfield). McGraw-Hill, New York, pp. 13-21.

Staff Training

C. A. GARFIELD

Professor, Cancer Research Institute, University of California, San Francisco, USA
and Founder and Chairman of the SHANTI Project, Berkeley, California, USA
106 Evergreen Lane, Berkeley, California 94705, USA

INTRODUCTION

People have thought about life and death since Neanderthal times.
The fact that "Living with Death" was a feature story of Newsweek
(May 1, 1978), and Time (June 5, 1978) two of the most popular maga-
zines in the United States indicates the extent to which dying and
death have become concerns to the lay public as well as to health
professionals--a surprising development for a culture so often described as death denying. There are a number of reasons for this
increasing awareness. Recent advance in innovative medical technology are significantly altering the nature of dying, often compel-
ling the terminally ill to confront years of chronic illness before
the actual moment of death. In addition, many post-industrial
Americans are alienated from traditional family, religious and community supports. The results are increased loneliness, anxiety, and
self-doubt. Feifel (1977) observes that it is a historic phenomenon
that consciousness of death becomes more acute during periods of
social disorganization, when individual choice tends to replace automatic conformity to consensual social values.

> With the advent of the H-bomb, physical science has presently
> made it possible for us all to share a common epitaph. Not
> only descendance in social immortality but history as well is
> being menaced. Time along with space can now be annihilated.
> Even celebration of the tragic will be beyond our power.
> Death is becoming a wall. (Feifel, 1977)

Death also has become more difficult to deal with because of its ex-
pulsion from daily life. Dying and death are now the responsibility
of the "professional," i.e. physician, nurse, clergymen, funeral
director. Unfortunately, many of us use our technical expertise as a
defense against our own death related anxieties.

CARE OF THE DYING

As physicians, nurses, and allied professionals perfect their skill
at providing care and support for the terminally ill, we must continually be aware of the enormity of the emotional trauma confronting

257

our dying patients and their families. It is interesting to realize the word "care" derives from the Gothic <u>kara</u>, which means "to lament, to grieve, to experience sorrow, to cry out with." Nouwen (1974) notes that "we tend to look at caring as an attitude of the strong toward the weak, of the powerful toward the powerless, the haves toward the have nots." We often experience great discomfort when we are invited to enter into someone's pain before we have done something about it. But distanced concern appears strangely antithetical to the basic component of caring, namely, empathy, the more express-ive German translation of which is "einfuhlung" meaning "to feel one-self into." Nouwen continues with the observation that

> when we honestly ask ourselves which persons in our lives
> mean the most to us, we often find that it is those who "in-
> stead of giving much advice, solutions, or cures, have chosen
> rather to share our pain and touch our wounds with a gentle
> and tender hand. The friend who can be silent with us in a
> moment of despair or confusion, who can stay with us in an
> hour of grief and bereavement, who can tolerate not knowing,
> not curing, not healing and face with us the reality of our
> powerlessness, that is the friend who cares."

In as emotionally charged an environment as exists in most of our contact with seriously ill patients and their families, attempts at decreased emotional involvement are frequently experienced by patients as painful abandonment. These attempts to remain "object-ive" are born of the notion that to become emotionally accessible to one's patients implies a loss of scientific objectivity, a com-promising of rational judgment, and a decrease in the time-effective management of one's "caseload." When communicated to our students and younger practitioners, this bias serves largely to disallow authentic human communication between helper and patient and prevents the next generation of health providers from mastering the art as well as the science of patient care.

To understand the nature of effective support for dying patients and their families, health providers must:
1. Realize that role models appropriate to laboratory
    science are largely inappropriate to the effective
    emotional support of patients and families facing life-
    threatening illness. That is, we <u>are</u> emotionally in-
    volved with our patients and we need to be able to dis-
    cuss this involvement with our patients and our colleagues
    in order to maximize the supportive nature of these
    basically interdependent relationships.
2. Recognize that the psychosocial aspects of patient care
    require a great deal more than "hand holding." Almost
    without exception, physicians who take the psychological
    and social issues surrounding life-threatening illness
    seriously can develop a real mastery of this increasingly
    important aspect of patient care.
3. Examine carefully our own attitudes concerning death and
    the dying patient and realize what when it comes to a
    subjective understanding of the nature of the dying
    process, most patients know a great deal more than those
    who care for them.

As health professionals, we are often involved in situations in which

we are like lifeguards watching our patients flounder in the water
several hundred yards off shore. Perhaps the distressed person does
not know how to swim or, knowing how, simply does not have enough
strength to make it to shore.

> Our professional lifeguards, it seems, do not know how to
> swim themselves. To be sure, they have been given extensive
> training in many life-saving techniques, all of which they
> have tested in the children's pool. They know how to row a
> boat; they know how to throw out a ring buoy; they know how
> to give artificial respiration. But they do not know how to
> swim themselves. They cannot save another because, given
> the same sircumstances, they could not save themselves.
> (Carkhuff and Berenson, 1967).

Many of our attempts to understand the emotional realities of dying
patients and their families are doomed to failure because we base our
approaches on a set of faulty operational assumptions:
1. We rely on summary information about the patient's
    emotional world, that is, notes in the chart or brief
    word-of-mouth explanations.
2. Our values as health professionals are most often
    firmly rooted in middle-class thinking, making it
    difficult to comprehend cross-cultural variation in
    value systems.
3. We are unable to effectively incorporate or interpret
    experiential and behavioral extremes in a meaningful
    fashion.
4. We have great difficulty in dealing with emotional
    expression, for example, extreme anger, long-term
    depression, etc. The somewhat presumptuous yet
    frequently invoked assessment of the patient's chosen
    form of expression as "inappropriate affect" is often
    a signal of our own inability to cope.
5. We attempt to deal reasonably with what is most often
    --from the patient's perspective-an unreasonable life
    situation.

Our efforts to ignore or disqualify emotional expression, make decisions on the basis of cursory and most often superficial data, and
eliminate extremes from the dying patient's emotional life are
usually perfectly reasonable yet superficial. Our effectiveness will
increase in direct proportion to our capacity to acknowledge the
great range of quite normal emotional responses to life-threatening
illness and the complexities of psychological functioning and assessment. Increased effectiveness results when we continue to be present
to our patients in spite of the fact that the greater portion of
their psychological functioning remains a mystery to us.

Feelings about death and the process of dying, like feelings about
human sexuality, are very intimate concerns that most people are unwilling to share with those constrained by the scientific rigors of
a tightly designed research protocol. As one elderly man dying of
lung cancer stated, "I'll be damned if I share my feelings about
dying and death with anyone who makes two-minute U-turns at the foot
of my bed." To date, no research or systematic clinical observation
has verified any preprogramed set of stages in the dying process;
that is, researchers and practitioners have not empirically ident-

ified any set of linear, unidirectional, and invariant stages. Certainly many patients who are dying exhibit denial, anger, bargaining, depression, and occasionally acceptance (Kubler-Ross, 1969), but it is inaccurate to suppose that all individuals, regardless of belief system, age, race, culture, and historical period, die in a uniform sequence. It is more likely that existing theoretical frameworks become self-fulfilling prophecies imposed by health professionals who may coerce the dying person into conforming with a powerfully suggestive typology. All too frequently I have heard health professionals talk about "forcing a patient to move from stage three (bargaining) to stage four (depression) because the patient's condition was deteriorating so fast that he or she might not have time to reach stage five (acceptance). To needlessly add one more ponderous agenda to a patient's already heavily burdened psyche is an injustice to all concerned. Out of respect and appreciation for Elisabeth Kubler-Ross and her work, I must note that she has made this point many times herself. With regard to all our theoretical models, I am reminded of Aristotle's observation: "Dear is Plato, but dearer still is truth."

In my own research, the major issues identified by the dying patient are first, that he will become quietly isolated because of a decrease in communication resulting from the unwillingness of those responsible for his care to maintain the openness and emotional support essential for him to live out his life with some hope and participation in meaningful relationships; second, that he will be subjected to painful, uncomfortable, and demanding procedures that might prolong existence without prolonging a desirable quality of life, and that the disease will force him to endure intense, chronic pain seemingly without end; and finally, that loss of control of bodily, interpersonal, and cognitive functions will compel him to confront a terrifying and alien set of experiences, stripped of all decision-making powers.

I have found the following outline useful in determining and meeting the psychosocial needs of terminal patients.
  1. With the assistance of the patient, define the major
     areas of emotional distress.
  2. Respond to the patient's requests for information with an
     honest, complete, and accurate presentation of the major
     aspects of illness and treatment.
  3. Inform the patient's family of the status of his health
     so that family members can assume their rightful status
     as members of the treatment team.
  4. Make it possible for the patient to be aware of staff
     expectations concerning treatment, patient-staff relation-
     ships, etc., and conversely for the staff to be aware of
     patient expectations.
  5. Always compare your perceptions of the patient and his
     situation with those of your colleagues. It is hazardous
     to make unilateral judgments about another person's
     emotional reality.
  6. Remember that psychosocial evaluation, like medical
     appraisal, is a continuous process. Two innovations that
     have proven successful in maintaining ongoing evaluation
     are (a) the institution of interdisciplinary psychosocial
     rounds, the specific purpose of which is to evaluate staff
     success in meeting the emotional needs of all patients
     (the option of inviting patients to talk to staff about

how to best care for them has been a successful aspect
of these rounds), and (b) the use of a psychosocial log
in which all health providers may record their feelings
and thoughts on various aspects of working with seriously
ill patients. This log can serve as a catalyst for
discussion during psychosocial rounds.

HOSPICE AND COUNSELING PROGRAMS

Two important and creative responses to the needs of dying patients
and their families have been the development of the hospice concept
and volunteer counseling programs modeled after the SHANTI Project in
the San Francisco Bay Area of the United States. Pioneered successfully throughout England and other European countries, the hospice is
seen by some as a major medical innovation in America and Canada.
SHANTI Project volunteers currently number more than one hundred and
are donating nearly 50,000 hours of counseling time per year. Both
hospice and the SHANTI Project offer opportunities for staff training
in the U.S., Europe and elsewhere.

Liegner (1974) notes that the key principle of hospice care is reduction of pain; by pain he means not only physical pain but also
psychic pain. The reduction of pain in a hospice is effected through
several strategies:
1. Polypharmacy--the practice of administering medication
    in doses adequate to keep the patient's pain always below
    the pain threshold;
2. Humane treatment and environment;
3. Psychological and pastoral counseling;
4. Special attention at the moment of death;
5. Social services for the bereaved.

Ideally, hospices rely on a core of dedicated staff and volunteers.
All health providers, physicians, nurses and auxiliary staff are encouraged to listen carefully to the patient and to share their observations with other staff in the hope of more successfully meeting
the physical and emotional needs of the patient.

Projects modeled after the SHANTI Project, often referred to as volunteer hospice programs, are appearing in many parts of the United
States and abroad. Requests for volunteer counseling, companionship,
and emotional support come from patients, family members, survivors
of a death, and members of the health professions. Volunteers provide services to clients free of charge with primary allegiance to
the client rather than to any single institutional setting. The project is committed to providing continuity of care for all clients;
thus, volunteers continue to work with their clients in the home,
general hospital or extended care facility. After a rigorous screen-
ing and selection process, SHANTI Project volunteers go through a
comprehensive training program and make a commitment to work at least
one year with the project for a period of eight to ten hours per
week. A training film for physicians and nurses on "Counseling the
Terminally Ill" focusing largely on the work of the SHANTI Project
has been produced under the sponsorship of the National Institute of
Mental Health. For further information:
   National Hospice Organization   SHANTI Project
   765 Prospect Street   106 Evergreen Lane
   New Haven, CT 06511, U.S.A.   Berkeley, CA 94705, U.S.A.

THE BASICS OF STAFF TRAINING

Guidelines for Delivering Bad News

Hogshead (1976) notes the following
"Every physician derives satisfaction from delivering good
news to a patient; and no physician that I know enjoys delivering bad news. Still, there are rare occasions when it
becomes necessary for the physician to disclose a fatal or
crippling diagnosis and prognosis to the patient. There is
no greater test of the physician's skill and courage than
this task of delivering medical bad news. Some physicians
delay or avoid this unpleasant task for fear of provoking an
emotional scene which they are ill prepared to handle, fear
of producing a serious depression or perhaps fear of losing
the trust and confidence of the patient. All of these are
valid possibilities which need to be considered.

There are as many ways of handling bad news conferences as
there are physicians. There is probably no 'right' way, and
no 'wrong' way to handle this. No thinking physician would
use the same stock techniques with every patient. Patients
are much too different and too sophisticated to be handled in
such a fashion. The particular method of delivering bad
news must be varied to meet the needs of the situation."

The following are some general guidelines developed by Hogshead
(1976) which I have expanded upon and found very helpful.

1. Keep it simple. There is a tendency to go into too
    many details and technicalities.
2. Ask yourself, "What does this diagnosis mean to this
    patient?" Such news is frequently very unsettling.
    It is often necessary to educate the patient gradually
    and gently regarding the diagnosis.
3. Meet on "cool ground" first. It is always easier to
    deliver bad news if you have some earlier relationship
    to the patient or his family, and have some notion of
    their background and possible reactions to the news.
    (Such news should always be communicated in as private
    a setting as possible.)
4. Don't deliver all the news at once. It is a good idea
    to try not to provide too much information at the first
    sitting. People have a marvelous way of letting you
    know how much they are able to handle. A useful approach
    is to ask the patient, "Is there anything else you'd
    like to discuss? I'd be glad to try to answer any
    questions you may have."
5. Wait for questions. A long pause will allow the question
    that tells you where to go next.
6. Do not argue with denial. A characteristic response in
    many patients is outright denial of the reality of the
    situation. No matter how illogical the denial, it is
    serving a purpose, and there is nothing to gain by
    battering down the denial with logic. This usually
    leads to loss of rapport with the patient. In general,
    the patient will "hear" the message when he is ready to
    accept it. It is sufficient that he has been told at

least once that condition"x" has been discovered.
7. <u>Ask questions yourself</u>. Ask the patient to tell you
   what you have told him, or ask him what it means. Valuable
   clarifications can result from gentle, clear questioning.
8. <u>Do not destroy all hope</u>. There are many ways of handling
   this, and it requires real tact and experience to be able
   to acquire the necessary skill. "Most people with this
   form of cancer are living longer but are not cured of
   their disease" is a useful kind of statement.
9. <u>Do not say anything that is not true</u>. This would be the
   cruelest blow of all.

The two main areas of serious concern to dying patients are (1) emotional and physical isolation and the threat of abandonment and
(2) extreme pain. The most cogent analysis of patient isolation and
abandonment I have read is that of Erikson and Hyerstay (1974), who
describe a hospital death with considerable accuracy. The need for
developing better palliation strategies has been discussed by LeShan
(1964) and Marks and Sachar (1973).

Pain Management

With the help of our colleagues at the hospices in Great Britain, we
are beginning to learn that patients may, at times, endure much
needless pain because of undereffective palliation strategies. Hospice physicians and patients claim that (1) effective pain management
strategies exist for almost all cancer patients, (2) patients can remain lucid <u>and</u> pain-free throughout most of the dying process, and
(3) addiction and habituation result from the ineffective administration of palliative drugs. There is no possible excuse for not
thoroughly investigating this important work. My own clinical experience has substantially borne out their validity (which does not
derive from the fact that British pain-killers contain heroin as the
active pharmacological ingredient since morphine is often the agent
of preference). In studying the psychopharmacological aspects of
pain, it is importnat to remember that making judgments about another
person's pain is an extremely hazardous proposition. Physicians must
use their patient's feedback as the most significant criterion. In
evaluating the effectiveness of pain-management strategies, to say,
as one professional did in reaction to a patient in extreme pain,
"He's not in as much pain as he says he is," is most unfortunate. In
general, physicians need to acknowledge as primary data the subjective reports of their patients and develop palliative strategies
based largely on this acknowledgment.

The Patient's Family

Dobihal (1974) has noted that the dying patient and his or her family
constitute the optimal unit of health care. It is extremely important for patients to live out and conclude family relationships in as
emotionally satisfying a way as possible. It can be very distressing
for critically ill persons and their families to be separated by the
treatment milieu and forced to limit or terminate their relationships. Dobihal offers the following suggestions to health professionals:

1. Train family members to participate in treatment.
2. Encourage them to do such things as continue to cook
   special meals for the patient.

3. Allow unlimited visiting so that the total family, including children, can spend time with the patient.
4. Provide special hospital space for patient-family meetings,
   as well as space for family members to live when the
   patient's death is imminent.
5. Provide special social and educational programs for the
   family and patient, and continue these programs, adding
   home visits for the family, after the patient has died.
   Research in preventive health indicates that the bereaved
   are much more susceptible to mental and physical trauma
   (including early death) than people not suffering from
   the loss of a close friend or relation.

MODEL FOR STAFF TRAINING

The following is an outline of the staff training program that I have
been privileged to conduct at healthcare institutions throughout the
United States and Europe. It has been developed in the context of
the SHANTI Project work with over 1900 dying patients during the past
five years (1975-1979).

The goals of the program are similar to those of Barton et al. (1972)
That is,
1. to facilitate gradual desensitization to the topic
   through the process of group interaction and discussion
   in order to promote staff understanding and appreciation
   for their personal feelings about death and dying.
2. to focus staff attention on the numerous and important
   medical, psychological and socio-cultural issues involved
   in order that they, as health professionals, might help
   the patient, the family, and the interpersonal milieu in
   which the patient's care takes place to reach a reasonable
   level of adaptation in the face of death. By focusing
   on these issues, the need for the health professional to
   develop a flexible approach based on an appreciation of
   the subtle and often unique means employed by patients,
   families, and care-giving personnel is emphasized.
3. to present and discuss with staff the perspectives of
   medical, nursing, mental health, and allied personnel
   who are involved in providing care for patients with life-
   threatening illnesses.
4. to encourage active consideration and discussion of
   ethical issues which, though often encountered in medical
   practice, are rarely discussed with staff in a way which
   allows them to begin to formulate and express their own
   positions and ideas.

The basic texts developed for this staff training and used as ongoing
references are PSYCHOSOCIAL CARE OF THE DYING PATIENT (Garfield,
1978) and STRESS AND SURVIVAL: THE EMOTIONAL REALITIES OF LIFE-
THREATENING ILLNESS (Garfield, 1979). Staff instruction can be conducted in interdisciplinary formats or with medical, nursing, or
allied professional staff exclusively.

OUTLINE OF STAFF TRAINING

Prior to the initial in-service training session, staff members read
Part Three: "Patients and Families Facing Life-Threatening Illness,"

(in Garfield, 1978) and Tolstoy's short story, The Death of Ivan Illych.

Week Number One

Introduction and patient presentation. A 29-year-old woman with widely disseminated breast cancer was interviewed by Dr. Garfield, and staff were encouraged to ask additional questions.

Week Number Two

Patient presentation. A 48-year-old man with lymphocytic lymphoma was interviewed by the class. His wife accompanied him to the session and spoke of her adaptation to his illness and the effect of his illness on their children.

Week Number Three

Patient presentation. A 56-year-old businessman with acute myelogenous leukemia discussed his adaptation to his illness with the class. He discussed the ways in which his life had changed and his efforts to develop a purposeful and meaningful life even in the face of a very limited life span.

Week Number Four

The perspective of the physician. After reading selections from (Garfield, 1978) Part Four: "Doctor-Patient Relationships," the staff listened to two senior physicians discuss their philosophy and approach to care of the dying patient.

Week Number Five

The perspective of the nurse. An oncology nurse, an intensive care nurse, and a pediatric nurse shared their perspectives on working with seriously ill and dying patients and their families.

Week Number Six

Readings from (Garfield, 1978) Part Five "Psychological Needs: Recognition and Action." The emotional needs of the patient and family. A clinical nurse specialist in psychiatric nursing and a psychologist shared their perspectives in caring for the dying and described the emotional problems evident for patients, families, and care-givers.

Week Number Seven

The perspective of the priest. A priest who counsels patients and families with life-threatening illness discussed the pastoral care of a patient during an extended illness.

Week Number Eight

Life-prolongation and patient survival. A case of a patient who was a candidate for the employment of a number of newly developed life-prolonging procedures was described and the multiple determinants of the decisions made were presented for discussion. This provided a

focal point for the discussion of ethical considerations in prolonging life.

Week Number Nine

An interview was done with a man who had open-heart surgery to discuss the ways of supporting life-threatening situations for cardiac
patients and an interview with a kidney dialysis patient to discuss
the physical and emotional demands imposed by survival by machine.

Week Number Ten

Grief and bereavement. Lindemann's paper "Symptomatology and Management of Acute Grief" was utilized to focus the attention of the group
on the phenomenon of grief. The class had the opportunity to discuss with one widow and one widower the various aspects of coping
with the loss of a loved one.

Week Number Eleven

Recent developments in palliation were presented during this session,
the latest developments in the use of Brompton's Mixture, etc., were
discussed. Also the emotional difficulties involved in the treatment
of patients receiving various palliative treatments over long periods
of time. A physician who was an expert in hospice palliative strategies and a staff nurse who worked frequently with this physician
offered their expertise on the issues involved in providing effective
relief from pain.

Week Number Twelve

Treatment of the elderly patient facing death. Two elderly patients,
one a 66-year-old man with a severe heart condition, and a 71-year-
old woman with pancreatic cancer discussed their situations with
staff, with special focus on the problems of the elderly.

Week Number Thirteen

Life-threatening illness in children. The parents of a 3-year-old
boy who had died of leukemia spoke with staff about their problems
coping with the death of their son. Interaction was encouraged
specifically around suggestions for better staff approaches. A
pediatric nurse who had cared for the child participated in the discussion.

Week Number Fourteen

Care of the terminally ill at home. The various aspects of caring
for dying patients at home were discussed including the use of the
patient's family and visits by health professionals.

Week Number Fifteen

Communication skills in the care of the dying patient. This session
offered a discussion of the art of delivering bad news as well as
the various communication skills involved in discussing diagnosis,
prognosis, etc.

Week Number Sixteen

Supporting the patient coping with pain, anger, depression, fear, and treatment side-effects.

Week Number Seventeen

Occupational stress and burnout. The emotional demands on the health provider were discussed in detail including concrete individual and institutional plans for alleviating occupational stress.

The specific purpose of this training is to suggest for medical, nursing, and allied health providers an effective model for dealing with the medical, psychological, and social issues involved in caring for dying patients. The focus was on the sequence of events generally encountered by the professional and dying patient from diagnosis through death. Basic issues in providing care were outlined to allow the health provider to acquire a working knowledge of the effective care of the dying patient.

The following resource material, presented in the form of an annotated bibliography, was used throughout the training.

ANNOTATED BIBLIOGRAPHY

Becker, Ernest. THE DENIAL OF DEATH. New York: The Free Press, 1973. In the first three chapters of this Pulitzer Prize winning work, the author develops the thesis that man's innate fear of death is a principal source of his activity. In brilliant fashion, he develops the notion that the suppression of our innate vulnerability provides our major source of energy. Although the remainder of the book covers such topics as mental illness and especially the psychoanalytic theories of Otto Rank, this initial section is one of the best analyses of the relationship among dying, death, and the human condition.

de Beauvoir, Simone. A VERY EASY DEATH. Harmondsworth: Penguin Books, 1969. An insightful and moving account of her mother's death. I recommend it for its accurate description of the inexorable humiliation of a proud woman during a dying process that was far more tortuous than easy. The daughter's conflicting experiences of anger and affection in the face of her mother's death are superb and constitute an expositon of some of the experiences of a prototypic survivor.

Feifel, Herman. NEW MEANINGS OF DEATH. New York: McGraw-Hill Book Company, 1977. This anthology is an update of the editor's influential work, The Meaning of Death, published in 1959. It examines the historical, sociological, psychological, developmental, and clinical aspects of death and dying. Some of the leaders in the field examine such topics as death and development through the life span meanings of death to children, death and the physician, nurses and the human experience of dying, preparation for death, death education, and the relationship of death to immortality, the law, and poetry. This is an interesting collection of papers suitable for students, academicians, and clinicians.

Garfield, Charles A. PSYCHOSOCIAL CARE OF THE DYING PATIENT. New

York: McGraw-Hill Book Company, 1978.   This anthology is directed
specifically at all physicians, nurses, and allied health professionals who work with dying patients and their families.   It is intended
as a resource text for clinicians to assist in identifying the
emotional needs of the dying patient and family and to suggest helpful ways of providing the necessary support.   A more ambitious intent
is to identify the entire area of basic emotional support for
patients and families as a legitimate and vital concern for any fully
competent health professional.   Topics include: guidelines for terminal patient care, patients and families facing life-threatening
illness, doctor-patient relationships, psychological needs of the
terminally ill, counseling the patient's family, bioethical issues,
and the development of the SHANTI Project and the hospice movement.

Garfield, Charles A.   STRESS AND SURVIVAL: THE EMOTIONAL REALITIES
OF LIFE-THREATENING ILLNESS.   St. Louis: Mosby Publishing Company,
1979.   This anthology is intended for physicians, nurses, and allied
health professionals who provide support for patients and families
facing life-threatening illness.   A basic premise of the book is that
one or more such supportive presences can markedly influence the
patient's level of stress, will to live, and possibility of survival.
The primary purposes of the book are: 1)   In the words of Terrence
Des Pres in his book The Survivor, "To understand the capacity of men
and women to live beneath the pressure of protracted crisis, to
sustain terrible damage in mind and body, and yet be there, sane,
alive, still human."   2)   To offer insights into the ways that emotional support may be instrumental in promoting quality of life, long-
evity, and, at times, survival.   3)   To examine closely the optimal
ways of providing emotional support to patients and families facing
life-threatening illness.   Topics include: psychosocial elements of
survival, the relation of social and psychological factors to illness, new dimensions in the alleviation of stress, emotional impact
on health professional and patient, personal encounters with life-
threatening illness, the chronically ill child, understanding pain
and suffering, and care of the dying patient.

Glaser, Barney, and Strauss, Anselm.   AWARENESS OF DYING.   Chicago:
Aldine, 1965.   The best of the sociological studies available on the
subject of dying.   The data gathered for this book came from considerable field work in a variety of hospital settings.   Perhaps the
most important theoretical concept is that of varying contexts of
awareness of death that exist in the hospital social system.   This
book will be of interest to hospital clinicians interested in understanding the impact of the hospital itself on staff, patients, and
families.

Kastenbaum, Robert, and Aisenberg, Ruth.   THE PSYCHOLOGY OF DEATH.
New York: Springer Publishing Company, 1972.   This book is one of
the most informative and interesting on the pyschology of death.   It
is a scholarly work combining original thought and the best research
and thinking available.   It contains enlightening analyses of historical, cultural, societal, developmental, and clinical issues involved in understanding the psychological aspects of dying and death.

Kubler-Ross, Elisabeth.   ON DEATH AND DYING.   New York: Macmillan
Publishing Company, 1969.   This popular work has had more circulation
than any other book in the field.   It is a caring and humane analysis
of the needs of the dying patient with practical advice for all those

who provide care. Although Dr. Kubler-Ross' "five stage" model has
been repudiated by most major thinkers in the field, this book should
be regarded as a helpful and compassionate guide for clinicians.

Lewis, C. S. A GRIEF OBSERVED. New York: Seabury Press, 1973. "No
one ever told me that grief felt so much like fear." So begins an
extraordinarily honest and revealing expose of the grief of this
well-known writer-philosopher. Originally written as a self-therapy
journal without plans for publication, this powerful little book
provides a superb first-hand account of the existential and emotional
plight of an individual who has lost the most important person in his
world. I highly recommend this book as a resource in providing a
humane balance to the more clinical literature on grief and bereavement.

Lund, Doris. ERIC. Philadelphia: J. G. Lippincott Company, 1974.
This book is the product of a mother's arduous task of writing about
the death of her 17-year-old son from acute leukemia. It is an in-
spiring and lovingly written story of a boy who challenged his illness and its insidious effects by living powerfully and creatively in
the face of death. It will be of assistance to those clinicians who
need to understand the plight of the parent in life-threatening illness and will provide a balance to the more detached clinical literature.

Parkes, Colin Murray. BEREAVEMENT. New York: Penguin, 1972. This
work is the result of a comprehensive study of adult grief and its
impact. It is a scholarly work of use to those interested in more
than a clinical distillation of grief reactions and their symptoms.
Included are suggestions for helping the bereaved and understanding
the psychological processes involved in coping with the loss of a
loved one.

Rosenthal, Ted. HOW COULD I NOT BE AMONG YOU? New York: Braziller,
1973. This is a collection of some extremely moving poetry and prose
from Ted Rosenthal, a Berkeley poet, who discovered at the age of 30
that he was dying of acute leukemia. He powerfully shares the
emotional realities confronting the dying patient by examining his
own reactions to the illness, human relationships, and life in general. At rock bottom, he becomes aware of the psychic outrageousness
of "ceasing to be" and the emotionally unfathomable question "How
could I not be among you?" This book is highly recommended for anyone attempting to understand the existential drama confronting the
dying patient.

Shneidman, Edwin. DEATHS OF MAN. New York: Quadrangle/New York
Times, 1973. An extremely well-written analysis of death including
some innovative ideas of considerable interest. This is a psychologically sophisticated work of interest to scholars and others interested in the impact and the implications of death for the human
psyche. The author includes some of his own concepts such as sur-
vivor-victims and their assistance by postvention; subintentioned
death, and the effects of megadeath.

Weisman, Avery. ON DYING AND DENYING. New York: Behavioral Publications, 1972. This scholarly work, based on some of the best research available, concentrates on the central role of denial in the
dying process. The book contains some excellent clinical case

material and is best suited for those with more than an elementary
understanding of psychological processes.

        REFERENCES

Barton, D., and others: "Death and Dying: A Course for Medical
    Students" in C. Garfield (ed.), Psychosocial Care of the Dying
    Patient, McGraw-Hill, New York, 1978.
Carkhuff, R. and B. Berenson: Beyond Counseling and Therapy, Holt
    Rinehart, and Winston, New York, 1967.
Des Pres, T.: "The Survivor, Oxford University Press, New York, 1976.
Dobihal, E." "Talk or Terminal Care," Connecticut Medicine, 38:364-
    367, 1974.
Erikson, R. and B. Hyerstay: "The Dying Patient and the Double Bind
    Hypothesis," Omega, 5(4):287-298, 1974.
Feifel, Herman, New Meanings of Death, McGraw-Hill, New York, 1977.
Garfield, C.: "The Impact of Death on the Healthcare Professional,"
    in H. Feifel (ed.), New Meanings of Death, McGraw-Hill, New York,
    1977.
Garfield, C.: Psychosocial Care of the Dying Patient, McGraw-Hill,
    New York, 1978.
Hogshead, H.: "The Art of Delivering Bad News," in C. Garfield (ed.),
    Psychosocial Care of the Dying Patient, McGraw-Hill, 1978.
Kubler-Ross, E.: "On Death and Dying, Macmillan, New York, 1969.
LeShan, L.: "The World of the Patient in Severe Pain of Long Dur-
    ation," Journal of Chronic Diseases, 17:119-126, 1964.
Liegner, L.: "St. Christopher"s Hospice, Care of the Dying Patient,"
    Journal of the American Medical Association, 234:1047-1048, 1974.
Lindemann, E.: "Symptomatology and Management of Acute Grief," Amer-
    ican Journal of Psychiatry, 101:141-148, 1944.
Marks, R. and E. Sachar: "Undertreatment of Medical Inpatients with
    Narcotic Analgesics," Annals of Internal Medicine, 78(2):173-126,
Nouwen, H.: Out of Solitude, Ave Maria Press, Notre Dame, Indiana,
    1974.

Goal Setting in Terminal Cancer

E. R. HILLIER and B. LUNT

Countess Mountbatten House, Southampton, UK

The term "goal setting" will be completely unfamiliar to most of you, which is why I shall begin by describing how we at Countess Mountbatten House came to approach dying patients in a way which may at first seem rather curious.

During the past few years a great deal of progress has been made in the management of patients suffering a number of other disabling conditions. These include the mentally ill, the elderly and infirm, and the mentally handicapped, all of whom have previously been in the back waters of medicine. These patients have been helped by the setting of short term treatment objectives aimed at achieving longer term objectives (goals) which have been set by the patient and his family. They are not set by the doctor, although he will usually need to guide and to help the participants make up this list of goals.

The characteristics of this approach to treatment include - first that these goals arise from a careful analysis of the patient's present problems and what he hopes to achieve; secondly, the treatment builds on whatever abilities, strength and resources are possessed by him and his family; thirdly, the goals must be positive rather than negative, they must build new patterns of activity and behaviour within the limits of the patient's disabilities. In other words, one is aiming for a moderate success rather than an ambitious failure.

With these methods in mind we approached the problems of dying patients and their families. Our reading of the literature on terminal care and the evidence of our own eyes showed a widespread problem of poor quality terminal care. This includes both poor symptom control, but also an obvious lack of help for patients and their families in coping with mental and emotional distress. On the other hand, there are several well-known centres of excellence where patients and their families are treated with sensitivity and great attention to detail, and where symptom control is excellent. This led us to ask two questions:

1. How do we explain this difference between centres of excellence and the general picture? What is it about hospices; what happens at hospices; what do the staff in hospices do which accounts for the difference in quality of care described by patients, relatives, researchers, journalists, and by almost all who find themselves in a position to make such a judgment?

2. How can we help those working elsewhere to improve the general picture so that it mirrors the quality of care attained in the centres of excellence?

Let us first consider the question: What is high quality terminal care? In looking at the day-to-day work of Countess Mountbatten House in Southampton, in talking to patients and staff there, and in reading about the activities of hospices, it appears that the successful care of their patients is achieved in a very similar way to the good quality care achieved for the other kinds of patients I already mentioned. Perhaps the reason is that the one thing all these different categories of patient have in common is that they are all people, and good quality care is achieved when we treat the person rather than the disease or symptom which people happen to have. What does this mean in caring for the dying? If one looks at a team of dedicated doctors, nurses, social workers and other staff caring success-fully for a person in the final stages of his or her life, one will see them dealing with that person with enormous sensitivity and great attention to detail. They will be doing these things:

1. Looking in detail at the person's problems, at their abilities and strengths, at the resources they have to call on and at the history of their problems and the ways they have found of dealing with them in the past.

2. Identifying, together with the patient, aspects of the patient's life which he wants changing from what is currently happening.

3. Deciding which of these have the highest priority.

4. Working out with the patient the specific goals to be worked on and in what order. By the term "goal" we mean what the patient will be doing as a result of our care and treatment which is different, and better than what he is doing now.

5. Breaking down distant goals into manageable parts or "short term goals" which build on the strengths and abilities of the patient or his family.

6. Plan and carry out the treatment programme.

7. Regularly assessing the progress of the patient in relation to his goals, and changing treatment accordingly.

8. Reviewing goals frequently as the illness progresses, and as the patient's and staff's understanding of the patient's abilities change. This may happen quickly, particularly if the patient is physically deteriorating. Under these circumstances the goals may change daily. Even the most static patient will probably need weekly review of the goals set.

The whole procedure of carrying out these steps is called "goal setting".

This description is rather different from the descriptions of the care of the dying patient usually found in the medical, nursing and social work literature. The difference is largely one of emphasis, but nevertheless it is a big difference. We read and have heard a lot about treatment - how to select appropriate treatment, how to implement it; which drugs to use under particular circumstances, and what side-effects to look out for. This is only right, for without descriptions of this kind by pioneers in the field we cannot expect others to learn and profit from their experience. But there is more to the care of the dying than expert execution of the treatment - there is also the framework within which decisions are made, treatment is planned, and care is given. It is that aspect of the care of the care of the dying that needs emphasis, because it is that which the experts must begin to teach to all the other people working with the dying, if we are to see any major progress in the kind of care offered to terminally ill patients the world over.

We are suggesting that one of the reasons for the excellent standard of care achieved in the hospices and continuing care units is that treatment is planned within the sort of goal-oriented framework just described. But because it is done intuitively, the goal setting is implicit rather than explicit, implied rather than described. It is being used haphazardly, and is not necessarily being used for all patients. One often finds oneself on a ward round saying "Now what are we doing for Mrs Jones?" A search through the notes begins in order to look for the reason for admission and to make a plan. Nobody has worked out what Mrs Jones' goals are. How often does one find in conversation with another member of the health care team that, although you know what you are trying to do for Mrs Jones, and are happy with progress, the person you are talking to has very little idea why they are treating the patient in this way, how they are supposed to tell if they are making progress, or if they are making enough progress. Your goal-setting was implicit, and it left others in the dark.

In any setting, to ensure a high quality of care it is necessary to have three things:

1. Communication between the different members of the team, which may include several doctors, social workers, occupational therapists, physiotherapists, as well as twenty or more nurses; and between all of these staff and the patient and his relatives. This means two-way communication about treatment goals, plans and progress.

2. Co-ordination between the activities of various members of staff.

3. Evaluation of the effects of treatment. Are goals being attained? If not, has one been either too ambitious or, alternatively, given the wrong treatment?

We suggest that one way to do this is to make the goal-setting an explicit, rather than an intuitive part of patient care. That is, to go through the seven steps listed earlier in a systematic way, to make the goals clear, and to write them down in the patient's notes so that they are there for all to see.

At Countess Mountbatten House we are trying to develop such a systematic approach and this is how we do it.

Identifying the Goals

To start with one needs to identify certain "goal areas". These are general problem areas which need improvement. Having done this, more specific goals can be set. For example, a goal area may be pain control. More specific goals in this general are may turn out to be that:

1. This particular patient wants to be sufficiently pain-free to sleep through the night, and

2. To be able to sit out of bed without pain for some part of the day.

So how do you go about identifying a patient's goal areas and the more detailed goals? First of all, of course, you do what you have always done: talk to the patient, find out the history of his illness and his background; find out about the family, and so on. Find out about the things which presently concern him. It can be helpful to have a checklist of aspects of a person's life, or situation, or functioning, in which problems or goals may appear, and towards the end of the first interview begin to structure the discussion round this checklist. Our check-list includes, at present, the following areas:

1. Symptoms
2. Self-care
3. Mobility
4. Sleep
5. Recreation/Leisure
6. Social Activities

7. Family Relationships
8. Work
9. Financial
10. Information about illness
11. Others

Patients are usually rather good at telling you their problems, and so one might well get problems described in many or all of these areas. Some will be very general: "I've never felt so ill in my life." Others will be insoluble anyway: "I've got terminal cancer." Many will be quite specific and potentially soluble. We note the problems down because they are likely to be a good guide to the areas where the patient has goals. They may well be relevant to how we go about helping the patient to attain his goals and they should tell us a lot about his understanding of the implications of his illness. However, the next and crucial step is to turn discussion away from the negatives and on to positives, to find out what the patient's goal areas are, what the immediate goals are within each goal area. Let us take an example.

We have a patient who is ill, probably pretty miserable, feeling fairly sorry for himself, and dwelling on his problems and difficulties because they are important to him. Our job is to help this patient clarify the kind of changes he wants in his life as it is at the moment, so that we know how to help him, and how to assess the effectiveness of our help. The patient may not have goals before we talk to him; he may say he just wants to die; he may say everything is fine; he may not understand what you are talking about. The process of goal-setting should be regarded , not just as a matter of finding out from the patient what he wants (though it is this), but also as counselling as part of the therapeutic process. It is an interaction in which we have a lot to contribute from our understanding of the illness and from our experience. It is an exchange which should leave both us and the patient feeling that there is something positive to work on, and all hope is not lost. We will probably be in a good position to judge what is possible to achieve tomorrow, the next day, in a week, or so on. The patient is in the best position to decide which direction he wants to go in, and the importance to be attached to each goal area.

In response to an initial question about the sort of changes they would like to see, people will often say "I want to be better", "To feel happier", or "Feel less depressed." These things can mean as many different things as there are different patients. We need some clarification. We must ask "What would you be doing if you were better, happier, or less depressed?" The answer might be "Well, I would be more independent" or "I would be getting on better with my wife." This sort of answer is a little more clear, but if we are to give this patient practical help we need to know exactly what this means for him. So we keep on clarifying, suggesting and prompting, until we find out what "independence" or "getting on better with his wife" means for this particular person at this particular time.

Here there may be useful clues from the patient's initial description of his problems. For one man, who had just gone home, independence meant washing and dressing without his wife's help and helping to prepare the vegetables for the evening meal. By setting these goals explicitly and discussing them with his wife, Mr G. hoped to prevent his wife making an invalid of him as she had done each time he went home from hospital in the past. Indeed his wife joined in keeping a diary of his success and in celebrating it.

The husband of a lady who was dying at home of cancer of the colon was doing almost all the nursing care his wife required, but was becoming increasingly unhappy about their relationship. Their only contact with each other was when she rang her buzzer to summon him and he left her as soon as he had done what she demanded. After a long discussion it became clear that, for him, "Getting on better with his wife" meant, among other things, talking together. He was loathe to talk about the past or the future for fear the subject would upset his wife, who knew she was becoming increasingly ill. On the other hand, his wife enjoyed talking about holidays they had had in the past, and wondered why her husband was becoming so uncommunicative. A short-term goal for this couple was to talk for a few minutes about past holidays when he took her evening meal upstairs.

Many of the goals will be distant. Some may be quite unattainable - in your opinion. After finding out what the goal areas are, the second aspect of goal-setting is to come to an agreement with the patient and any other people involved as to what is a realistic short-term goal to set within each of the goal areas. For this one needs to know the current state. One also needs to know the resources the patient has to call upon, what related abilities he has, what support he has from his relatives for attaining the goals, i.e. his strengths.   Then it is a matter of using professional judgement and experience in discussion with the patient to find a short-term goal which you think is attainable and which, above all, the patient agrees to. It is better to aim too low than too high, since the patient has probably had his fill of failure in the recent past as his illness has progressed, and an important part of maintaining morale (for staff as well as for the patient) seems to be to get some success in what you are trying to do, even if it is success on a modest scale.

In a goal area such as mobility, there may be a whole series of short-term goals in a programme geared to attaining a particular long-term goal for a patient. For example, mobility may be related to helping a patient join in the activities which are available in the ward, rather than lying in bed all day bored. This is the goal area which, explicitly stated, would read as follows:

"To improve mobility in order to help the patient take part in the ward activities."

Now the first three goals within this goal area are a progression from the patient being bedridden to being up and moving around independently in a wheelchair. Explicitly stated, these are:

Goal 1 is to sit up in bed with help from two nurses, and stay sitting up for two hours.

Goal 2 is to sit in the wheelchair in the day-room for the afternoon, the nurses to help the patient in and out of, and push, the wheelchair.

Goal 3 is to propel the wheelchair from the ward to the day-room, the nurses to help the patient in and out of the wheelchair.

Goal 4 is to practice using the electric wheelchair for fifteen minutes with help and instructions from a nurse.

The last goal is aimed at maintaining this independence despite the patient's increasing weakness, by changing the physical conditions under which he or she is expected to move about. Because this sequence of goals is related to enabling the patient to participate in ward activities, the emphasis is on promoting independent movement round the ward.

In another example, improving mobility may be related to the goal of getting to the lavatory. The emphasis is on enabling the patient to move from bed to bath-room with the minimum of delay, and with the minimum of assistance. The sequence

of goals begins as in the previous case. That is, the patient sits up in bed,
but progress then takes a different course, designed to make the patient stronger,
increase his confidence, and to attain as quickly as possible the goal of more
dignified and independent toileting.

Goal 1 to sit up in bed with the help of two nurses, and remain sitting up for
two hours.

Goal 2 to get up to use commode, with the help of two nurses.

Goal 3 is to get up to use commode, with the help of one nurse.

Goal 4 is to walk from the bed to the end of the ward with the help of two nurses
twice a day.

Goal 5 is to walk from the bed to the end of the ward with a Zimmer frame twice
daily with only one nurse in attendance.

Goal 6 is to walk from the bed to the bathroom twice a day with the Zimmer frame
with one nurse in attendance.

One of the reasons for setting explicit goals is to enable us to assess the
effectiveness of our interventions. For this purpose it is important that the
goals are as clear as possible, and are recorded in terms which can be reliably
assessed. One needs to ask oneself "How will I know whether the patient has
achieved this goal?" "What change will I see in him?" If, together, you can
answer this question, then you have successfully described the goal you wish to
attain.

The following simple examples illustrate the degree of specificity needed to
enable reliable assessment to take place.

1. Mr N. will talk to his wife about holidays they have enjoyed in the past for
at least five minutes when he takes her evening meal.

2. Miss P. will drink a bowl of soup for lunch without vomiting within half-an-
hour afterwards, provided she does not feel nauseated beforehand.

3. Miss B. will go home by Friday to collect some clothes, and the paper she needs
to make her Will.

4. Mr D. will sleep until 2 a.m. without waking in pain on any occasion, having
taken his medicine and gone to bed between 10 p.m. and 11 p.m.

In addition to describing who will do what, the goals also state the criterion of
success which the patient finds acceptable - go home by Friday, without waking in
pain, etc.

These examples should help to make clear some of the main aspects of the goal-
setting approach. But in conclusion there are three general points which may
clarify some of the issues on which a certain amount of confusion arises.

First, people often say "Goals are all very well for rehabilitation, but surely
they cannot be applied to people who are deteriorating, because they will always
be failing to achieve whatever goals are set for them?"

But much of terminal care is rehabilitation. It is enabling people to overcome
their disabling condition and to live in whatever way they wish. "Rehabilitation

goals" will often be made to re-equip a person with a skill - such as walking, eating, dressing, etc., which they will be able to use in the future in order to function effectively in their day-to-day living. The rehabilitation aspect of terminal care might also include helping a person to overcome his emotional response to his illness or to come to terms with it. For one of our patients a "coming to terms" goal was that he would be able to talk to the doctor about his illness without becoming distressed. For another person it might be starting to take an interest in dressing and grooming.

However, at some time rehabilitation loses significance. When someone's physical condition is deteriorating rapidly, that person may be losing skills and abilities. However, this does not mean that they have no aims or aspirations. The job now lies in identifying what the patient wants to do and is capable of doing (perhaps with much assistance) and helping him to do just that.

New goal areas may, and probably will, emerge at this state and things may change rapidly. Within the shortened time scale the goals become related not to re-establishing the ability to function, but related to what the person wants to do now, today, or in the next hour. Again, the goals may relate to emotional or spiritual matters, and the job in hand is to find out more specifically what the patient wants to do.

A second comment people often make is "Isn't this goal-setting approach just the same thing as problem oriented records?"

Goals are not necessarily just the opposite side of the coin to problems. They may be, but in the cases where this approach pays dividends, the goals are quite different from the problems. If you ask somebody what they would like "to be doing this afternoon" they may say "I'd like to go to Mass and then sit in the garden with my wife." There may well be things it is necessary for nurses to do or not do to allow this to happen.   However, if you ask that same person what his problems are, it is unlikely that he will say "I anticipate having difficulty in attending Mass and then going outside to sit in the garden with my wife." If you start from the point of view of problems alone, you will miss out many important ways of helping patients. An important point is that people produce very long, and sometimes endless, lists of problems. When, however, you ask them instead to describe their aims, or what they would be doing if the problems were solved, they often produce quite a short list. Table 1 shows the numerous problems and difficulties described by a particularly miserable lady.

TABLE 1   Problems

Pain in right shoulder	Difficulty in walking
Stiff right arm	Bored all day
Weight loss	Drousy during the day
Difficulty in swallowing	Insomnia
Poor appetite	Cannot concentrate
Cataract in right eye	Unable to knit
Cannot get dressed	

However, the list of goal areas was relatively short, simple and positive (Table 2):

TABLE 2   Goal Areas

Pain control (right shoulder)*	Get dressed
Improvement in shoulder*	Go home*
Start knitting*	Cook own meals
Write letters*	

Some of them were short-term goals and the last, to go home, was a long-term goal which in practice was highly unlikely to be attained. The asterisks indicate goals which immediate efforts were made to work on. In the case of the very distant goal of going home, this was to break it down into a sequence of steps, the first of which was to go home for an afternoon with some relatives - a goal that could be attained. However, the main point of this example is to illustrate the difference, in number and in kind, of the problems and the goal areas identified by simply asking the questions "What are your problems?" and "What do you want to do, what improvements do you want to see?"

Another important difference between problems and goals is that a list of problems doesn't necessarily indicate in what direction to move. An analogy is of somebody lost in the desert. The problem is most likely to be stated as "We're lost". The goal, if it could be identified, might be "We should be further to the West". The goal tells you what to do: you find out where West is and start walking. The problem just tells you bad news.

A third comment which has been made is "Isn't this just one more job to do which takes us away from really looking after our patients?" The case that I have presented here is that finding out patients' goals really is caring for patients. The most time-consuming part is talking to the patient, working out with him what the goals of treatment are, and checking that the list of goals really reflects the way he feels about how he wants help. After that you need to assess regularly whether the goals are being attained, whether they have changed through changing circumstances, and to modify the care and treatment accordingly. I hope that you will agree that doing these things is caring for the patient. The extra work arises from the discipline of doing this explicitly for your patients. Although this may take a little longer, it does save time in the long run.

At the beginning of this article two questions presented themselves when we began looking at the care of the dying. The first was: What is it about the hospices that makes them so different from the general picture of terminal care? We suggest to you that the attention to detail, the constructive approach, the focus on the patient's aims, and the evaluation of treatment in terms of its effects on the patient's ability to do the things he wants - in short, the characteristics of the goal-setting approach - are in fact the features which make the hospices stand out from the general pattern of care offered to people with a terminal illness.

The second question was: How can we help those working in other settings to do a similarly good job? We believe that this can only be done by describing the procedures and features which are special in the hospices in such detail that others can copy them. If it is right that the goal-setting approach is part of this, albeit at present an intuitive part, then we must describe exactly how it is done. This is precisely what we are researching at Countess Mountbatten House.

INDEX